Proton Therapy

FIRST EDITION

Proton Therapy

Indications, Techniques, and Outcomes

STEVEN J. FRANK, MD
Professor
Radiation Oncology
The University of Texas MD Anderson Cancer Center
Houston, Texas

X. RONALD ZHU, PhD
Professor
Radiation Physics
The University of Texas MD Anderson Cancer Center
Houston, Texas

ELSEVIER

1600 John F. Kennedy Blvd.
Ste 1800
Philadelphia, PA 19103-899

PROTON THERAPY: INDICATIONS, TECHNIQUES, AND OUTCOMES ISBN: 978-0-323-73349-6

Library of Congress Control Number: 2020932479

Content Strategist: Robin Carter
Content Development Manager: Ellen Wurm-Cutter
Content Development Specialist: Sara Watkins
Publishing Services Manager: Deepthi Unni
Project Manager: Janish Ashwin Paul
Design Direction: Bridget Hoette

Last digit is the print number: 9 8 7 6 5 4 3 2 1

DEDICATION

This book is dedicated to all of our patients and their loved ones who have entrusted us with their cancer care with proton therapy.

LIST OF CONTRIBUTORS

Houda Bahig, MD
Department of Radiation Oncology
Division of Radiation Oncology
The University of Texas MD Anderson Cancer Center

Andrew J. Bishop, MD
Department of Radiation Oncology
Division of Radiation Oncology
The University of Texas MD Anderson Cancer Center

Bouthaina S. Dabaja, MD
Department of Radiation Oncology
Division of Radiation Oncology
The University of Texas MD Anderson Cancer Center

Joe Y. Chang, MD, PhD
Department of Radiation Oncology
Division of Radiation Oncology
The University of Texas MD Anderson Cancer Center

Seungtaek L. Choi, MD
Department of Radiation Oncology
Division of Radiation Oncology
The University of Texas MD Anderson Cancer Center

Prajnan Das, MD, MS, MPH
Department of Radiation Oncology
Division of Radiation Oncology
The University of Texas MD Anderson Cancer Center

Steven J. Frank, MD
Department of Radiation Oncology
Division of Radiation Oncology
The University of Texas MD Anderson Cancer Center

Michael T. Gillin, PhD
Department of Radiation Physics
Division of Radiation Oncology
The University of Texas MD Anderson Cancer Center

Daniel R. Gomez, MD, MBA
Department of Radiation Oncology
Memorial Sloan Kettering Cancer Center

David R. Grosshans, MD, PhD
Departments of Experimental and Radiation Oncology
Division of Radiation Oncology
The University of Texas MD Anderson Cancer Center

Archana S. Gautam, MSc
Department of Radiation Oncology
Division of Radiation Oncology
The University of Texas MD Anderson Cancer Center

G. Brandon Gunn, MD
Department of Radiation Oncology
Division of Radiation Oncology
The University of Texas MD Anderson Cancer Center

Jillian R. Gunther, MD, PhD
Department of Radiation Oncology
Division of Radiation Oncology
The University of Texas MD Anderson Cancer Center

Stephen M. Hahn, MD
Division of Radiation Oncology
The University of Texas MD Anderson Cancer Center

Karen E. Hoffman, MD
Department of Radiation Oncology
Division of Radiation Oncology
The University of Texas MD Anderson Cancer Center

Yoshifumi Hojo, PhD
Department of Radiation Physics
Division of Radiation Oncology
The University of Texas MD Anderson Cancer Center

Emma B. Holliday, MD
Department of Radiation Oncology
Division of Radiation Oncology
The University of Texas MD Anderson Cancer Center

Heng Li, PhD
Department of Radiation Oncology and Molecular Radiation Sciences
Johns Hopkins University

Yupeng Li, MS
Department of Radiation Physics
Division of Radiation Oncology
The University of Texas MD Anderson Cancer Center

Zhongxing Liao, MD
Department of Radiation Oncology
Division of Radiation Oncology
The University of Texas MD Anderson Cancer Center

Lillie L. Lin, MD
Department of Radiation Oncology
Division of Radiation Oncology
The University of Texas MD Anderson Cancer Center

Steven H. Lin, MD, PhD
Department of Radiation Oncology
Division of Radiation Oncology
The University of Texas MD Anderson Cancer Center

Radhe Mohan, PhD
Department of Radiation Physics
Division of Radiation Oncology
The University of Texas MD Anderson Cancer Center

Quynh-Nhu Nguyen, MD
Department of Radiation Oncology
Division of Radiation Oncology
The University of Texas MD Anderson Cancer Center

Matthew Palmer, MBA, BA
Chief Operating Officer
MD Anderson Proton Therapy Center
The University of Texas MD Anderson Cancer Center

Arnold C. Paulino, MD, FACR, FASTRO
Department of Radiation Oncology
Division of Radiation Oncology
The University of Texas MD Anderson Cancer Center

Falk Poenisch, PhD
Department of Radiation Physics
Division of Radiation Oncology
The University of Texas MD Anderson Cancer Center

Narayan Sahoo, PhD
Department of Radiation Physics
Division of Radiation Oncology
The University of Texas MD Anderson Cancer Center

Li Wang, MD, PhD
Department of Experimental Radiation Oncology
Division of Radiation Oncology
The University of Texas MD Anderson Cancer Center

Wendy A. Woodward, MD, PhD
Department of Radiation Oncology
Division of Radiation Oncology
The University of Texas MD Anderson Cancer Center

Richard Wu, MS
Department of Radiation Physics
Division of Radiation Oncology
The University of Texas MD Anderson Cancer Center

Xiaodong Zhang, PhD
Department of Radiation Physics
Division of Radiation Oncology
The University of Texas MD Anderson Cancer Center

X. Ronald Zhu, PhD
Department of Radiation Physics
Division of Radiation Oncology
The University of Texas MD Anderson Cancer Center

PREFACE

Proton therapy has been used to treat cancer patients since the early 1950s; however, technologic advancements in proton therapy delivery with spot scanning and treatment planning systems are rapidly evolving, making it more accessible for the management of solid tumors. In this first edition of *Proton Therapy: Indications, Techniques, and Outcomes*, we aim to communicate the most up-to-date advancements in radiobiology, indications, literature, management approaches, treatment planning, quality assurance, and outcomes after proton therapy by disease site. Education and training in proton therapy are more important now than ever before, as systems become smaller and more cost-effective, resulting in greater access for community hospitals and their multidisciplinary oncology teams.

The radiobiology of proton therapy and its relative biological effectiveness versus conventional x-rays (RBE) will continue to be a dynamic field of interest based on the DNA damage and repair mechanisms in individual tumor cell lines as well as the acute and late effects on normal tissues. Specifically, multifield optimization intensity-modulated proton therapy (MFO-IMPT) provides a great opportunity for understanding how best to exploit the linear energy transfer (LET) of protons at the distal edge of the Bragg peak to our advantage.

Proton therapy quality assurance and management of uncertainties during treatment planning and treatment delivery will continue to be a hallmark of medical physics. Robust planning, robust analysis, and robust optimization are important tools during the proton therapy treatment planning process. Deeper understanding of the variations of stopping power and their effects on adaptive real-time planning is an exciting opportunity to further advance patient care.

Clinical outcomes by disease site are carefully examined in each clinical chapter, and a special section on head and neck cases is included that photographically documents the full cycle of proton therapy care. Finally, the current indications for proton therapy at The University of Texas MD Anderson Cancer Center are a clarified, as well as opportunities for the advancement of proton therapy in future indications.

We thank all of the authors and dedicate this first edition of *Proton Therapy: Indications, Techniques, and Outcomes* to the late James D. Cox, MD, whose leadership and vision became a clinical reality in 2006 when the first cancer patient was treated with proton therapy at The University of Texas MD Anderson Cancer Center.

Steven J. Frank, MD, FACR, and
X. Ronald Zhu, PhD, FAAPM

ACKNOWLEDGMENT

We would like to acknowledge Christine F. Wogan, MS, ELS, of MD Anderson's Division of Radiation Oncology, for her substantive editorial efforts.

TABLE OF CONTENTS

SECTION I

Introduction

CHAPTER 1

Principles of Radiobiology

Li Wang ■ Steven J. Frank

Introduction

Radiotherapy is used as one of the major treatment modalities for patients with malignant diseases at different disease stages. Currently, the most common radiation choice for the majority of cancers is photon (x-ray)-based intensity-modulated external beam radiotherapy. Notably, recent advances in technology and basic and clinical research have facilitated the safe delivery of more effective and noninvasive radiotherapy for malignant diseases using charged particles, including intensity-modulated proton therapy. Proton beams deliver most of their energy at the distal edge of their range (the Bragg peak), which leads to an increase of the radiation doses to the clinical targets and minimization of the irradiation dose to adjacent normal tissues. Moreover, photon beams are categorized as low linear energy transfer (LET), whereas proton beams, especially in the spread-out Bragg peak (SOBP), which majorly contains Bragg peaks, are categorized as high LET. Thus in addition to the physical dose distribution advantage, proton therapy also presents distinct biology advantages compared with photon radiation. Even though the biological features of tumors and normal tissues after photon radiation have been extensively studied, the biological responses of tumors and normal tissues to proton radiation are far from clear. The biological properties of proton beams that differ significantly from those of photons will be summarized in this chapter. Particular emphasis is placed on relative biological effectiveness (RBE), DNA damage, and repair effects induced by protons, proton beam–induced cell death mechanisms, the impact of proton beams on tumor immune responses, and the influence of proton beams on tumor angiogenesis.

DNA Damage and Repair

DNA DAMAGE

DNA is the critical target of radiation. Photon radiation induces DNA damage by the direct action of deposing beam energy to DNA. Photon radiation also induces DNA damage by the indirect action of forming reactive species near the DNA, primarily by turning a water molecule into a free radical (hydroxyl radicals, OH).[1–3] Photon radiation causes many types of DNA damage, including single-base damage and single-strand breaks (isolated), and clustered base damage and double-strand breaks (DSBs) (clustered within a few DNA helical turns).[4] Most single-strand breaks can be repaired normally. However, repair is more difficult, and erroneous rejoining of broken ends in DSBs may result in significant biological consequences. Failure of DNA DSBs repair results in induction of mutations, chromosome aberrations, cell death, or even possibly in malignant cell transformation.[4–6] It is believed that the complexity of DNA damage is the determining factor for the consequent cellular response to radiation.

Although photon radiation–related DNA damage and repair researches have been conducted extensively, the DNA damage and repair as a consequence of proton radiation remain poorly understood. Similar to that of photon radiation, it has been proven that the indirect effect of proton beams plays a major role and causes a large proportion of DNA damage compared with the direct effect of proton beams.[1,7–9] However, Monte Carlo simulations have indicated that the average number of DNA damages per cluster tends to increase with the increasing of the radiation beam LET, which implies a higher level of DNA damage complexity induced by proton beams versus by that caused by photon beams.[1,4] These mathematical model prediction results have been verified by several other studies by testing DNA plasmids or cell lines. Using DNA plasmids pBR322 or T7 as testing material, the direct damage effect of proton beams to DNA was proven to generate more DSB clusters compared with non-DSB clusters compared with photon beams.[7,10] Similar observations were also demonstrated in cell-based studies. An increased complexity of DNA damages and slower DNA damage repair kinetics were observed in the human skin fibroblast AG01522 cells at the distal end of the SOBP after proton radiation.[11] Other than this, large foci, which represent the DSB clusters, were also found more commonly in Chinese hamster ovary (CHO) cell lines CHO10B2 and irs-20 after proton radiation compared with photon radiation.[12] The more severe DNA damage caused by proton beams were also proven by another study on the thyroid-stimulating hormone–dependent Fischer rat thyroid cells.[13] The authors found more free-end DNAs 1 hour after proton radiation than photon radiation, which means a more rapid DNA damage repair in the cells exposed to photon beams than those exposed to proton beams. They further verified their results by finding a higher rate of micronucleus formation and the presence of larger micronuclei in cells treated by proton beams than those cells treated with photon beams.[13] Persistent DNA damage was also observed in different head and neck cancer cell lines after exposure to proton beams versus exposure to photon beams.[14] However, conflicting results were observed in a study using the DNA plasmid pBR322. In this study, the authors did not find a difference in the amount of the clustered DNA damage induced by proton beams compared with photon beams in either the liquid or in the dry samples.[4]

DNA DAMAGE REPAIR

Because DNA DSBs are the key lesion leading to severe biological consequences in cells exposed to photon radiation, it is meaningful to study DSB and its processing after cells are exposed to proton beams. Because the DNA damages induced by proton beams are with higher complexity than those induced by photon beams, the repair of the damaged DNA caused by proton beams may be different from the repair of damaged DNA caused by photon beams. Compared with the extensively studied DNA damage repair mechanisms after photon beam exposure, the study of DNA damage repair after proton beam radiation is limited, and mechanisms underlying the DNA damage repair are still to be uncovered.

There are two major distinguished DSB repair pathways[15–17](Fig. 1.1): homologous recombination (HR) and nonhomologous end joining (NHEJ). NHEJ is active throughout the cell cycle and is the predominant repair pathway for photon radiation–induced DSBs in mammalian cells.[15,18] The roles of HR and NHEJ in DNA damage repair in response to proton versus photon beams have been studied.[15] In this study, the CHO cells AA8, CHO9, UV5, Irs1sf, and XR-C1 with different Rad51 (a protein related to HR[15,17]) and DNA-PKcs (a protein related to NHEJ[15,17]) status were exposed to proton or photon beams. Cell survival and DSB repair were evaluated after radiation. The authors found that when compared with wild-type cells, Rad-51-deficient or suppressed cells have a higher proton versus photon radiation response rate; however, DNA-PKcs-deficient cells have not shown a different response rate to proton versus photon radiation when compared with wild-type cells. Moreover, delayed DSB repair was also found in the Rad-51-deficient cells after proton radiation. The authors concluded that HR is preferentially required for proton beam–induced DSB repair.[15] A similar phenomenon was also found in human lung adenocarcinoma (A549) and human glioblastoma (M059K and M059J) cells.[19] In this study, after blocking DNA-PKcs, a higher level of delayed DSBs repair and a more

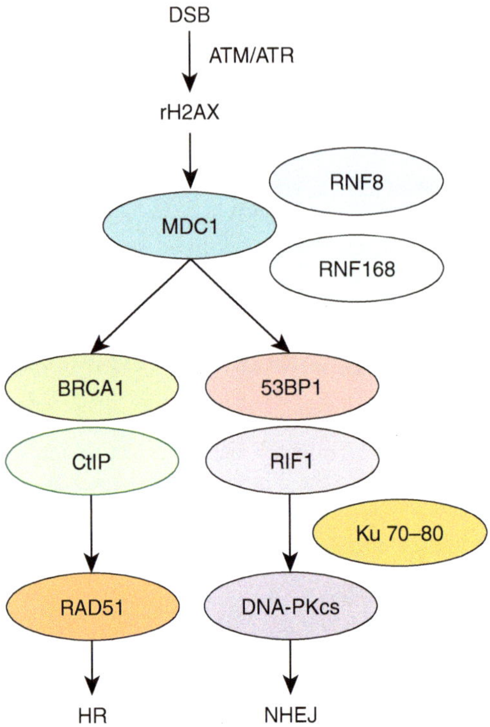

Fig. 1.1 Double-strand break *(DSB)* repair pathways *ATM,* Ataxia-Telangiesctasia mutated; *ATR,* ataxia telangiectasia and Rad3 related; *HR,* homologous recombination; *NHEJ,* nonhomologous end joining.

profound radio response was observed after cells were exposed to photon versus proton beams. On the other hand, depleting RAD51 led to an enhanced response of A549 cells to proton beams. The authors claimed a preference of HR versus NHEJ in proton beam–induced DSB repair.[19] On the contrary, conflicting results were reported by others.[12] In one study, the authors compared the DSB repair of the DNA-PKcs wild-type CHO cell line CHO10B2 with its derived radiosensitive mutant cell line, the DNA-PKcs-deficient cell line irs-20 after cells were exposed to photon and proton beams.[12] Irs-20 cells presented more persistent DSBs compared with CHO10B cells after cells were exposed to both photon and proton beams. A dependence on the DNA-PKcs in repairing DSBs caused by both proton and photon beams was verified.[12] In another study involving the DNA-PKcs wild-type CHO cell line CHO10B2, Ku80-mutated CHO mutant cell XRS-5, DNA-PKcs null V3 cells, Rad51D-mutated 51D1 cells, and 14 cell lines derived from V3 cells with complementary human DNA PKcs containing amino acid substitutions at specific positions, the cell responses to proton beams versus photon beams were not correlated with the status of DNA-PKcs or RAD51; thus, no preferential DSB repair pathway of HR or NHEJ was observed in proton beam–induced DSB repair.[18] Other than the previously mentioned, a study using cervical cancer HeLa cells claimed that the higher cell response rate of proton beams versus photon beams in the SOBP is in an Artemis protein–dependent manner. Because Artemis protein is a member of the NHEJ pathway, this result reflects the dependency of the repair of proton beam–induced DSBs on NHEJ.[20] Some other studies also demonstrated the preference of the NHEJ pathway in the repair of DSBs induced by proton beams.[21,22] This evidence includes the activation of Ataxia-Telangiesctasia mutated (ATM, contributing to NHEJ[23]) and DNA-PKcs but not ataxia telangiectasia and Rad3 related (ATR) by proton beams in human lung adenocarcinoma A549 cells[21] and the induction of ATM by proton beams in human prostate cancer PC3 cells.[22]

Taken together, the overall DNA damage caused by proton is different than that of photon beams, at least to a certain extent. However, the repair mechanisms of the DSBs induced by proton beams are still unclear. Future studies specifically investigating the DNA repair pathways of proton beams will translate the findings into biology-based rationales of treatment selection between proton- and photon-based radiation and the combination of therapies that targeted specific signal pathways.

Cell Death

One of the severe consequences of the failure of DNA damage repair induced by radiation is cell death. The mechanisms of photon radiation–induced cell death are intensively studied. Photon radiation is known to kill cancer cells via apoptosis, necrosis, autophagy, mitotic catastrophe, and senescence.[24–28] However, the mechanisms by which proton radiation induces cell death are unclear.

CELL MITOTIC CATASTROPHE

Extensive evidence demonstrated that mitotic catastrophe is the major mechanism of cell death in solid tumors in response to photon radiotherapy.[24,26] However, the role of cell mitotic catastrophe in response to proton beam radiation is unclear. We uncovered that mitotic catastrophe was the dominant mechanism of cell death in both human papillomavirus (HPV)–related and HPV-unrelated human head and neck squamous carcinoma cells after proton beam radiation at 4, 24, 48, and 72 hours after radiation (Fig. 1.2). Moreover, the results demonstrated that compared with photon beams, a 4-Gy dose of proton radiation led to a higher level of mitotic catastrophe in these cells. The more pronounced cell mitotic catastrophe induced by proton beams versus photon beams suggests that combining therapy targeting the DNA damage repair pathway may promote cell death differently after proton radiation compared with photon radiation.

CELL SENESCENCE

With emerging evidence, cellular senescence is increasingly being recognized as one of the most important mechanisms in photon radiation–induced tumor suppression.[26,29,30] Similar to that observed in photon radiation, we found that senescence was also a major type of cell death induced by a 4-Gy dose of proton beam radiation in HPV-related and HPV-unrelated human head and neck squamous carcinoma cells at 4 and 6 days after exposure (Fig. 1.3). More importantly, compared with photon beams, proton beams led to a higher proportion of cells undergoing senescence in these cell lines. Based on the above facts, the role of combination treatment that interferes with cell senescence pathways may influence cell responses to proton beams versus photon beams differently and warrants further investigation.

CELL APOPTOSIS

Apoptosis plays a modest role in the response of many solid tumors to photon irradiation. To date, little is known about cell apoptosis after they are exposed to proton radiation. The study result from one group[31] indicated that compared with photon beams, proton beams led to a greater level of cell apoptosis at 48 hours after radiation in H460 and A549.[21,31] Similarly, a study (16 in DNA damage literature) using patient-derived glioma stem cells to compare proton beam with photon beam irradiation indicated that proton beams induce more cell apoptosis and lead to more cell apoptosis–related caspase-3 activation and poly(adenosine diphosphate [ADP]-ribose) polymerase (PARP) cleavage. Other than the higher incidence of cell apoptosis after

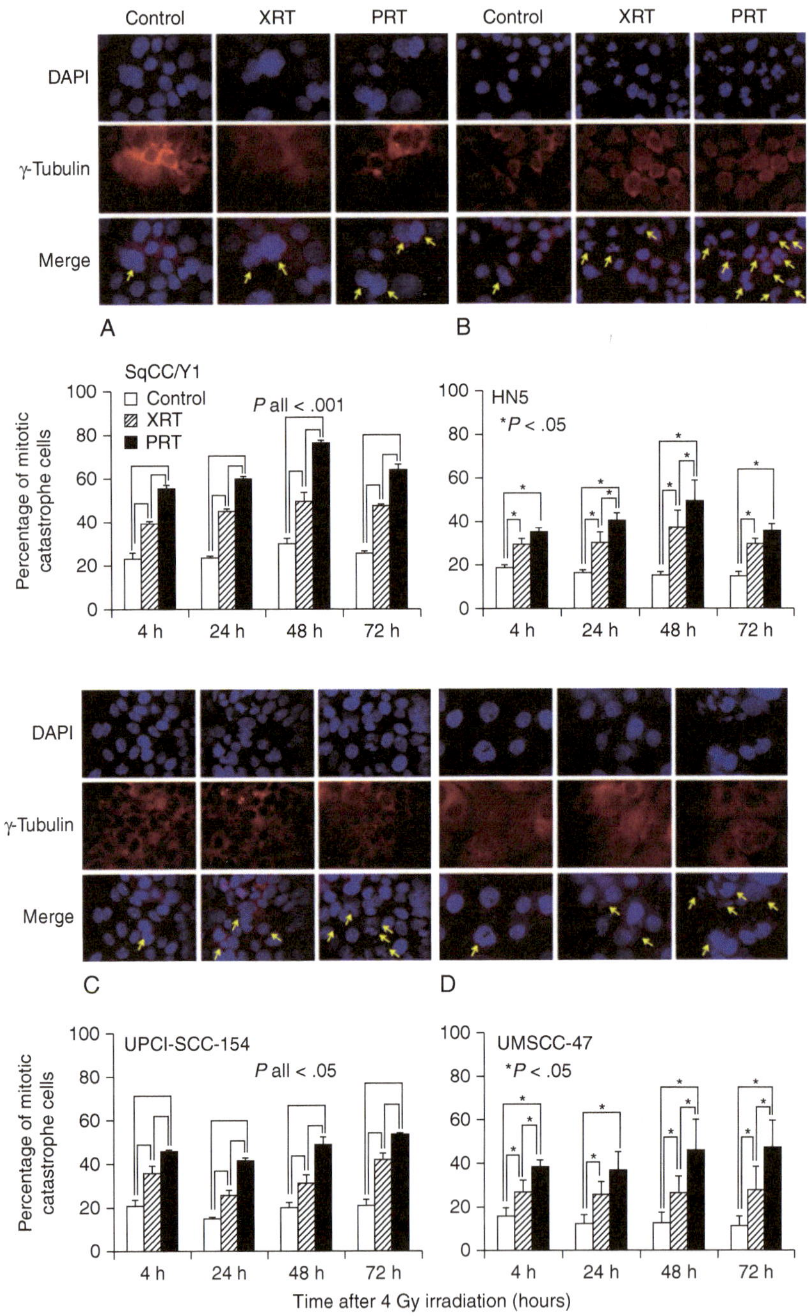

Fig. 1.2 Mitotic catastrophe in head and neck squamous cell carcinoma cell lines after exposure to photon *(XRT)* versus proton *(PRT)* irradiation. Two human papillomavirus (HPV)–negative cell lines (SqCC/Y1, panel A; and HN5, panel B) and two HPV-positive cell lines (UPCI-SCC-154, panel C; UMSCC-47, panel D) were tested. Cells were fixed, permeabilized, blocked, and incubated with anti-γ-tubulin (primary antibody) and Texas Red (secondary antibody) to visualize immunoreactivity; DNA was stained with 4′,6-diamidino-2-phenylindole. Immunoreactions were visualized with a Leica Microsystem at ×100 magnification.

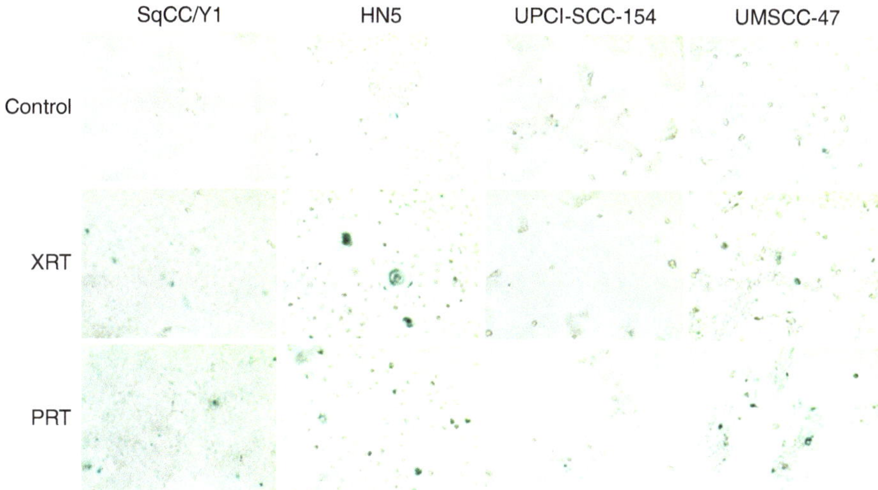

A

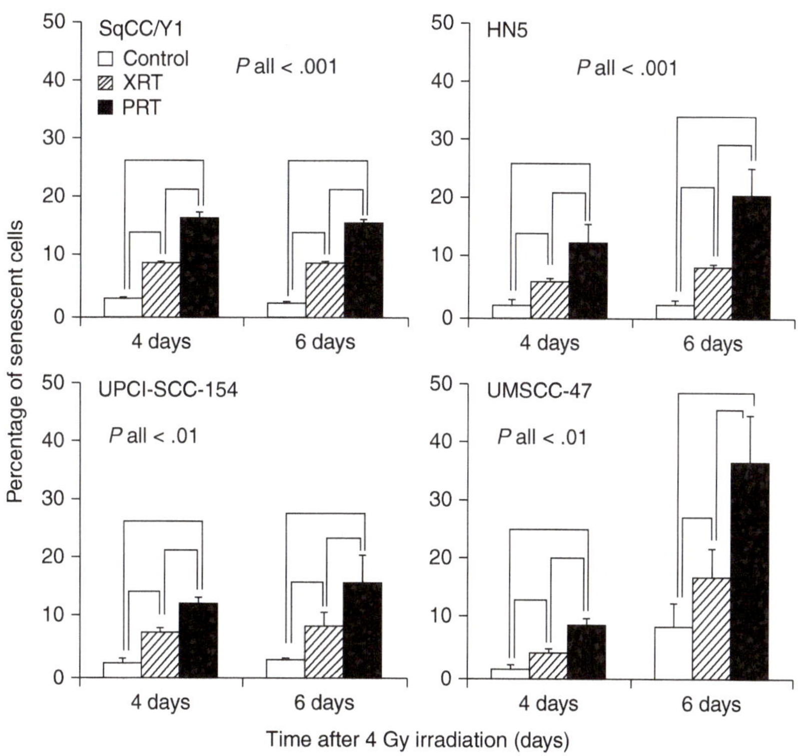

Fig. 1.3 Senescence in head and neck squamous cell carcinoma cell lines after exposure to photon *(XRT)* versus proton *(PRT)* irradiation. Two human papillomavirus (HPV)–negative cell lines (SqCC/Y1 and HN5) and two HPV-positive cell lines (UPCI-SCC-154 and UMSCC-47) were stained with senescence-associated β-galactosidase (SA-β-gal) and analyzed 4 days and 6 days later. (A) Photographs of senescent cells at 6 days after irradiation. Cells were photographed with an optic microscope at ×20 magnification. Cells staining positive for SA-β-gal show blue cytoplasmic staining.

proton beam versus photon beam radiation, studies from other groups also revealed the time point differences of the cell apoptosis occurrence between photon versus proton beam radiation. One group from Italy[32] exposed the prostate adenocarcinoma cell line PC3 to photon and proton beams. They found that the peak of PC3 cells undergoing apoptosis was reached at 8 hours after proton irradiation compared with 48 hours for photon irradiation. Differently, a study from Germany on HeLa cells indicated that during the maximum observation time of 48 hours, the proportion of apoptotic cells induced by proton beams increased with time.[33] Other than the above direct evidence of cell apoptosis induced by proton beams, indirect evidence of cell apoptosis–related signal pathway changes were also generated. One study[21] demonstrated significantly more upregulation of proapoptotic gene, *Bax*, and downregulation of antiapoptotic gene, *Bcl-2*, at 12 hours after lung cancer A549 cells were exposed to proton beams compared with those cells exposed to photon beams. However, our study in HPV-related and HPV-unrelated human head and neck squamous carcinoma cells showed a different result (Fig. 1.4A). Both photon and proton beams only induced limited cell apoptosis, and no difference was observed in the proportion of proton beam–induced cell apoptosis versus that induced by photon beams. Because both proton beams and photon beams can cause DNA damage and DNA damage is a major pathway by which radiation causes apoptosis, strategies to target apoptosis pathway to enhance proton beam or photon beam–induced tumor cell apoptosis may be another effective strategy for enhancing the antitumor activity of radiation.

CELL NECROSIS

Necrosis typically occurs after a large dose of photon radiation,[27,34] but it has also been observed in cancer cell lines and patient tumor tissue–derived cancer cells after a single 4-Gy or 6-Gy dose of photon irradiation.[35] Comparing the proportion of cells undergoing necrosis in four HPV-related and HPV-unrelated human head and neck squamous carcinoma cell lines after a single 4-Gy dose of proton or photon beam radiation, we found that proton and photon beams only led to significantly increased necrosis in one HPV-unrelated cell line 48 hours after radiation, and no differences were found between proton versus photon beams (Fig. 1.4B). Mechanistic studies of tumor necrosis have identified several molecular targets that mediate necrosis after treatment.[34–36] Interfering with those molecular targets may be another new approach to promote both proton and photon beam–induced necrotic cell death and may be a potential to enhance radiosensitivity.[34,35]

In summary, mitotic catastrophe and senescence are the major types of cell death induced by both photon and proton beams, and proton beams kill more cells by either mechanism than photon beams. Individual cancer patients with different gene mutation statuses may derive different levels of benefit from targeted therapy that interferes with different cell death–related pathways according to whether the radiotherapy is photon or proton based. Further mechanistic and in vivo studies may open a new avenue of improving tumor control with proton or photon radiation and lead to novel, individually optimized combination treatment plans consisting of molecular-targeted therapy combined with proton or photon beams for cancer patients with tumors of different biological features.

Relative Biological Effectiveness

Proton therapy has shown promise to protect normal tissues in the treatment of malignant diseases such as pediatric cancers,[37] central nervous system and skull base tumors,[38–40] ocular melanoma,[41,42] and head and neck cancers that are near critical structures[43–45] and are difficult to treat with surgery or conventional photon radiation.[46,47] However, because of variations in the RBE of protons in different types of cells or tissues,[48,49] whether the dosimetric advantages of proton

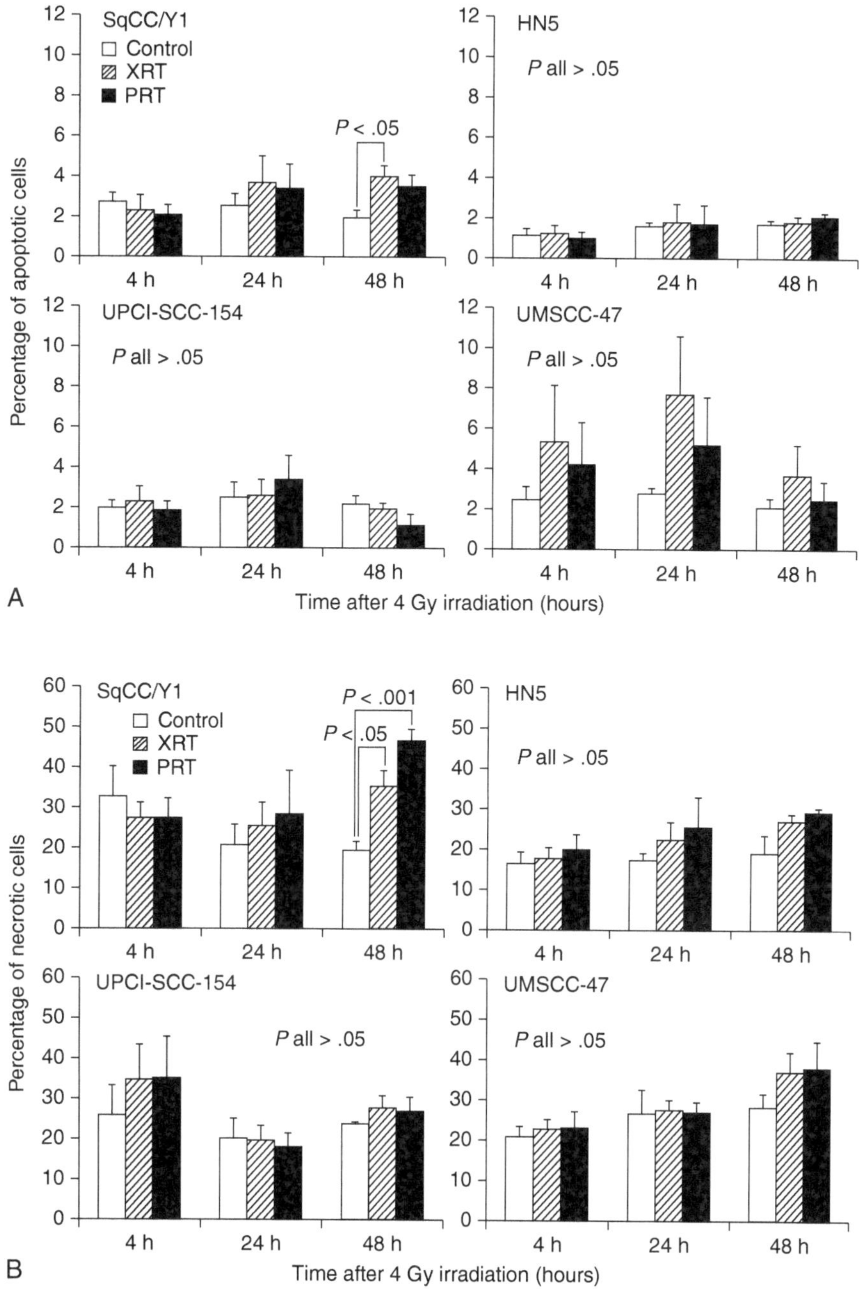

Fig. 1.4 Necrosis and apoptosis in head and neck squamous cell carcinoma cell lines after photon *(XRT)* or proton *(PRT)* irradiation. Two human papillomavirus (HPV)–negative cell lines (SqCC/Y1 and HN5) and two HPV-positive cell lines (UPCI-SCC-154 and UMSCC-47) were subjected to terminal deoxy-nucleotidyltransferase (TdT) dYTP nick-end labeling (TUNEL) and incubated with fluorescein isothiocyanate (FITC)-conjugated annexin V and propidium iodide and analyzed by BD Accuri C6. Percentages of necrotic or apoptotic cells were quantified with FlowJo V10 software. (A) Quantification of apoptotic cells. (B) Quantification of necrotic cells.

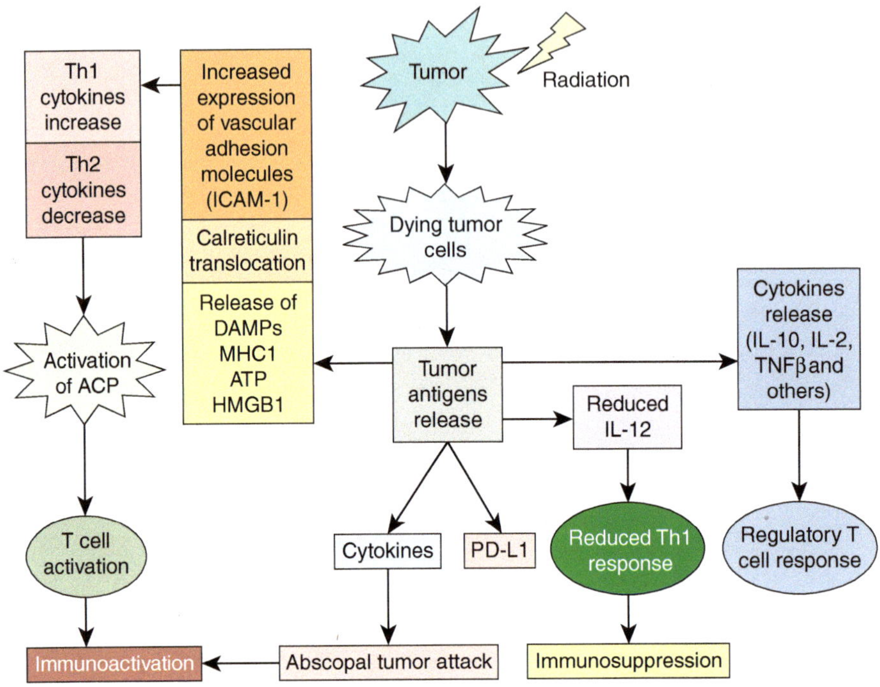

Fig. 1.5 Immune response changes after x-ray-based radiation. *ATP,* Adenosine triphosphate; *DAMP*, damage-associated molecular pattern; *HMGB1*, high mobility group box-1; *IL*, interleukin; *PD-L1*, programmed death-ligand 1. (Summarized based on Diegeler S, Hellweg CE. Intercellular communication of tumor cells and immune cells after exposure to different ionizing radiation qualities. *Front Immunol*. 2017;8:664 and Ebner DK, Tinganelli W, Helm A, et al. The immunoregulatory potential of particle radiation in cancer therapy. *Front Immunol*. 2017;8:99.)

beams can be translated into demonstrable clinical benefits of normal tissue protection and tumor control for these cancers remains unclear.

Currently, clinical use of proton beams is based largely on the experiences that are derived from photon beam radiation. However, the difference in the energy deposition patterns of photon beams and proton beams means that equal doses of proton or photon beam radiation do not produce equal biological effects; one type of radiation may be more effective at killing cells than the other one. The RBE of proton beams is defined as the ratio of the doses required for photon versus proton beams radiation to produce the same level of biological effectiveness, such as cell killing or DNA damage.[50,51] The RBE of proton beams has been recognized as variable values. The RBE is determined by a number of physical and biological factors, such as proton beam energy, depth, radiation dose, radiation fraction size, radiation fraction number, cell or tissue types, and the end points.[47,52–57] The advantages of proton versus photon beams only can be presented in the case of accurately assured higher/equal target volume dose and lowered surrounding normal tissue dose in proton radiation. Therefore an accurate proton beam RBE is required in proton beam radiation.

In current clinical practice, the RBE of proton therapy has been assumed to be 1.1 regardless of tumor type, beam energy, and treatment planning differences.[49] This RBE value was mainly derived from preclinical experiments with normal cells or early-reacting normal tissues rather than cancer cells or tumor xenografts.[53–55] Moreover, these experiments also demonstrated a big range of RBE at the middle of SOBP (ranging from 0.9 to 2.1 for in vitro experiments and from 0.7 to 1.6 for in vivo experiments).[52] Thus, use of this constant RBE without considering differences in tumor biology or the effects of fractionation increases the extent of clinical dose uncertainties for tumor and normal tissues associated with proton therapy, the nature and extent of which are largely unknown but are crucial to the safe and effective use of proton therapy.

More importantly, emerging evidence has established the increased RBE values in regions of high LET at the distal falloff of most proton beams, which are normally located within the target volume.[58–60] Thus, special attention should bring in treatment planning of proton beam radiation to avoid locating organs at risk to the distal portion of SOBP, which might induce normal tissue complications at the distal field edges. Furthermore, because in vivo study also found a trend that late-responding tissues may have higher RBE values compared with early-responding tissues,[61] more attention should be placed on the observation of late normal tissue response in those patients who accepted proton beam radiation in the clinical setting.

In summary, because of the uncertainties of the RBE in proton beam radiation, more studies on the clinically relevant dose range in the response of different normal tissues or tumor types in animals are needed.

Immune Response

Accumulated evidence has demonstrated that photon beam radiation not only can control tumor by local tumor irradiation but can also influence tumor growth by the effects of photon radiation on the activation and suppression of the immune system (Fig. 1.5).[62–64] To avoid the immunosuppression effect and to enhance the immunoactivation effect of photon radiation, the impact of photon radiation on the immune system is under extensive study currently to investigate the possibility of radiation and immune therapy combination to improve cancer treatment outcomes.

IMMUNOACTIVATION EFFECT OF PHOTON AND PROTON BEAMS

It has been demonstrated that photon radiation can influence tumor immune response through different mechanisms, which include direct effects and indirect effects. Photon beams can directly influence both immune cells and tumor cells to impact the tumor suppression effect of radiation. One of the important mechanisms of the activation of tumor immunity by photon radiation is that photon beams can turn tumor cells into in situ vaccine to facilitate tumor cell immune recognition by inducing the expression of different molecules on the surface of the tumor cells, increased expression of adhesion molecules, death receptors, stress-induced ligands, and immune cell stimulatory molecules.[65–71]

The direct damage caused by photon beams in tumor cells can lead to an increased expression of major histocompatibility complex I, which can facilitate the immune cells to recognize the tumor cells and initiate immune response to the tumor cells.[62,72] The important factor of photon beam–related immune activation is the presence of damage-associated molecular patterns (DAMPs) in tumor cells after irradiation. Calreticulin (CRT), adenosine triphosphate, high mobility group box-1 (HMGB1), and type I interferons are major factors in the DAMPs.[27,73,74] Photon beam radiation can induce the translocation of CRT to the tumor cell surface.[65,67] CRT is a critical molecule that is involved in immune recognition to increase sensitivity of tumor cells to T cell killing.[65,75] A similar phenomenon was also observed after different types of tumor cells were exposed to proton beams.[65,67] When human prostate cancer cells (LNCaP), human breast cancer cells (MDA-MB-231), human lung cancer cells (H1703), and chordoma cells (JHC7) were exposed to 200-MeV proton beams or photon beams of a dose of 8 Gy irradiation, increased expression of surface molecules that are involved in immune recognition, such as HLA-ABC, CEA, MUC-1, and ICAM-1, was observed after both photon and proton beam exposure; an increased cell-surface CRT expression and cytotoxic T lymphocytes–mediated tumor cell lysis was demonstrated.[67] However, unlike those of photon beams, the changes of other members in DAMPs in tumor cells after exposure to proton beams were absent and need to be uncovered.

INDIRECT IMMUNOACTIVATION EFFECT OF PHOTON AND PROTON BEAMS

Other than the previously mentioned direct immunoactivation effect by photon beams, it also has been established that photon beams can also induce the bystander effect, where a nontargeted effect is observed in unexposed cells that are nearby the irradiated cells. The bystander effect is the result of the direct exchange of cytokines via gap junctions between the irradiated cells and the unexposed cells. These cytokines are produced by tumor and immune cells that are exposed to photon beams. This nontargeted effect is an important factor to influence the immune system.[62] Another photon radiation–induced nontargeted effect that contributes to tumor regression at a site distant from the local radiation through recruiting immune cells to the tumor and by activating immune cells at the tumor site is the abscopal effect.[62,65,76–81] Even though the above radiation-induced interactions of immune cells and tumor cells after photon beams radiation are extensively studied, the above effects of proton beams are largely unknown and warrant further investigation.

IMMUNE SUPPRESSION EFFECT OF PHOTON AND PROTON BEAMS

Other than the discussed immune activation effect, photon irradiation is also known to have immune suppression effects. This immune suppression effect may be as a result of direct cell killing or a functional suppression of immune cells.[73] Dendritic cells (DCs) are antigen-presenting cells that can present tumor-derived antigens to tumor-specific cytotoxic T cells and can result in the local and systemic antitumor immune responses.[65,81–85] It has been demonstrated that, after exposure to photon beams, the functions of DCs to activate lymphocytes and to produce immune-activating cytokine interleukin 12 (IL-12) were suppressed.[73,86] These changes caused by photon beams may suppress the immune response to tumors. Proton beams were expected to have less direct suppression of immune response based on the physical feature of proton beams, where less normal tissues are included in the radiation compared with photon beams, and less immune cells will be exposed to proton beams. More in vitro and in vivo studies are needed to uncover this phenomenon.

Aside from the direct inhibition of immune cells, photon beams also can suppress different types of immune cells through in situ secretion of cytokines by the damaged cells.[65,87] IL-10 is a cytokine that can suppress immune response by reducing antigen presentation, inhibiting Th1 responses, reducing NK cell cytokine expression, and thus suppressing functions of monocytes and macrophages.[62,88] The release of cytokines IL-10 after the exposure of photon beams was observed, and subsequently, the interferences of DCs maturation were demonstrated.[73] Proton beams were reported to influence immune suppression cytokines differently compared with photon beams by several studies. In a study using two human head and neck cancer cell lines (CAL33 and CAL27), the authors tested the inflammatory cytokines IL-6 and IL-8, both of which play important roles in tumor microenvironment, tumor angiogenesis, tumorigenicity, tumor metastasis, and immune suppression. The study results indicated that compared with photon beams, proton beams downregulated the proinflammatory gene IL-6 expression. On the other hand, photon beams upregulated the proinflammatory gene IL-8 expression; however, no similar gene regulation was observed in proton beams.[89] Another study also demonstrated that proton beam exposure can lead to reduced levels of IL-6 and IL-8 both in vitro and in vivo.[90,91] The cytokines transforming growth factor β (TGF-β) and prostaglandin E2 (PGE2) both lead to immune suppression through multiple mechanisms, including increasing the ratio of immune suppression cell Treg cells.[73,92,93] It was reported that photon beam exposure can cause an increased expression of TGF-β and PGE2, whereas the influence of proton beams on the expression of these cytokines is unknown and deserves to be uncovered.

The programmed death-ligand 1 (PD-L1) is an immune checkpoint molecule that plays an important role in tumor immune tolerance and is therefore induced to tumor formation and tumor progression.[89,94] It has been demonstrated that photon beams can induce an upregulated expression of PD-L1 in different types of tumor cells by different studies.[73,89,95] However, the impact of proton beams on the expression of PD-L1 is conflicted and needs further clarification.[65,67,89]

In summary, based on these facts, using immune therapy that includes strategies to promote activation or recruitment of immune cells, injection of nonirradiated endogenous immune cells, administration of cancer-specific antibodies, cytokines, cancer vaccines, and immune checkpoint inhibitors,[65,96] in combination with photon radiation, may achieve a better tumor treatment outcome and is worth further investigation. Currently, immune therapy in combination with photon radiation is under clinical investigation.[62,97] However, the influence of proton beams on tumor immune response is based on limited studies with single, high-dose irradiation, which is different from the clinical setting of proton therapy. Moreover, preclinical study of immune therapy in combination with proton therapy is absent. Therefore, the effect of immune therapy in combination with proton therapy is unknown and needs to be further uncovered.

Angiogenic Signal Pathway

Numerous studies have demonstrated that vascular endothelial growth factor (VEGF) is a major factor in promoting tumor angiogenesis and lymphangiogenesis to promote tumor growth and metastasis.[89,98] Multiple studies have demonstrated that photon beams can cause significantly upregulated VEGF in different cancer cells.[99–101] Moreover, other cytokines that are related to tumor angiogenesis, such as IL-6[102–104] and IL-8,[105,106] were also found to be upregulated by photon beams. On the other hand, in a study using head and neck cancer cells, compared with cells exposed to photon beams, a significantly lower expression of VEGF was observed in cells exposed to proton beams.[89] Notably, the inhibition of angiogenesis was also observed after proton beam exposure.[107] After exposure to proton beams, decreased levels of VEGF, IL-6, and IL-8 were found both in vitro and in vivo.[66,91,108,109]

Taken together, these findings demonstrated that compared with photon beam radiation, proton beam radiation may have a special impact on tumor angiogenesis and lymphangiogenesis, indicating that proton beams might be particularly effective in the control of tumor progression and metastasis compared with photon beams. Further studies are warranted to clarify these points.

Conclusions and Remarks

Photon beams, including x-rays and γ-rays, are the most widely used type of ionizing radiation in cancer radiotherapy. The biological consequences of photon beams to tumors and normal tissues are extensively studied and relatively well established. Proton beam therapy is currently gaining importance worldwide based on its advantageous physical features, such as sparing normal tissues, which makes it particularly suitable for tumors that are located close to critical normal structures. Proton beam radiation is increasingly used as an advanced alternative radiotherapy modality. However, the knowledge of the biological effects of proton beams is very limited. Comparative studies of proton versus photon beam radiation will provide new biological insights of radiotherapy and facilitate translational studies that are aimed at personalized combination therapy to improve treatment outcomes and decrease treatment-related toxicities for patients with different malignant diseases. Further studies aimed at investigating the tumor-specific RBEs will decrease the treatment dose uncertainties of proton beam radiation. More investigations of proton beam radiation biology to uncover the many remaining unknowns, including DNA damage responses, gene expression, cell death mechanisms, immune response, angiogenesis, cell cycle regulation, and hypoxia response, are warranted.

References Available Online.

CHAPTER 2

Principles of Proton Beam Therapy

Radhe Mohan

Introduction

The potential of physical characteristics of protons for cancer treatments was first recognized by Wilson in 1946.[1] During the following four decades or so, proton accelerators at various physics laboratories around the world were adapted for clinical purposes. Examples of such facilities include the University of California Berkeley; the Harvard Cyclotron Laboratory in Cambridge, Massachusetts; Uppsala University, Sweden; Dubna, Russia; and Chiba, Japan. Physics laboratory-based particle therapy facilities are designed for physics applications and, as such, are not suitable for clinical applications. This led to the establishment of hospital-based proton therapy facilities. The first among these was at the Loma Linda University Medical Center, California,[2] in 1990, followed by Massachusetts General Hospital-Harvard University in 1999, the MD Anderson Cancer Center (MDACC) in Houston, and the University of Florida in Jacksonville, both in 2006. Since then, the number of proton therapy centers in the United States and around the world has grown dramatically. According to the Particle Therapy Co-Operative Group (PTCOG) website (http://www.ptcog.ch), as of March 2018, there were approximately 27 proton therapy facilities in operation in the United States and nearly 70 around the world. As of December 2016, 150,000 patients worldwide had been treated with protons.

Along with the rapid growth in the number of proton centers, the technology has continued to evolve. Whereas up until the last decade most of the proton treatments were carried out using passively scattered beams, the new treatment centers are now being equipped almost exclusively with scanning beam systems. These systems provide much greater flexibility to optimally shape dose distributions. Accelerators and gantries continue to become more compact and have greater functionality and lower cost. The treatment delivery control systems are becoming more sophisticated, allowing proton therapy systems to deliver superior treatments more efficiently.

Furthermore, ongoing research over the last dozen years is resulting in improved understanding of the sensitivity of protons to inter- and intrafractional anatomy variations, range uncertainties, setup uncertainties, and the unique biological effects of protons. This knowledge is being incorporated into the development of intensity-modulated proton therapy (IMPT) methods to optimize biologically effective proton dose distributions to achieve higher and higher therapeutic ratios. Accuracy of dose distributions is being improved with the introduction of Monte Carlo techniques and made practical with the development of fast Monte Carlo methods. Clinical trials, many of them randomized protons versus photons, are being conducted to evaluate the relative clinical and cost-effectiveness of protons.

In principle, protons have a much greater therapeutic potential than has been realized to date. Although the technology has improved substantially and we have made significant strides in improving our understanding of physical, biological, and clinical aspects of proton therapy in the recent past, considerable additional research and development are needed to maximally exploit the potential of proton therapy. Sections later describe the principles underlying proton therapy, the current state of the art and its limitations, ongoing research and development to advance the state of the art, and the long-term promise of radiotherapy with protons.

Physical Characteristics of Protons

The rationale for the use of protons to treat cancers is built upon their unique physical characteristics. These characteristics allow the production of radiation dose distribution patterns that conform more tightly to the shape of the tumor target and avoid normal tissues to a greater extent. The physical characteristics of protons also lead to biological effects that are, in general, quite different from those of the traditional radiation treatment modalities. Taken together, the physical and biological properties of protons offer a substantially higher therapeutic ratio.

Protons interact with matter primarily through Coulomb interactions with atomic electrons, Coulomb interactions with nuclei, and nuclear interactions. As a proton traverses the medium, it slows down continuously. The energy deposited by it per unit distance (called the linear energy transfer, or LET) increases until all of its energy is depleted, and it comes to essentially an abrupt stop. Thus, in a uniform medium, for example, a water phantom, a monoenergetic beam of protons leads to the formation of the characteristic Bragg curve (Fig. 2.1).[3] Because protons are much heavier than electrons, Coulomb interactions with electrons do not deflect them appreciably from their original path. However, Coulomb scattering from nuclei, although it occurs much less frequently, leads to larger-angle scattering and contributes to a substantial lateral spreading of proton beams. It leads to the widening of proton beam penumbra, especially when the protons have slowed down near the end of their range. Interactions of protons with nuclei occur with even lower probability and mainly at higher energies and lead to large-angle scattering and the production of secondary particles, including neutrons.

These properties of protons have a profound impact on the biological and clinical effects. Protons ionize more densely than photons. The density of ionization increases with increasing LET as they slow down as a function of depth. This, in turn, causes continuously increasing biological damage (e.g., more complex and clustered DNA damage), thus continuously increasing relative biological effectiveness (RBE) as a function of depth. The RBE is a complex function with physical and biological parameters. It is briefly dealt with in the section on Proton Biological Characteristics. More details can be found in Chapter 1 and in the literature, including some cited at the end of this chapter. The variations in RBE can be exploited to enhance the biologically effective dose differential between the target and normal tissues.

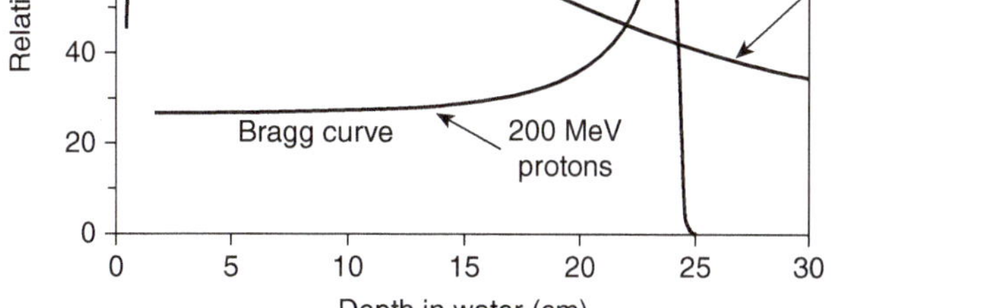

Fig. 2.1 Depth-dose curves for a 200-MeV proton beam: both unmodulated and with a 5 cm spread-out Bragg peak *(SOBP)*, compared with a 16-MV x-ray beam (for 10 × 10 cm^2 fields). The curves are normalized in each case to 100 at maximum dose. *SSD,* Source-to-skin distance. (Modified from Mohan R, Grosshans D. Proton therapy—present and future. *Adv Drug Deliv Rev.* 2017;109:26-44.)

In addition, protons have a lower entrance dose compared with photons (except in the entrance buildup region, see Fig. 2.1) and virtually no dose beyond the end of their range. Thus theoretically, they can be used to produce considerably more "compact" dose distributions (smaller "low-dose bath"). Such dose distributions can, in general, spare large volumes of normal tissues for the same target dose (see the section on Proton Therapy Planning and Plan Evaluation and Chapter 5 for more details.). Recent recognition of additional value of such compact dose distributions is their potential to mitigate radiation-induced lymphopenia (RIL), which is widely recognized to be a significant prognostic indicator of adverse outcomes.

It should be noted that although sharp falloff of dose at the end of the range of protons is critical to the improved patterns of dose distributions, it also has potential negative ramifications. It renders proton dose distributions, compared with photon dose distributions, more vulnerable to intrafractional changes in anatomy due respiratory motion and other physiological functions, and to interfractional variations in anatomy because of such factors as weight gain or loss, tumor shrinkage, setup variations, and so on. Special efforts are required to minimize uncertainties thus introduced and to address residual uncertainties.

Proton Biological Characteristics

A common misconception about proton therapy is an inherent assumption that, for the same physical dose delivered to a tissue, the biological and clinical effects of protons and photons are identical except that protons are 10% more biologically effective. In other words, the RBE of protons is a constant of 1.1. In reality, as protons interact with the tissues in the body (and matter in general), they traverse very differently and in a more complex manner. As a consequence, they have very different biological and clinical effects. They should be considered a different form of drug, perhaps many different forms of drug, depending on their physical parameters and the dose delivered. It is crucial that practitioners of proton therapy understand and appreciate these differences to apply proton therapy more effectively.

BIOLOGICAL EFFECTS IN THE CURRENT PRACTICE OF PROTON THERAPY

Appropriately, the clinical practice of proton therapy is based on our vast clinical experience with photon therapy. Such extrapolation requires that we understand the biological effects of the protons relative to photons. Extensive in vitro and in vivo studies have been carried out in the past to measure the biological effectiveness of protons relative to photon irradiation (i.e., the RBE). Paganetti et al. have summarized these data in two articles.[4,5] They argued that, considering uncertainties in the data, the use of an average value would be appropriate. In the current practice of proton therapy, the proton RBE is simplistically assumed to be a constant of 1.1 for all tumors and tissues, independent of dose and LET. However, the past experiments, the foundation of RBE of 1.1, were carried out under a broad range of inconsistent and underreported conditions and had large uncertainties in the results. Most of these experiments were conducted at high doses per fraction (5–8 Gy) and at points in the middle of large (~10 cm), spread-out Bragg peaks (SOBPs) of relatively high-energy protons. Moreover, the data were measured for only for a relatively small number of cell lines, tissues, and end points. Thus, it is not surprising that most of them yielded a value in the neighborhood of 1.1.

It is increasingly being recognized now that RBE is variable and a complex nonlinear function of dose per fraction, LET, tissue and cell properties, and other factors. Ignoring such variability may have a significant adverse impact on outcomes and could limit the effectiveness of proton therapy. Nevertheless, the RBE of 1.1 continues to be used clinically. To justify this practice, many have argued that no adverse responses have been reported attributable to this choice. However, "absence of evidence is not evidence of absence" of the effect. It is quite plausible that uncertainties in treatment planning and delivery processes could have masked the effect. As more and more patients are treated, unforeseen recurrences and toxicities are now being reported.[6–8] Among them is the report of Gunther et al., who compared rates of postradiotherapy changes in magnetic resonance (MR) images in pediatric ependymoma patients treated with photon and proton therapy. They found that a greater proportion of proton therapy patients versus IMRT patients (43% vs. 17%) developed postradiation MRI changes and at earlier times (3.8 months [median] vs. 5.3 months [median]). The grade and incidence of image intensity changes were also greater for protons than for photons. Other examples include reports of Weber et al.[9] and Mizumoto et al.,[10] who have reported serious neurological toxicities for patients treated with proton therapy.

Although there may be multiple contributing factors involved in such failures, the assumption of RBE of 1.1 may be among the important ones. The remedy chosen, applicable mainly to passively scattered proton therapy (PSPT), has been to avoid beam directions pointing toward the critical normal structures, such as brain stem or spinal cord, or to block the protons from reaching the critical structure. These approaches are ineffective for IMPT because the dose distributions per beam are highly heterogeneous. Another approach used has been to reduce the prescription dose. For instance, realizing the potential for increased brainstem necrosis, which can have profound clinical consequences, Indelicato et al.[7] have opted to reduce the prescription doses.

LABORATORY AND CLINICAL STUDIES TO QUANTIFY PROTON BIOLOGICAL EFFECTS ACCURATELY

Realizing the large gaps in knowledge of the biological effects of protons, multiple efforts are being mounted to conduct high-precision, high-accuracy in vitro and in vivo experiments. Examples of the studies already published include the works of Guan et al.,[11] Chaudhary et al.,[12,13] and Liu et al.[14,15] Guan et al., for instance, using specialized equipment designed using Monte Carlo simulations and scanning monoenergetic proton beams, showed that RBE varies substantially, especially around the Bragg peak, reaching values of up to 3 or 4 in the distal falloff region (Fig. 2.2).[16] Chaudhary et al. reported similar behavior for different cell lines. In addition, Liu et al.[14,15] showed that, for a set of 17 different lung cancer cell lines, the RBE deviates substantially from 1.1, even in the middle of the SOBP. They attributed their findings to, in part, Fanconi anemia/Breast Cancer gene (BRCA) pathway defects. Interestingly, although the dose-averaged LET value in the middle of the SOBP is low, there is a wide spectrum of energies and LET values at mid-SOBP. It is plausible that using dose-averaged LET as a surrogate of biological effect is not warranted. In general, proton biology is more complex, and continued further investigations are needed. (More details may be found in Chapter 1.)

DEDUCING PROTON RELATIVE BIOLOGICAL EFFECTIVENESS FROM CLINICAL RESPONSE

Translating laboratory in vitro and in vivo data directly into clinical practice, especially because most of the data are for clonogenic cell survival, is questionable. One could attempt to deduce it from the proton versus photon clinical response data. Unfortunately, data available are insufficient and have a high degree of uncertainty, which is likely to obscure the real properties of RBE. Nevertheless, it would be useful to refine the laboratory data–based models to fit clinical response differences between protons and photons. For instance, one may fit a normal tissue complication probability model to photon data and proton data separately. The differences in the model fits may be attributable to RBE. Then, assuming dose distributions for both protons and photons are calculated accurately (e.g., using Monte Carlo techniques), the RBE model parameters may be adjusted (optimized) so that they fit proton and photon data fit simultaneously.

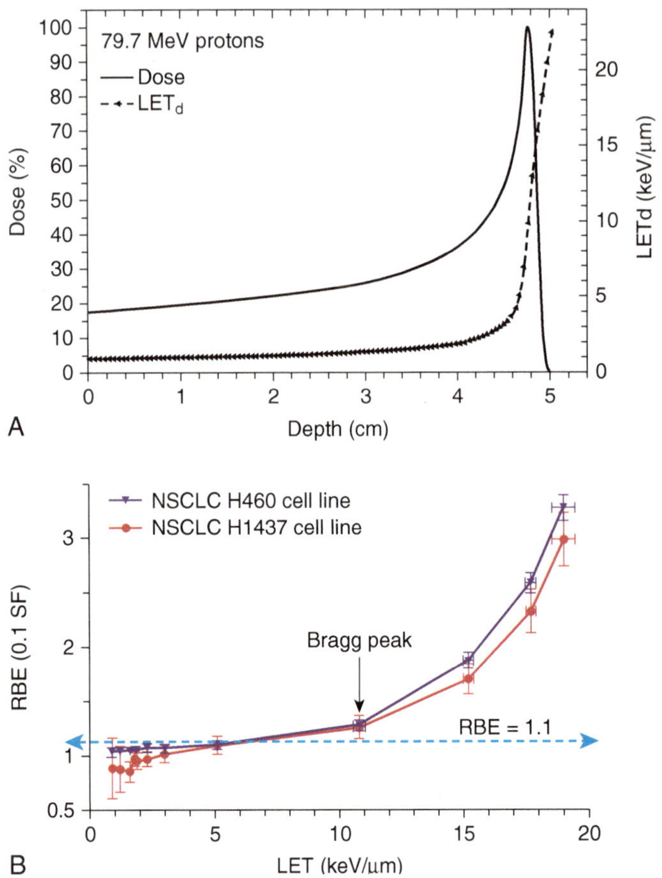

Fig. 2.2 (A) Depth-dose and linear energy transfer *(LET)* curves for an 18 cm × 18 cm scanned 79.7-MeV proton beam. (B) Measured relative biological effectiveness *(RBE)* as a function of LET along the path of the same beam in water-equivalent material. Note that the RBE increases essentially linearly up to the Bragg peak and then rapidly and nonlinearly in the distal falloff. *NSCLC*, Non–small-cell lung cancer. (A, From Guan F, Peeler C, Bronk L, et al. Analysis of the track- and dose-averaged LET and LET spectra in proton therapy using the geant4 Monte Carlo code. *Med Phys.* 2015;42:6234-6247. B, From Guan F, Bronk L, Titt U, et al. Spatial mapping of the biologic effectiveness of scanned particle beams: towards biologically optimized particle therapy. *Sci Rep.* 2015;5:9850.)

Using a different approach, Peeler et al.[17] analyzed the data of Gunther et al.[6] mentioned earlier to determine if the pre- and postradiotherapy image changes were associated with higher LET and hence attributed to a deviation of proton RBE from 1.1. They showed that the probability of image change is a function of dose as well as LET and that the dose for 50% probability of change in image voxel intensity is a function of LET. Their results suggest that increased LET contributes to a higher incidence of imaging changes within the brain tissue, indicative of radiation damage with increasing RBE. Extracting RBE from treatment response data, although challenging, is more clinically relevant.

MODELING OF PROTON BIOLOGICAL EFFECTS

Improved knowledge of RBE could be used to enhance optimality and clinical effectiveness of treatment plans. This can be realized most suitably using IMPT, which affords the highest degree of control over achievable dose distribution patterns. Predictive RBE models may be incorporated into the criteria of optimization of IMPT dose distributions to direct higher RBE protons into the target volume and away from normal tissues. RBE models may also be used to compute biological effects to evaluate given dose distributions to aid in clinical decision making. Such models can also be highly valuable in comparing competing treatment plans as well as proton dose distributions with photon dose distributions. Numerous models to predict RBE have been published.[18–27] However, they tend to be simplistic, assuming that RBE is a linear function of dose-averaged LET, and do not adequately fit most recently published radiobiology data. Research is taking place to develop novel models and to improve the accuracy of the current models to predict RBE. For further discussion of RBE models, the reader is referred to an article by Mohan et al.[28] and to references cited earlier.

Proton Therapy Delivery System

For clinical applications, protons are accelerated with cyclotrons or synchrotrons to therapeutically relevant energies, typically from 70 to 250 MeV. The energy or the sequence of energies needed are determined by the minimum and maximum depths of penetration required to irradiate the target volume.

An accelerated proton beam entering the treatment delivery head (i.e., the "nozzle") is very thin and has depth dose characteristics shown as the Bragg curve in Fig. 2.1. As such, it is not suitable for treating three-dimensional, arbitrarily shaped tumor targets. It must be broadened longitudinally and laterally and shaped to conform to the target shape. There are two main approaches to achieve this: (1) passive scattering to deliver PSPT, and (2) magnetic scanning of "beamlets" of protons of a sequence of initial energies to deliver IMPT. The latter is much more powerful technique to produce desired patterns of dose distributions. As mentioned, most of the treatments with protons to date have employed PSPT. However, nearly all the new installations are now based on scanning beam technology.

PROTON ACCELERATORS

In general, protons for radiotherapy applications are accelerated using cyclotrons or synchrotrons; each type has advantages and disadvantages. Cyclotrons produce a continuous stream of protons. In theory, they are more compact and have higher beam intensity. Protons are accelerated to the maximum of the energy of the cyclotron (e.g., 230 MeV), and the required lower energies are achieved by electromechanically inserting energy degraders in the path of protons. Synchrotrons, on the other hand, accelerate batches of protons to the desired energy. Once a batch has reached the required energy, it is extracted and transmitted via the "beam line" to the treatment room. The extraction may occur over a variable period of time from 0.5 to 4.5 seconds or longer, depending on the application. An additional 1 to 2 seconds are required to allow for resetting of the acceleration system between extractions and changing energy. Generally, the advantages of synchrotrons include greater energy flexibility, smaller energy spread, and lower power consumption. Regardless of the acceleration mechanism, the extracted narrow monoenergetic beam is magnetically guided through the beam line to the treatment room into the nozzle mounted, in most cases, on a rotating gantry. At most treatment facilities, a single accelerator serves multiple rooms. However, vendors are now offering single-room systems.

In typical scanning beam treatments with synchrotrons, depending on the depth of the target, a large number (~20–50) of energy layers may need to be scanned. If a field is large, multiple cycles may be required for the same energy layer, and for small fields, unused protons may be discarded. Considering that each cycle takes about 6 seconds or more, including the change in energy, the total time to deliver a fraction may be quite long. Newer systems are being designed to have higher dose rates and faster energy changes. Moreover, they permit multienergy extraction in which the energy is reduced from a maximum in a series of steps to allow scanning along the depth of the target.

For scanning beam treatments with cyclotrons, the energies of scanning beams from energy layer to energy layer are changed using high-precision movements of a fast energy degrader.

PASSIVELY SCATTERED PROTON THERAPY

For PSPT, the lateral and longitudinal spreading of the thin beam entering the nozzle is achieved with a combination of a rotating modulation wheel and one or two scatterers. This combination produces a SOBP, a uniform, cylindrically shaped dose distribution with a relatively low dose proximally and a rapidly falling dose distally. To conform the dose distribution laterally to the shape of the target volume, an aperture, typically made from blocks of brass of sufficient thickness (2−8 cm) to absorb incident protons of the highest energy, is used. To create a dose distribution that conforms to the distal shape of the target, the SOBP is shaped further by using a range compensator made of a nearly water-equivalent material. Because the SOBP width for a passively scattered beam is designed to be constant across the entire field, passive scattering provides no control over dose distribution proximal to the target. For a target with a highly irregular distal edge, this may lead to a substantial excess volume of high dose proximal to the target.

SCANNING BEAMS

A considerably clinically more effective approach is to shape the beams using magnetic scanning of thin beamlets of protons. Multiple beams incident from different directions, each comprising the scanning beamlets of sequences of energies, may be used to produce the desired pattern of dose.

Protons in a beamlet incident on a patient or a phantom are very nearly monoenergetic and are distributed essentially as a narrow Gaussian function of position relative to the beamlet's central axis. The lateral dimension of a beamlet is expressed in terms of the full width at half maximum (FWHM) of the Gaussian, or its σ. A smaller FWHM is desirable because it allows for a sharper penumbra and a greater control over dose distributions. In air, higher-energy proton pencil beams have a smaller FWHM than the lower-energy ones. Typically, the smallest achievable FWHMs in air for the highest energies (220−250 MeV) range from 7 to 12 mm (or σ of 3–5 mm), depending on the vendor and the machine model. Once the pencil beam enters a medium, such as a phantom or a patient, the FWHM increases substantially, especially near the end of the range of protons.

Magnetic scanning of beamlets provides greater flexibility and control for creating the optimum conformal proton dose distribution. In addition, the elimination of mechanical shaping devices (such as apertures and compensators) saves the cost of fabricating them and the time required for the insertion of these devices, obviates the need to enter the treatment room between fields, and makes the treatments more efficient. Most importantly, scanned techniques allow the delivery of IMPT, potentially the most effective form of proton therapy. The positions and intensities (in terms of monitor units) for a matrix of spots within the target volume for each scanned beam are determined by the treatment planning system to achieve the acceptable or the best possible approximation of the desired dose distribution.

Proton scanning beams have been in use for patient treatments at the Paul Scherrer Institute since 1996, where a one-dimensional scanning of proton pencil beams of different energies in the patient's transverse plane is used. The other dimension is achieved by moving the couch along the patient's longitudinal axis. The first use of two-dimensional scanning occurred in May 2008 at MDACC, where it is now used routinely. Recognizing the potential of scanning beams, most new proton therapy installations primarily or entirely employ scanning beams. Further research and development of this technology are continuing.

For scanning beams, proximal and lateral field shaping is achieved by limiting the positions of the spots to within the target regions only. Presumably, there is no need for an aperture. However, because of the substantial size of the pencil beam spots, consideration is now being given to the use of dynamic apertures that can change their shapes layer by layer.

More details on treatment delivery issues may be found in Chapter 6.

Proton Therapy Planning and Plan Evaluation

These issues are discussed in detail in Chapter 5. However, some comments are in order and may be helpful in appreciating the differences in processes and techniques for protons and photons. Planning and evaluation also often require different types of tools.

We reiterate the statement that protons are more sensitive to intrafractional anatomy motion, interfractional anatomy changes, and setup variations. Moreover, although they have a finite range and a rapid dose falloff at the end of the range, there is uncertainty in range, which is a function of depth of penetration. In addition, heterogeneities in the path of protons and their shifts relative to the beam direction perturb dose distributions in the tumor in a complex manner. On the other hand, rigid shifts in patient position along the beam direction have virtually no impact on dose distribution. Thus, the traditional concept of PTV margin for photon therapy to ensure that the clinical target volume (CTV), in the face of uncertainties, receives the prescribed dose with high probability does not apply to the beam direction. The solution applied for PSPT is to assign margins to distal and proximal edges of the tumor along each beam's direction to design the target volume. Further, to mitigate the perturbation of dose within the tumor, the compensator used to conform the dose distribution to the distal edge of the target is "smeared." Such solutions are not applicable for IMPT. In IMPT, dose distributions in the target for each of a group of beams are highly heterogeneous, which match with each other in a way that there is a homogeneous dose distribution. The perturbations caused by sources of physical uncertainties lead to a loss of match and, therefore, to heterogeneity in the target dose.

For both PSPT and IMPT, respiratory motion is accounted for by defining an internal motion-incorporated volume, and dose distributions are computed assuming the body to be a rigid representation of the average of phases of four-dimensional computed tomography (4D CT). In common with photon therapy, it is further assumed that, if the tumor motion is less than a certain threshold (e.g., 5 mm), there is no need for any special motion management intervention, such as breathhold or respiratory gating. In fact, it has been shown that the perturbation of dose distribution depends not just on tumor motion but also on the respiration-induced changes in the path of protons.[29] Thus the decision regarding whether to use special motion management steps should be based on changes in dose distribution over the breathing cycle, for instance, from end-inhale to end-exhale.

Uncertainties mentioned in the paragraphs above mean that the dose distribution actually received by the patient is different from what a clinician sees on the treatment plan and uses to make treatment decisions. Such differences are greater for protons than for photons. Solutions to address this problem have been developed in the recent past and are being implemented in commercial treatment planning systems. Among them is robust evaluation of treatment plans to assess their resilience in the face of uncertainties. Dose distributions are recalculated for a set of expected uncertainty scenarios, and bands of dose-volume histograms (DVHs) for all scenarios are graphed and used to assess the suitability of a plan. Often, the "worst-case" scenario for the CTV coverage is chosen because it corresponds to the use of planning target volume (PTV) for photons. Note that PTV is meant to ensure that the CTV is covered with a prescribed dose with high probability. In other words, the PTV DVH represents the worst-case DVH for the CTV. Robustness evaluation is applicable to both PSPT and IMPT. It is also applicable to photons but generally is not considered necessary.

For IMPT, it also possible to render dose distributions as less sensitive uncertainties by using a process called robust optimization, in which the intensities of beamlets are optimized to maximize the probability of CTV coverage and normal tissue sparing under all uncertainties simultaneously.[30–37] For IMPT of disease sites affected by respiratory motion, 4D robust optimization is a solution. In it, IMPT is optimized to achieve the desired tumor and normal tissue constraints simultaneously for all uncertainty scenarios as well as for all respiratory phases.[37]

Although robustness evaluation and robust optimization make dose distributions more reliable in terms of what a patient receives, they do not necessarily improve the optimality of the plan. In fact, making robustness requirements more stringent in robust optimization may degrade the optimality. Thus it is important to reduce uncertainties using such techniques as in-room volumetric imaging for treatment setup and more frequent adaptive replanning to account for interfractional anatomy changes. Another source of uncertainty for proton therapy is the approximations in computed dose distributions. It is important that the CT images used for dose calculations be obtained with dual-energy CTs, which have reduced artifacts and provide image data that can be converted more accurately to stopping power ratios, the quantities that are required for proton dose calculations. Moreover, the analytic proton dose calculation models implemented in commercial treatment planning systems are inadequate, and it is necessary to resort to Monte Carlo systems or their faster versions being developed. Monte Carlo systems are also more appropriate for computing proton LET values and energy spectra needed for computing variable RBE values.

Although many of the steps mentioned may also be useful for photons, they are essential for protons.

Incorporating Variable Relative Biological Effectiveness in Evaluating and Optimizing Proton Dose Distributions

As emphasized previously, a unique aspect of protons is their biological properties. The proton RBE models being developed can be used to calculate biologically effective (RBE-weighted) dose distributions. Such dose distributions may be particularly useful to assess whether the variable RBE might have played a role in unforeseen toxicity or local failure. However, it is essential that, to isolate the biological effect that may be responsible, uncertainty in computed dose distributions need to be minimized to the extent possible.

RBE models may also be incorporated into IMPT optimization criteria to, in principle, produce a higher biologically effective dose within the target and lower within the surrounding normal tissues. Note that the primary rationale for using protons is their characteristic Bragg curve. Because the variable RBE-weighted dose at the Bragg peak is 30% to 40% higher than the entrance dose compared with the physical dose, it would seem that the incorporation of variable RBE into the IMPT optimization criteria may lead to a greater differential between target and normal tissue doses compared with the use of a constant RBE of 1.1. However, there has been some resistance to the use of variable RBE models for this purpose, citing uncertainty in the models as the reason. This is true; however, it can be argued that even the rudimentary models would lead to superior biologically effective dose distributions compared with the assumption of RBE of 1.1.

An alternative strategy has been proposed to include terms based on LET in the optimization criteria to push the LET to higher levels in the target volume to lower levels in normal tissues.[38,39] The rationale is that LET distributions can be calculated accurately. However, LET may not be an adequate surrogate of biological effect, and, ultimately, accurate RBE models will need to be incorporated (Fig. 2.3).

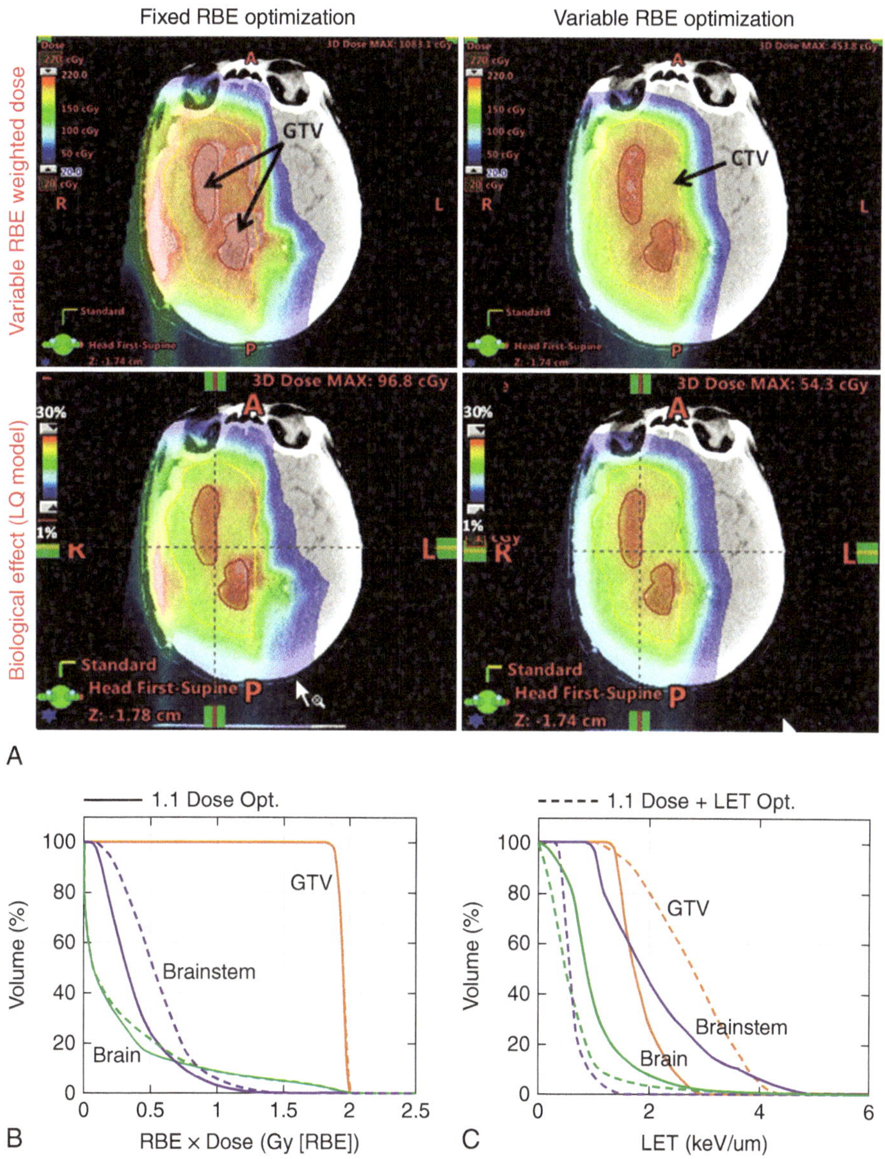

Fig. 2.3 (A) Comparison of a glioblastoma intensity-modulated proton therapy (IMPT) plan optimized using criteria defined in terms of fixed relative biological effectiveness *(RBE)* (RBE = 1.1) versus the plan optimized using criteria defined in terms of variable RBE. The variable RBE was computed using the Wilkens and Oelfke model.[17] The top two panels display dose distributions in terms of variable RBE-weighted dose, whereas the bottom two panels display biological effect in terms (one surviving fraction) calculated using the linear-quadratic model. Panels (B) and (C) compare a pediatric brain tumor IMPT plan optimized based on criteria defined in terms of RBE 1.1-weighted dose versus a plan based on same criteria plus additional terms that control linear energy transfer *(LET)* in the target and normal structures. Panel (B) compares the RBE 1.1-weighted DVHs for the GTV, brainstem, and normal brain, whereas panel (C) compares the corresponding LET-volume histograms. This figure demonstrates that significant increases in LET values in the tumor and a significant reduction in normal structures are possible. Of course, achievable biological effect gain depends on the geometric configuration anatomic of structures and may necessitate trade-offs. *GTV,* Gross target volume; *LQ,* linear quadratic. (From Mohan R, Peeler CR, Guan F, et al. Radiobiological issues in proton therapy. *Acta Oncol.* 2017;56:1367-1373.)

Current Research and Development Activities, Future Prospects, and Summary

Proton therapy is potentially highly effective; however, outcomes compared to photons have not met expectations so far. To improve the state of the art, numerous advancements have taken place during the last decade or so through research and developments carried at academic institutions. Many of the technical advancements, inspired by clinical needs, have also been carried out at the industry level. Considerably more advancement is required and is possible to exploit the full potential of this promising modality.

Research is going on in improving our understanding of the clinical response to different patterns of proton dose distribution patterns. In addition, in vivo and in vitro experiments are being carried out to improve our understanding of the biology of protons. Efforts are being made to extract biological effect information from clinical response data, which may be combined with laboratory biological effects data to develop novel predictive models. These models are being incorporated into the evaluation and optimization of dose distributions. Among the future goals is to test the validity of these models and their effectiveness to enhance the therapeutic ratio prospectively with clinical trials and in routine practice.

Advancements are also being made on the technology front to develop more compact accelerators and gantries and to make the delivery systems more efficient and accurate. New features being developed include smaller spot sizes, faster energy changes, and multienergy extraction to facilitate repainting of the proton dose.

There is progress in developing proton therapy systems for imaging treating patients in a sitting or upright position with horizontal beams (see, for instance, http://www.chicagoprotoncenter.com/whats-new/). Such systems may require much less shielding and may be considerably less expensive. Treatments with them may be suitable, even preferable, for a substantial subset of patients. They may lend themselves for real-time MR-imaging based proton therapy.

A recent finding on the mitigation of RIL may have a profound effect on enhancing the value of protons. High-grade RIL is widely recognized as a prognostic factor for adverse outcomes. Lin and his colleagues[40,41] have confirmed the association of grade 4 RIL with poor survival among esophageal cancer patients treated with protons and photons. They have further shown statistically significant differences in survival between patients treated with protons and photons. They attributed this difference to differences in mean body dose, that is, more compact dose distributions of protons. In-depth analyses of data on lymphocyte depletion with proton and photon therapy is beginning with the goal to establish a more precise correlation between RIL and dose patterns in lymphocyte-bearing organs and other factors responsible for incidence and severity of RIL. The knowledge gained will be used to develop RIL models. Such models, when incorporated into IMPT optimization criteria, may further significantly reduce the severity and incidence of RIL, making proton therapy more effective and the treatment of choice for many more patients.

Thus, with the progress being made on many fronts, we believe that the future of proton therapy is bright and secure.

References Available Online.

SECTION II

Physics and Treatment Planning

CHAPTER 3

Clinical Commissioning of Pencil Beam Scanning for Intensity-Modulated Proton Therapy

X. Ronald Zhu ■ Falk Poenisch ■ Narayan Sahoo ■ Michael T. Gillin

Introduction

In radiation oncology, "clinical commissioning," or simply "commissioning," refers to the process that takes place after a machine has passed acceptance tests but before the first patient can be treated.[1] Commissioning tasks for proton therapy include but are not limited to the following: (1) calibrating the computed tomography (CT) scanner for proton therapy; (2) acquiring beam data and establishing and validating the beam model in the treatment planning system (TPS); (3) commissioning the radiation delivery system, including end-to-end testing with the electronic medical record (EMR) system to be used; (4) building a comprehensive quality assurance program with machine-specific and patient-specific components; (5) establishing a safety program and meeting regulatory requirements; (6) developing operational procedures; and (7) training staff members who will plan and deliver the treatments.[1,2] Many of these tasks can be started long before the beam becomes available on the machine, including calibrating a CT scanner, evaluating immobilization devices, and training and practice for proton therapy treatment planning. Some vendors also use the term *commissioning* to describe the process of tuning and adjusting the machine to prepare it for acceptance testing after the equipment is installed; we recommend that this process be referred to as *technical commissioning* to distinguish it from the subject of this chapter, which is "clinical commissioning."

The purpose of acceptance testing is to determine if the machine satisfies the contractual and performance specifications and pertinent safety requirements.[1] Acceptance testing can be performed entirely by qualified medical physicists, by vendor representatives, or by some combination of both. However, determining whether the machine is acceptable and ready for clinical commissioning is the responsibility of medical physicists. Because some acceptance and commissioning tests overlap, in such cases, the results of the two sets of tests can be shared to save time.[2] However, the goals of acceptance testing and commissioning are different, and the two processes cannot be combined into one. The focus of this chapter is on steps 1, 2, and 3 from the first paragraph, that is, calibrating the CT numbers (Hounsfield units [HUs]) for proton therapy, establishing and validating the beam model to be used for the TPS, and commissioning the treatment delivery system.

Calibration of Computed Tomography Numbers for Proton Therapy

As is the case for photon-based radiation therapy, kilovoltage (kV) x-ray CT images are currently used to create models of patients and treatment plans for proton therapy. For photon dose calculations, calibration needs to be established between the CT number and electron density; for proton dose calculations, the CT number is related to the proton stopping power. One common approach used for calibration is the stoichiometric method,[3,4] the main steps of which are as follows[3]:

1. Measure the CT numbers of some tissue substitutes of known chemical composition and physical density. (An example of tissue substitute inserts, with their compositions and physical density, is given in table 3.1 of Schneider et al.[3])
2. Use linear regression to fit the measured CT numbers of the tissue substitutes to Eq. (3.1) to determine the coefficients, A, B, and C, which characterize the cross-sections for the photoelectric effect, coherent scattering, and incoherent scattering, respectively, of the kV x-ray beam interacting with the phantom and the insert[4]:

$$HU_{SC} = \rho_e^{rel}(A\tilde{Z}^{3.62} + B\hat{Z}^{1.86} + C) \quad [3.1]$$

   where HU is the CT number and $HU_{SC} = HU + 1000$ is the scaled CT number; ρ_e^{rel} is the electron density relative to water; $\tilde{Z} = [\sum \lambda_i Z_i^{3.62}]^{1/3.62}$, $\hat{Z} = [\sum \lambda_i Z_i^{1.86}]^{1/1.86}$, λ_i, is the fraction of number of electrons per unit volume for element i; and Z_i is the atomic number of element i. An example of calculated scaled HU versus measured scaled HU is shown in Fig. 3.1.
3. Compute the CT numbers of various reference tissues as given in the International Commission on Radiological Protection (ICRP) Report 23[5] by using Eq. (3.1) with the coefficients determined in step 2.
4. Compute the relative linear stopping power (RLSP) for the same ICRP tissues by using an approximation to the Bethe-Block formula[3,4]:

$$RLSP = \rho_e^{rel} K \quad [3.2]$$

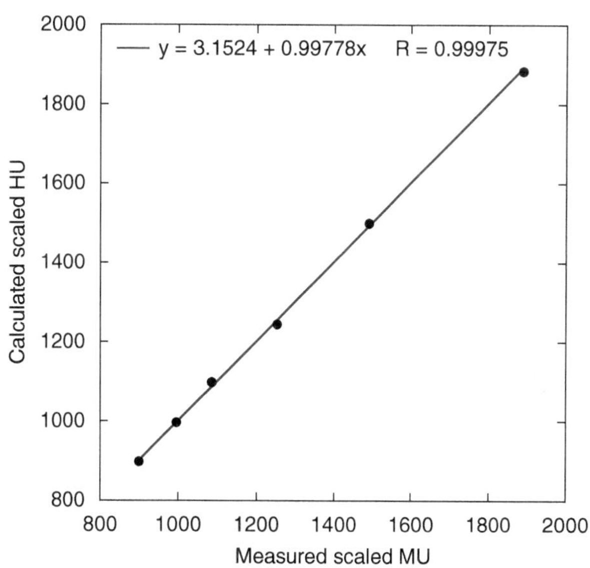

Fig. 3.1 Example of calculated versus measured scaled Hounsfield units (*HUs,* where a scaled HU = HU + 1000) of tissue-substitute materials of known composition and density. *MU,* Monitor unit.

where $K = \left\{\log\left[\frac{2m_ec^2\beta^2}{I^t(1-\beta^2)}\right] - \beta^2\right\} \Big/ \left\{\log\left[\frac{2m_ec^2\beta^2}{I^w(1-\beta^2)}\right] - \beta^2\right\}$, m_e is the mass of electron, c is the speed of light, βc is the speed of the proton, and I^t and I^w are the mean ionization potentials of the tissue and water, respectively. Among the physical quantities in Eq. (3.2), the mean ionization potentials have the largest uncertainties and therefore are the largest contributor to uncertainties in the proton stopping power. Notably, RLSP is proportional to the relative electron density, ρ_e^{rel} with the factor of K, which is the ratio of the Bethe-Block formula between tissue and water. Although the Bethe-Block formula for stopping power depends on the proton beam energy, the ratio K is a very slow-varying function of energy and is almost independent of β for the range of proton energy relevant to proton therapy. In fact, the largest difference between 175-MeV and 100-MeV proton beams is about 0.2% for cortical bone. For human tissues, the values of K are within 0.95 to 1.03.[3] The difference in K is caused by the different mean ionization potentials of tissue and water; the effect is reduced because of the logarithm dependence of the mean ionization potential.

5. Create the final calibration curve with appropriate fit through the data points (stopping powers vs. CT numbers). An example of a calibration curve is shown in Fig. 3.2.

In step 1, measurement of the CT numbers of tissue substitute inserts should involve placing the inserts at the center of the phantom with two different sizes, with the smaller size representing the head and the other larger one representing the body (Fig. 3.3). The average CT number of each tissue substitute insert from the head and body phantom should be used to reduce the beam-hardening effect.[4] The CT-number-to-stopping-power curve established by the stoichiometric method reflects the ICRP reference values for human tissues.[5] Because nonbiological materials used for immobilization devices (such as acrylic) may not fall on the calibration curve,[3,4] the proper CT number must be associated with the correct stopping power value assigned to the

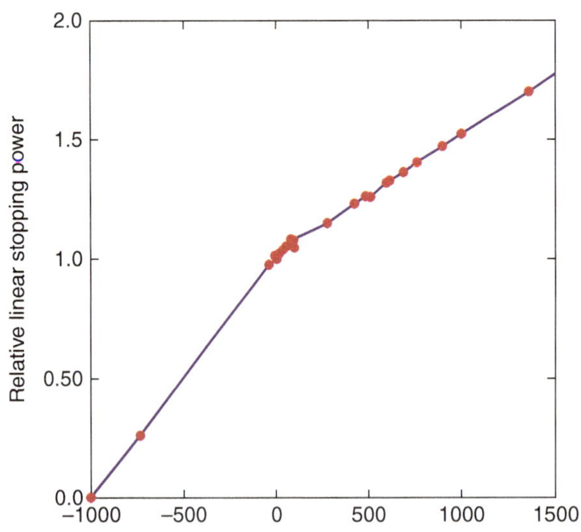

Fig. 3.2 Example of a computed tomography (CT) number (Hounsfield unit [*HU*]) versus relative linear stopping power calibration curve for a 120-kV CT scanner, derived by the stoichiometric method.

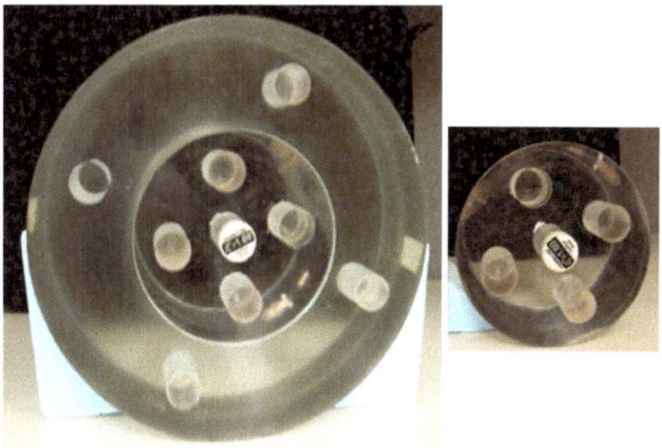

Fig. 3.3 Phantoms used for computed tomography number calibration for proton therapy. The large phantom at the left represents the "body," with a diameter of 32 cm, and the smaller one at the right is the "head" phantom, with a diameter of 16 cm. The "head" phantom is a part of the "body" phantom and can be inserted into the "body" phantom.

nonbiological material such that the water-equivalent thickness (WET) value is correct during the treatment planning process. (Examples of common nonhuman tissue materials encountered in proton therapy are listed in table 14.2 of reference[2].) It is also recommended to validate the CT number to RLSP calibration using a biological tissue sample.[4]

Detectors and Measurement Techniques

Dosimetric quantities to be measured during commissioning are used to meet the following overall goals: (1) define the monitor units (MUs), dose-monitor linearity, and output calibration; (2) define the dose and spot position accuracy; (3) provide beam data for the TPS; (4) verify the TPS; and (5) establish the quality assurance program.

IONIZATION CHAMBERS

Both Farmer-type cylindrical and parallel plate chambers are used for measurements in passive scattering beam and pencil beam scanning (PBS) proton therapy. The general principle is that Farmer-type cylindrical chambers are used for measurements in uniform, low-dose gradient regions, and parallel plate chambers are used for measurements involving high-dose gradients (e.g., depth dose measurements). For the correction factor, P_{ion}, for the recombination losses of these ionization chambers in proton beams, one should carefully determine which published formula, such as ones by International Atomic Energy Agency (IAEA) TRS-398,[6] are most appropriate for a particular beam condition. For example, Sahoo et al. found that for synchrotron-based PBS, the two-voltage formula for the continuous beam was the most appropriate.[7] Also, for higher instant-dose-rate beams such as those in some cyclotron-based PBS systems, the normal bias voltage of 300 V may not be high enough to keep the P_{ion} lower than 1.01, and thus, a higher bias voltage, such as 400 V, may be necessary. The polarity correction factor and temperature and pressure correction factors should also be determined when using these ionization chambers.

INTEGRAL DEPTH DOSES: MEASUREMENTS AND CORRECTIONS

The data required for the TPS include the integral depth dose (IDD) for each energy and the in-air lateral dose profiles. The IDD is defined as the integral of dose for a single spot over a very large plane normal to the beam direction (i.e., the total dose deposited at a specific depth and has the unit of Gy-mm^2/MU), otherwise known as the Bragg curve.[8] The detectors used for IDD measurements are large parallel-plate ionization chambers such as the PTW Bragg peak chamber (BPC) (model 34070, PTW-Freiburg, Germany), which has an effective radius of 4.08 cm and a nominal sensitive volume of 10.5 cm^3.[9] The effective measurement point for the BPC is at the inner surface of the front window, which has a WET value of 0.4 cm. Measuring the IDD with the BPC scanning in a three-dimensional water tank requires an electrometer with an extended dynamic range. The synchrotron pulse signal can be conveniently used to trigger the water tank scanning system.

A parallel plate chamber with radius $R \geq 3\sigma_{spot} = 3\sqrt{\sigma_{air}^2 + 2(0.0307R)^2}$ is recommended for accurate measurements of IDD, where $\boldsymbol{\sigma}_{spot}$ is the largest spot size for the beams to be measured, σ_{air} is the in-air spot size, and R is the range of the proton beam. The term $2(0.0307R)^2$ in the expression above represents the contribution of multi-Coulomb scattering within the patient to the beam size. The radius of the BPC may not be large enough to capture the entire low-dose envelope[10] because of multiple Coulomb scattering and nuclear interactions, and so correction factors based on Monte Carlo (MC) simulations may be needed.[9,11] The correction factor can be defined as $C(E,d;r_1,r_2) = \frac{IDD_{MC}(E,d;r_2)}{IDD_{MC}(E,d;r_1)}$, where IDD_{MC} is the MC-calculated IDD at a depth of d, E is the energy of a pencil beam, r_1 is the radius of the BPC, and r_2 is the radius of virtual ionization chamber used by simulation and should be sufficiently large to ensure the accuracy of the IDD_{MC}. For example, an r_2 value of 20 cm was used for the PBS system at the University of Texas MD Anderson Cancer Center; the measured and corrected IDDs and correction factors at a depth of 2 cm as a function of energy for the MD Anderson pencil beams are

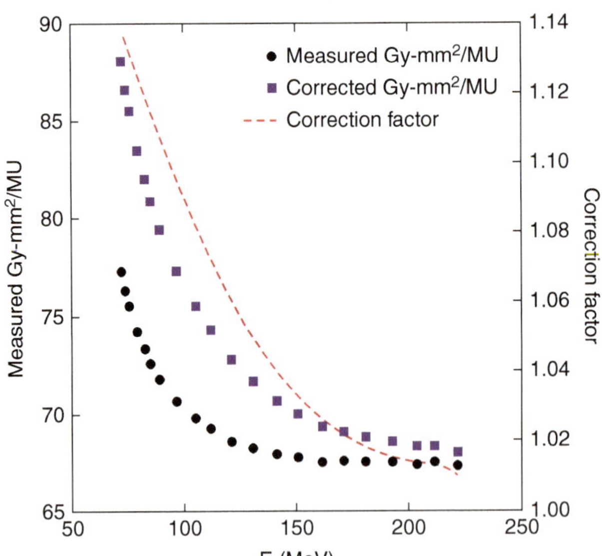

Fig. 3.4 Integral doses in Gy-mm^2/MU at the depth of 2 cm as a function of energy. Circles are measured integral doses; squares are corrected integral doses, and dashed line is the correction factors. *MU*, Monitor unit. (From Gillin MT, Sahoo N, Bues M, et al. Commissioning of the discrete spot scanning proton beam delivery system at the University of Texas M.D. Anderson Cancer Center, Proton Therapy Center, Houston. *Med Phys.* 2010;37:154-163.)

shown in Fig. 3.4. The correction factors ranged from 1.01 to 1.14 from the highest to the lowest energies. Notably, these correction factors would be different if the measurements were done at different depths.[11] For the pencil beam with energy of 221.8 MeV at MD Anderson, for example, the BPC could underestimate the IDD by as much as 7.8% at a depth of about 18 cm.[12] The measured IDD is determined by $IDD_{meas}(E, d; r_1) = M(E, d; r_1)\, N_{D,W}K_q\ \pi r_1^2$, where $M(E, d; r_1)$ is the corrected ionization chamber reading, $N_{D,W}k_q$ is the calibration factor multiplied by the beam quality factor, and πr_1^2 is the sensitive area of the BPC. Notably, no traceable national calibration standard has been established for the BPC chamber. Rather, users must determine $N_{D,W}k_q$ through cross-calibration with an ionization chamber calibrated by the Accredited Dosimetry Calibration Laboratory in a field with a uniform dose distribution.[9] The dose uniformity within the sensitive volume of the BPC would affect the accuracy of $N_{D,W}k_q$ value. A preliminary report of a difference in the values of $N_{D,W}k_q$ determined for cyclotron and synchrotron beams suggested a possible dose rate dependence.[13] This observation should be further investigated.

LATERAL PROFILES

In-air lateral profiles are also required as input data for the TPS. In-phantom lateral profiles can be useful for verifying the TPS model for multiple Coulomb scattering and nuclear interactions. Small ionization chambers and two-dimensional (2D) detectors such as scintillation detectors and films can be used for such measurements, as discussed in the following paragraphs.

Ionization Chamber Detectors: The Size Effect

Small cylindrical chambers such as the PTW pinpoint chambers (models 31023 and 31022, PTW-Freiburg, Germany) are often used for lateral profile measurements. Notably, the finite dimensions of the sensitive volume of these chambers could broaden the measured profiles, and thus, details about each detector should be available, and the smaller dimension of the detector should be used along the scanning direction. For example, the PTW model 31023 has a sensitive volume with a diameter of 2 mm and length of 5 mm, so the detector should be scanned along the direction of the 2-mm diameter. The concern would be if the 5-mm length would affect the measurement results. Fortunately, as long as the profiles to be measured can be represented by a separable function $F(x,y) = f(x)g(y)$, as is the case for the PBS system (each spot can be approximately represented by a 2D Gaussian function), it is easy to show that the length of 5 mm does not have any effect on the measured profiles. The PTW 31022 model is a "3D" chamber with a sensitive volume with a diameter of 2.9 mm and length of 2.9 mm. According to the argument provided above, the 31023 model should be the model of choice for measuring the lateral dose profiles because it has a smaller diameter—as long as the scanning is done along the direction of the diameter. Nevertheless, the detector size effect should be verified with much higher-resolution detectors, such as film and scintillation detectors, especially for small spots on the new generation of PBS nozzles.

Two-Dimensional Scintillation Detectors and Films

When ionization chambers are not the most appropriate detectors for lateral profile measurements, an alternative is to use 2D detectors such as scintillation detectors[14,15] and Gafchromic films.[16,17] For both types of detectors, the detector responses must be verified in terms of linearity and calibration with dose and dynamic range. The linear energy transfer dependence of the scintillation detectors and Gafchromic films due to quenching effects should be well understood when using these detectors.[15,17,18] One group has reported using a scintillator-based detector (Lynx, IBA Dosimetry, Schwarzenbruck, Germany) for in-air lateral profile measurements during clinical commissioning of a PBS system.[14]

Treatment Planning System

A TPS comprises various modules for the process of treatment planning; one such module, the beam model configuration, is one of the most important in commissioning a TPS. Tasks involved in commissioning a dose model include acquiring input data, configuring dose models, and validating those dose models.

PROTON DOSE ALGORITHMS

Both primary and secondary particles contribute to the absorbed dose from a proton beam. Primary protons are those that only undergo elastic interactions with electrons and elastic proton-nucleus scatterings in the medium; secondary particles are generated through nonelastic nuclear interactions and include secondary protons and other fragments (e.g., deuterons, tritons, alphas, and neutrons).[19] Multiple Coulomb scattering originates mainly from the patient, the range shifter propagating in the air gap to the patient, and some devices within the beamline. Nuclear interactions mainly occur in the patient, creating a beam "halo" attributed to large-angle inelastic nuclear fragments. Most of the dose models available in commercial planning systems are analytical algorithms, often called pencil algorithms,[20–27] although MC-based algorithms[28] have become available in recent years.

An analytical algorithm by Schaffner[20] using the notations of Zhu et al.[11] is described briefly below. The 3D dose distribution is written as a convolution of the 3D fluence, $\Phi_{E_k}(x, y, z)$, and the dose distribution of a beamlet (i.e., dose kernel), $D_{E_k}^{Beamlet}(x, y, d(z))$:

$$D(x,y,z) = \sum\nolimits_{E_k} \sum\nolimits_{Beamlet_j} \Phi_{E_k}\left(x_j, y_j, z\right) D_{E_k}^{Beamlet_j}\left(x - x_j, y - y_j, d(z)\right) \qquad [3.3]$$

where $d(z)$ is the WET of position z along the beamlet direction. The beamlet dose distribution (also known as the dose kernel) is assumed to have radial symmetry and can be written as

$$D_{E_k}^{Beamlet}\left(r, d(z)\right) = \frac{1}{\rho w}\left[S_{pp}\left(d(z)\right)K_{lat,pp}\left(r, d(z)\right) + S_{sp}\left(d(z)\right)K_{lat,sp}\left(r, d(z)\right)\right], \qquad [3.4]$$

where $r = \sqrt{x^2 + y^2}$ is the radial coordinate in the transverse plane, ρ_w is the density of water, and $S(d)$ is the weighted stopping power at the position of the z-axis with a WET of $d(z)$; the subscript pp indicates primary protons and sp secondary particles, such that $K_{lat,pp}$ and $K_{lat,sp}$ describe the lateral dose distributions of primary and secondary particles, respectively.[11,22–24] The secondary particles deposit energy outside the primary proton beam; therefore, the low-dose envelope from these secondary products, also known as the nuclear "halo" dose, is expected to have a broad lateral distribution.[10,19,29]

TYPICAL INPUT DATA REQUIRED BY THE TREATMENT PLANNING SYSTEM

Input data required by a TPS consist of in-air lateral profiles at three to five different positions from the isocenter and the IDD for each proton beam energy. If a range shifting device is used, an additional data set with the range shifter is also required. Detectors and measurement techniques for obtaining the input data were discussed in the previous sections. MC-simulated data that are validated by measurements can be used as the required import data. An example of MC-generated import data for the MD Anderson PBS beamline is shown in Fig. 3.5. MC-generated IDDs, IDD_{MC}, should be calibrated by the measured IDD, IDD_{meas}, at a reference depth:

$$IDD\left(E, d; r_2\right) = \frac{IDD_{MC}\left(E, d; r_2\right)}{IDD_{MC}\left(E, d_{ref}; r_2\right)} \times IDD_{meas}\left(E, d_{ref}; r_1\right) \times CF\left(E, d_{ref}, r_1, r_2\right) \qquad [3.5]$$

where E is the energy of the beam, d is the depth, r_1 and r_2 are the radii of the parallel plate chamber used for measurements and simulations, respectively, and CF is the correction factor. For example, $r_1 = 4.08$ cm for the BPC, $r_2 = 20$ cm, and $d_{ref} = 2.0$ cm were used for commissioning the MD Anderson pencil beam system. Notably, the dose gradients on the IDD curve are high at the depth $d_{ref} = 2.0$ cm for low-energy beams. Ensuring accurate dose measurements requires attention to the accuracy of the WET of the measurement depth. Alternatively, shallow depths such as 1.0 cm could be considered for this measurement.

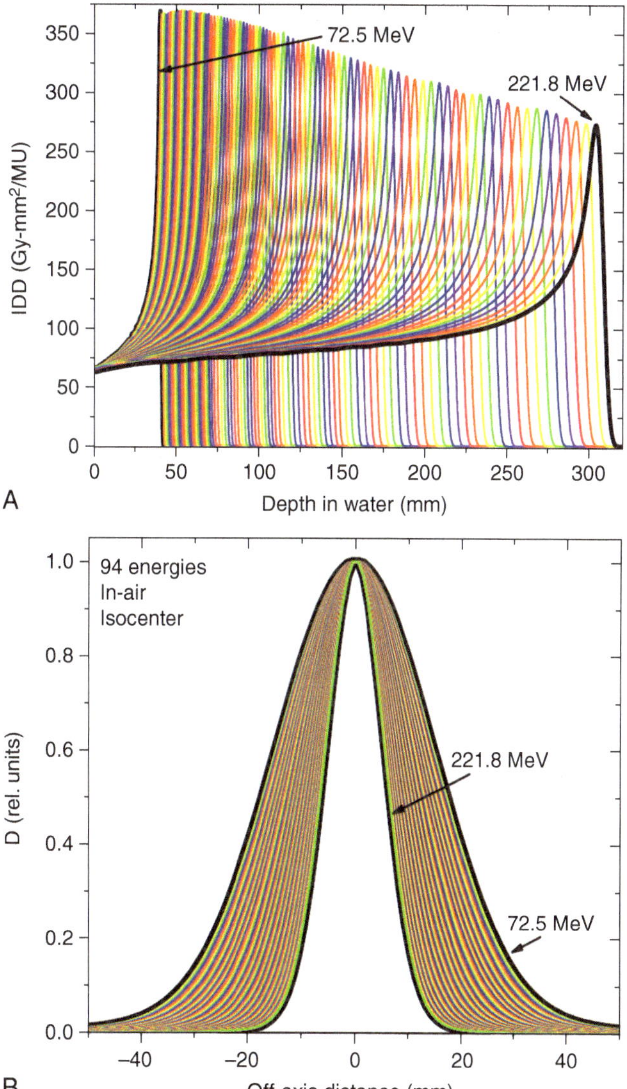

Fig. 3.5 (A) Integral depth doses *(IDDs)* for all 94 energies in units of Gy mm²/monitor unit *(MU)* generated using Monte Carlo (MC) simulations and MC simulation-generated lateral in-air dose profiles at different positions ($z = 0$, ± 10, ± 20 cm, $z = 0$ is defined at the isocenter): (B) for the pencil beam with energy of 221.8 MeV, and

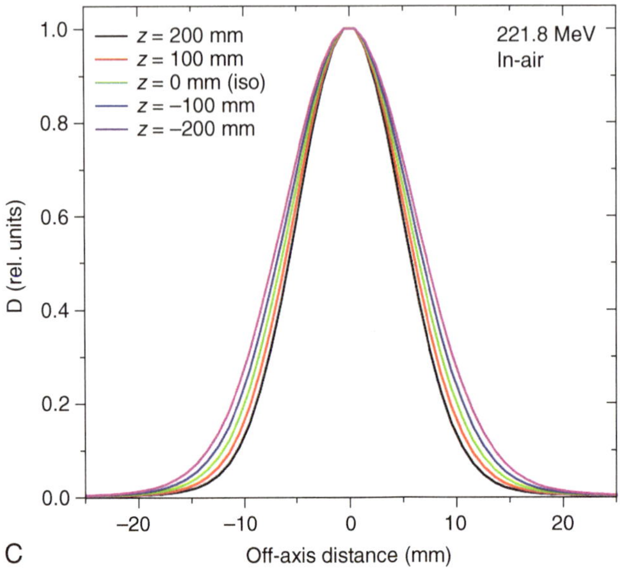

C

Fig. 3.5 cont'd, (C) for all energies. (Modified from Zhu XR, Poenisch F, Lii M, et al. Commissioning dose computation models for spot scanning proton beams in water for a commercially available treatment planning system. *Med Phys.* 2013;40:041723.)

Eq. (3.5) can be understood as follows: the ratio of IDD_{MC} normalizes the MC-generated IDD at the reference depth, and the $IDD_{meas} \times$ CF term converts normalized MC-generated IDD to units of Gy-mm^2/MU. This approach, based on absolute dose per MU, is equivalent to the approach based on the absolute dose per particle used by other institutions.[30]

BEAM MODEL CONFIGURATION

One of the most challenging tasks in configuring a beam model for PBS is to be able to accurately calculate the lateral dose profiles, especially the low-dose envelope resulting from multiple Coulomb scattering and nuclear interactions. For high-energy (≥150 MeV) pencil beams, the low-dose envelope is dominated by secondary particles created in the patient, whereas for low-energy (<150 MeV) pencil beams, the low-dose envelope is dominated by primary particles elastically scattered both in the beamline and inside the patient.[19] Pedroni et al.[29] observed a low-dose envelope several centimeters away from the center of a single pencil beam during beam delivery through a homogeneous phantom. This low-dose envelope could contribute up to 15% of the total dose delivered in a treatment using the scanning beam technique. Although possible, accurate direct measurements of low-dose profiles in-air and in-phantom to relative dose levels that are a factor of 10^4 lower than the central axis dose remain challenging.[10] Even when measurements of the low-dose envelopes can be obtained, independent verification confirming the accuracy of the dose model is desirable. In their original study, Pedroni et al. first used concentric square frame delivery patterns and measured the dose to the center of the scanning patterns to experimentally determine the characteristics of the low-dose envelope.[29] Based on a similar idea, field size factor measurements at the center of the scanning patterns were used to determine the low-dose envelopes for carbon ions by Inaniwa et al.[31] and for protons by Sawakuchi et al.[10] Later, Clasie et al. adapted concentric circles, with increasing circumference of the circle amplifying the small contributions of secondary particles, for the same purpose.[30] Field size factor measurements, including a schematic illustration of the experimental setup, are shown in Fig. 3.6. The

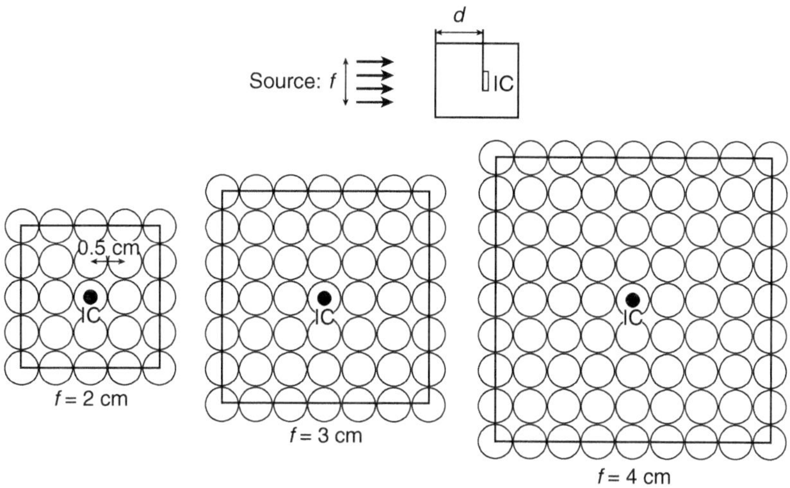

Fig. 3.6 Illustration of field size factor experiments. *Top*, The experimental setup. The surface of the water phantom was located at the isocenter plane. The ionization chamber *(IC)* was placed on the central axis at a fixed depth *d* and irradiated with various monoenergetic square fields of dimension *f* (*bottom*). The spacing between the centers of adjacent pencil beams was fixed at 0.5 cm at the isocenter plane. (From Sawakuchi GO, Zhu XR, Poenisch F, et al. Experimental characterization of the low-dose envelope of spot scanning proton beams. *Phys Med Biol.* 2010;55:3467-3478. © Institute of Physics and Engineering in Medicine. Reproduced by permission of IOP Publishing. All rights reserved.)

square fields were created by the superposition of a number of spots of monoenergetic pencil beams. Additional information about the influence of the low-dose envelope of an individual pencil beam can be determined through this type of measurement. The field size factors were measured at several depths for selected pencil beam energies that covered the entire range of available energies.

In the TPS beam configuration module, the phase space parameters were initially determined by fitting input data to an analytical formula, and then the calculated field size factors were compared with measured ones. The phase space parameters were iteratively adjusted to obtain the best possible agreement between the calculated and measured field size factors.[11] For example, in the initial implementation, the fluence of a pencil beam was modeled as a single Gaussian function. Our calculations and measurements demonstrated that a single Gaussian function could not accurately describe in-air lateral profiles for an individual pencil beam for the scanning nozzle at MD Anderson.[10,12,19,32] The TPS vendor therefore implemented a double-Gaussian fluence model to account for the pencil beam fluence due to the contributions of large-angle scattering from the devices within the scanning nozzle.[11] However, the parameters for the second Gaussian of the double-Gaussian fluence model had to be artificially adjusted, which contradicted the original intent to obtain better agreements between calculated and measured field size factors and led some to suggest the presence of deficiencies in the implementation of the dose kernel of the pencil beam algorithm in the commercial TPS.[11] Comparisons of calculated versus measured field size factors of square fields with field sizes of 2 cm × 2 cm to 20 cm × 20 cm are illustrated in Fig. 3.7. For a depth of 2.0 cm and a deeper depth near the Bragg peak, the calculated field size factors deviated from the measured values by 3.4% to 7.2% for the single Gaussian fluence model and by 1.0% to 1.9% for the double Gaussian fluence model. For the highest energy (221.8 MeV), a comparison for an intermediate depth of 23.2 cm is shown in Fig. 3.7G, where the nuclear "halo" effect was expected to be larger (indeed, the largest percentage differences in the field size factors were 16.9% for the single-Gaussian and

3.5% for the double-Gaussian fluence models). These results further suggested that the dose kernel implemented in the commercial TPS was limited. An efficient method to determine phase space parameters for the same commercial TPS was reported by Shen et al.,[33] who implemented an in-house dose kernel based on the same algorithm as that used in the commercial TPS and determined the phase space parameters by comparing the calculated in-house kernel with the measured field size factors outside the TPS at several depths of selected energies.

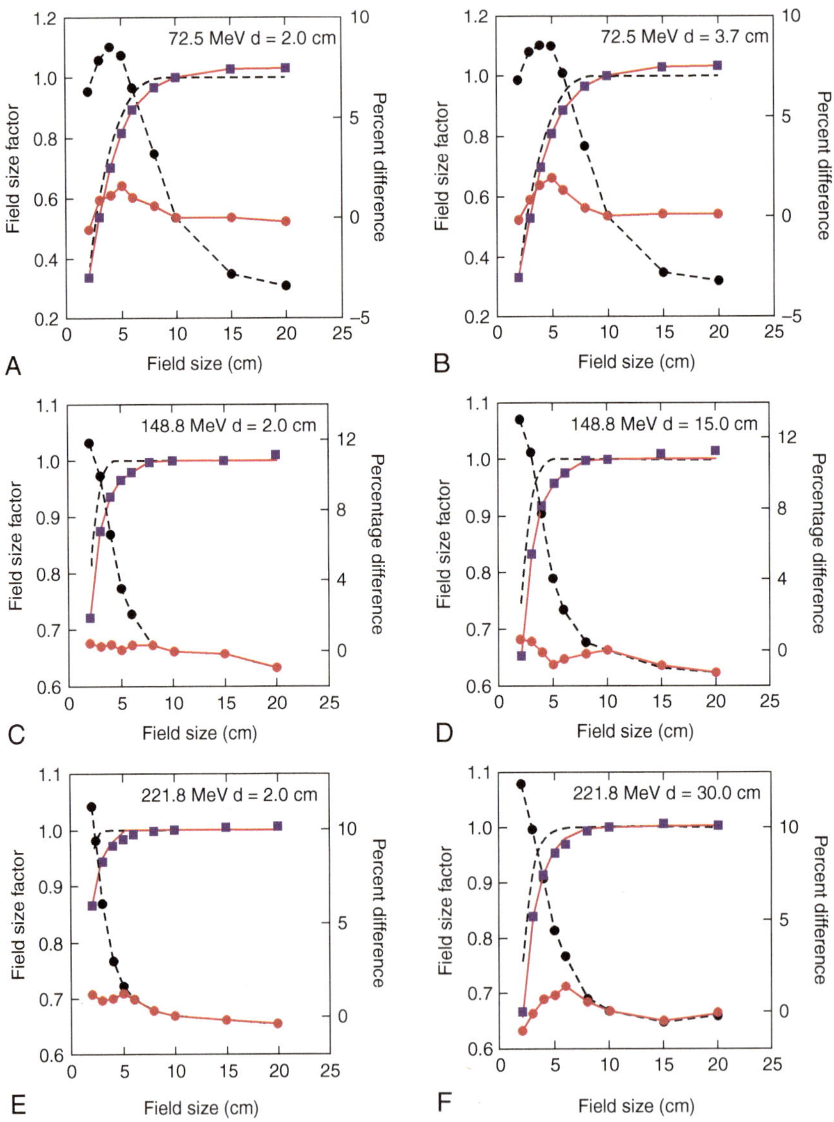

Fig. 3.7 Comparisons between calculated (single-Gaussian *[SG]* and double-Gaussian *[DG]* fluence models) and measured field size factors of square fields. Positive values in percentage differences represent calculated field size factors that are larger than measured ones. For field size factors, the dashed lines indicate SG; solid lines, DG; and squares, measured. For percent differences, dashed lines with circles indicate SG and solid lines with circles, DG. (A) and (B) for energy of 72.5 MeV (4.0 cm range) at depths of 2.0 and 3.7 cm; (C) and (D) for energy of 148.8 MeV (15.2 cm range) at depths of 2.0 and 15.0 cm; and (E) to

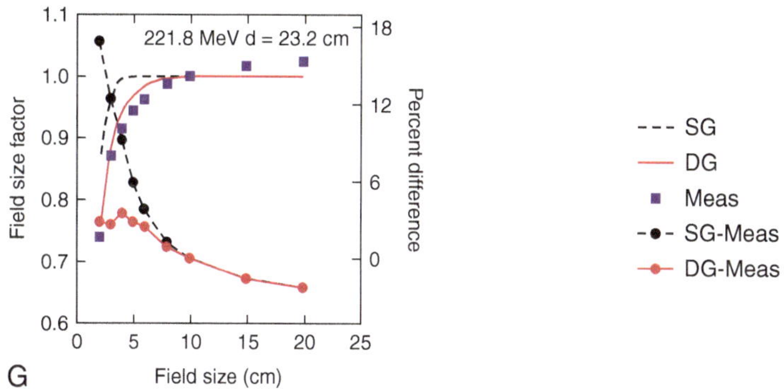

Fig. 3.7 cont'd, (G) for energy of 221.8 MeV (30.6 cm range) at depths of 2.0, 30.0, and 23.2 cm, respectively. *Meas,* Measurement. (Modified from Zhu XR, Poenisch F, Lii M, et al. Commissioning dose computation models for spot scanning proton beams in water for a commercially available treatment planning system. *Med Phys.* 2013;40:041723.)

Notably, commercial TPSs may provide a depth-dose normalization table to allow the user to scale the calculated absolute dose to obtain better agreement, if necessary. For MD Anderson pencil beams, the depth dose normalization table values were 2.2% to 3.9% larger than the ideal value.[11]

VALIDATING THE BEAM MODEL

Water Phantom

Verification measurements in the volumetric dose distributions can be used to verify the beam model, including absolute point doses in the center of the spread-out Bragg peak (SOBP) and field, absolute depth doses along the central axis, relative lateral dose profiles along the center of the SOBP, and 2D dose distributions in selected plans perpendicular to the beam incident direction for selected SOBPs. All absolute point doses at the center of the fields, including depth doses, can be measured as a function of nominal field size (ranging from 2 cm × 2 cm to 20 cm × 20 cm, for example), the width of the SOBP (e.g., 2–20 cm), and the range of the highest proton energies (e.g., 6–30.6 cm) in the same way as measurement of the field size factors. For example, differences between the calculated and measured absolute point doses (mean ± standard deviation) at the center of the field and the SOBP were 0.0% ± 0.6% (range: −1.9% to 1.2%) for the MD Anderson pencil beams.[11] Comparisons of calculated versus measured doses at various depths are shown in Fig. 3.8 and lateral profiles in Fig. 3.9.

Patient-Specific Plan Measurements

Before the first patient is treated, PBS plans should be generated for several patients who were previously treated (e.g., prostate, central nervous system, and esophagus) to evaluate the entire PBS planning, dose validation, and delivery process. Patient-specific measurements can include point doses, depth doses, and 2D measurements in the planes perpendicular to the beam incident direction for each field at several depths. Details of patient-specific quality assurance programs are given in Chapter 6 and elsewhere.[34,35]

Treatment Delivery System

Proton therapy based on PBS technology has been available at The MD Anderson Proton Therapy Center since May 2008. The delivery system consists of a synchrotron accelerator and scanning nozzle (Hitachi, Ltd., Tokyo, Japan) and an EMR system (Elekta AB, Stockholm,

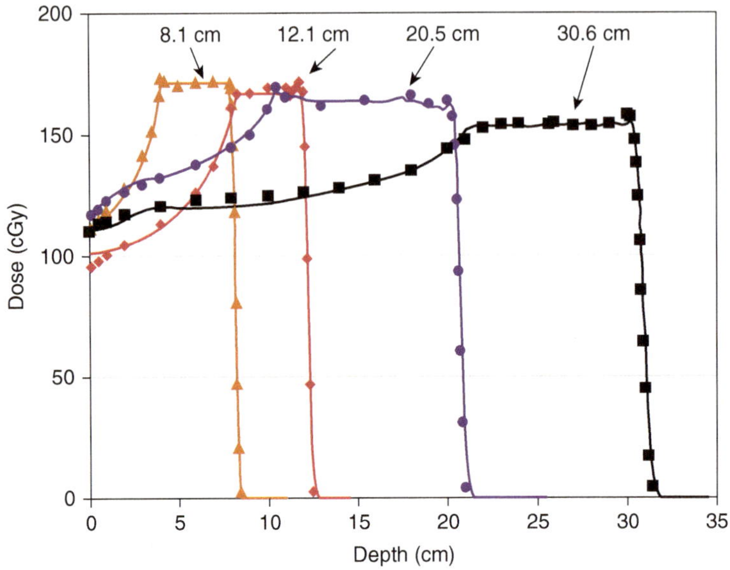

Fig. 3.8 Comparison of the depth doses calculated using the double-Gaussian fluence model and measurements along the central axis of proton fields with a nominal field size of 10 cm × 10 cm for four different proton ranges with spread-out Bragg peak width of 10 or 4 cm. (From Zhu XR, Poenisch F, Lii M, et al. Commissioning dose computation models for spot scanning proton beams in water for a commercially available treatment planning system. *Med Phys.* 2013;40:041723.)

Sweden).[36] To deliver a clinical beam, the plan is uploaded from the TPS in the format of the digital imaging and communication in medicine (DICOM) standard for ionizing radiation therapy to the EMR and then downloaded to the accelerator control system.[9]

A spot-scanning proton beam delivers dose on a spot-by-spot basis in a separate and distinct pattern on a 3D grid. In the direction of beam travel, the dose grid is determined by the available energies from the accelerator and specified by the treatment plan from the TPS. For the same energy, the location of a spot is controlled by changing the magnetic field strength of X and Y scanning magnets. In the X-Y plan, the spot positions can be defined by the user, either by using the TPS for testing and clinical cases through the EMR or, for physics testing, by creating them manually. Basic parameters in the delivery of the spot scanning treatment fields include the range (i.e., the proton energy) of the spot, the location of the spot, the size of the spot, and the dose delivered per spot. Also, given the current multivendor environment, the integrity of the information transfer between different systems must be ensured. The following description of commissioning the delivery system at MD Anderson largely follows that of Gillin et al.[9]

INTERLOCKS

The major interlocks, including the dose monitor, spot position monitor, the minimum and maximum spot MUs, and the bending magnetic field, should all be tested to ensure the safe and accurate delivery of scanning beam proton therapy.

Dose Monitor

Dose monitors are used to determine the MUs of each spot and the total MUs for the field. Of the two dose monitors, main and subdose, the main dose monitor is primarily used to determine

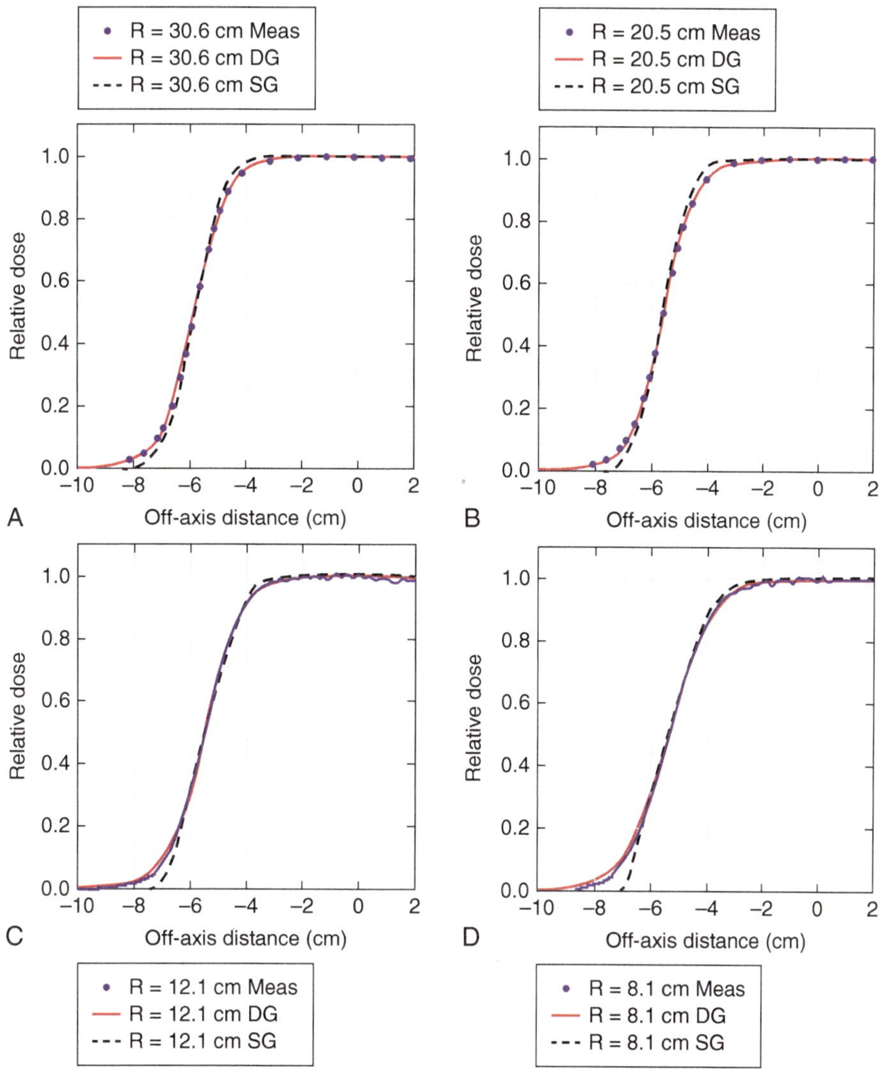

Fig. 3.9 Comparison of calculations from the double-Gaussian *(DG)* and single-Gaussian *(SG)* fluence models with measurement of in-plane lateral dose profiles at the center of the spread-out Bragg peak (SOBP) for four different proton ranges and SOBP widths of 10 cm or 4 cm. Dots indicate measured data; solid lines, double Gaussian model calculations; and dashed lines, single-Gaussian model calculations. (A) Range = 30.6 cm, SOBP = 10 cm; (B) range = 20.5 cm, SOBP = 10 cm; (C) range = 12.1 cm, SOBP = 4 cm; and (D) range = 8.1 cm, SOBP = 4 cm. *Meas,* Measurement. (From Zhu XR, Poenisch F, Lii M, et al. Commissioning dose computation models for spot scanning proton beams in water for a commercially available treatment planning system. *Med Phys.* 2013;40:041723.)

when each spot and each field have delivered the planned MUs; the subdose monitor is a backup if the main dose monitor fails. The interlocks can be tested simply by disconnecting the main or the subdose monitor to see if the beam is terminated by the connected dose monitor. It was found that when only one spot was delivered when the main or subdose monitor was not functioning properly.

Spot Position Monitor

The spot position monitor is unique for scanning beam delivery and serves as an independent verification of the spot position in the X and Y directions. If the planned spot positions deviate from the delivered positions by a certain threshold (e.g., 2–3 mm), the beam delivery should be terminated for the field. If the beam delivery does not abort in such cases, the user should require that the vendor fix the problem. The interlocks can be tested by disconnecting either the X or Y channel from the spot position monitor; if the interlock is active, then only one spot will be delivered upon disconnection of the X or Y channels.

Minimum and Maximum Spot Monitor Units

The limits of spot MUs are established based on the ability of the scanning nozzle to deliver each spot safely and accurately. For example, the maximum spot MU was established based on the maximum dose to be delivered when the location and size of the spot were verified. The minimum MU per spot was set such that the spot dose was greater than the expected delayed dose (or leaked dose). The interlocks of the minimum and maximum spot MU can be tested by programming fields with spots that have MUs less than the minimum or more than maximum values. For example, for the current scanning nozzle at the MD Anderson facility, the minimum spot MU is 0.005, and the maximum spot MU is 0.04 MU; doses were confirmed to be delivered when the unit was programmed for MUs greater than 0.00465 and less than 0.0429 per spot. These values are consistent with the designed tolerance of the spot MU.

Bending Magnetic Field Interlock

The bending magnetic field in the scanning nozzle is used as the final verification of the energy of each proton beam. For MD Anderson's scanning nozzle, the tolerance for the difference in the actual bending magnet field strength and the expected value before an interlock is activated is 0.006 T, which corresponds to an energy value of approximately 1.4 MeV. A simple test involving two separate runs, each containing two energies, was done in treatment mode to test whether the bending magnetic field strength was being properly checked by the delivery system. For the first run, normal values of the bending magnet were used, and for the second run, a change in the bending magnet field strength was introduced for the second energy. The delivery was aborted with an interlock after one spot was delivered for the second energy. This test was done in the service mode of the accelerator control system (as opposed to treatment mode).

CALIBRATION

Definition of Charge per Monitor Unit

The interaction of the protons with the wall of the monitor chamber and the air in the chamber in the nozzle results in the production of ionic charges, which are collected by the chamber. A single MU merely represents a certain amount of charge that is collected by the main dose monitor. Its relation to dose distribution depends on the energies and locations of spots. An MU is directly proportional to the number of protons passing through the dose monitor for each energy. The amount of charge in the main dose monitor, in terms of the number of counts defining an MU, has been arbitrarily defined for a reference condition using the IAEA TRS 398 protocol.[6] At MD Anderson, a uniform dose of 2.17 Gy is delivered to a 1-L volume of water centered at the isocenter by using pencil beams of 18 energies between 178.6 and 221.8 MeV (corresponding to proton ranges of 21.0–30.6 g/cm^2 and a nominal SOBP width of 10 cm), 10 cm × 10 cm field size, 8-mm spot spacing, and a total of 217 MUs. The calibration point is in the center of SOBP. Alternatively, a calibration point can be selected that is near the entrance of a uniformly spaced single energy layer spot pattern.[2] The second method has advantages when a uniform SOBP such as the one described above is not available.

Dose Monitor Linearity

The charge collected in the dose monitor for each spot is usually small. For example, for the scanning nozzle at MD Anderson, the charge collected for the minimum MU per spot is about 100 pC, and that for the maximum MU per spot is about 800 pC. With such small charges being collected, it is important to be able to confirm the linearity of the dose monitor. Two methods can be used to determine the dose monitor linearity: the first is to measure a single spot with different MUs ranging from the minimum to maximum MU per spot by using a large ionization chamber such as the PTW BPC. The weakness of this method is that the uncertainty of such measurements may be large because of the small MU per spot. The second method is to use a pattern with the same total MU (e.g., 10 MU) but consisting of different spot MUs (e.g., 250 spots each with 0.04 MU, 1000 spots with 0.01 MU per spot, and 2000 spots with 0.005 MU per spot) to determine any difference in the measured doses. Both methods have been used at MD Anderson.

DOSIMETRIC PARAMETERS OF SPOTS

Basic parameters in the delivery of the PBS treatment fields include the range (i.e., the proton energy), location, size of the spot, and the dose delivered per spot.

Energies, Range, and Depth Doses

The energy is the most fundamental quantity for a proton beam, dictating the range of the beam in a given medium. The energy for PBS is usually selected based on the need to create a uniform dose to a volume, and that choice reflects the physics of pristine Bragg peaks. The range of a proton beam is defined as the depth of 90% of the dose distal to the Bragg peak; for example, the MD Anderson PBS nozzle has 94 energies available, with range intervals between 0.1 and 0.6 g/cm^2. When the PBS nozzle at MD Anderson was commissioned, time constraints dictated that only 11 of 94 depth dose curves were measured to verify the measurements of all 94 energies obtained during the acceptance tests.[9] The measured ranges were within 1 mm of the measurements for the acceptance tests.

Spot Position and Size

The spot positions are controlled by two scanning magnets. The variation in the magnetic field strength during "beam-on" is within ±0.1% of the maximum current, which is equivalent to ±0.5-mm beam position stability at the isocenter. Owing to beam optics and accelerator characteristics, the spot may be not circular in the transverse X-Y plane for beams generated by synchrotrons. A spot can be characterized, at least in part, by measuring its full width at half maximum (FWHM) in air and at various depths. An example of an in-air spot size in terms of FWHM as a function of energy is shown in Fig. 3.10. Examples of lateral profiles in-air and in-phantom, both measured by using a pinpoint ionization chamber, are shown in Figs. 3.11 and 3.12. An example of spot position verification using Gafchromic film is shown in Fig. 3.13.

END-TO-END TESTING

Finally, the entire process, from treatment planning to EMR to treatment delivery, should be tested. Should a situation be encountered in which the DICOM definitions are slightly different among systems produced by different vendors, the vendors should be required to work together to provide the necessary consistency for treating patients safely. In-house software tools can be

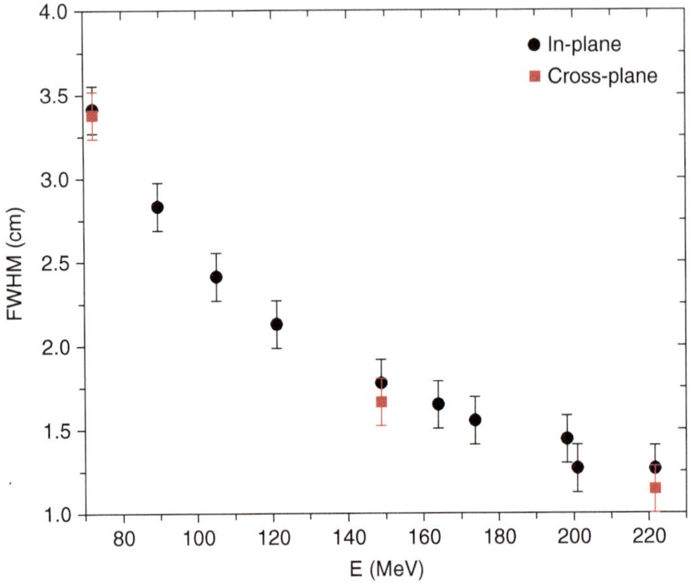

Fig. 3.10 In-air spot sizes in terms of their full width at half maximum *(FWHM)* of lateral profiles of single pencil beams at the isocenter plane as function of proton nominal energy *E*. (From Gillin MT, Sahoo N, Bues M, et al. Commissioning of the discrete spot scanning proton beam delivery system at the University of Texas M.D. Anderson Cancer Center, Proton Therapy Center, Houston. *Med Phys.* 2010;37:154-163.)

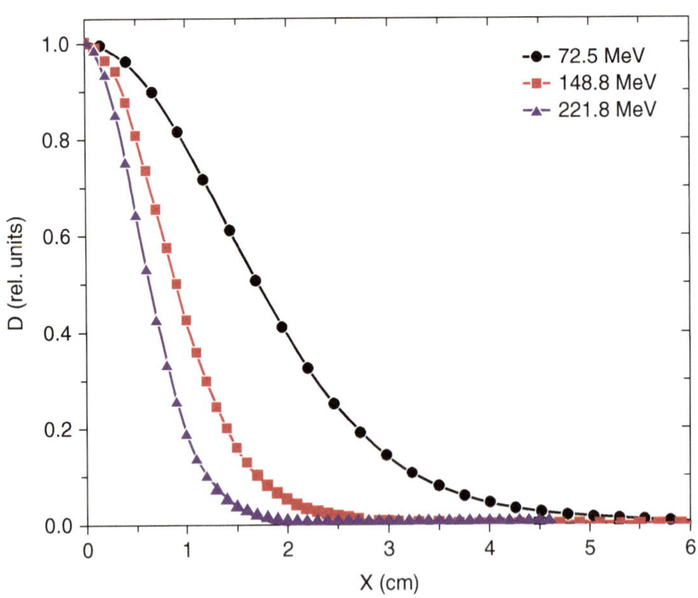

Fig. 3.11 In-plane half-lateral profiles of single pencil beams at the isocenter plane in air for energies of 72.5 MeV, 148.8 MeV, and 221.8 MeV. Measurements were obtained with a cylindrical ionization chamber. Model 31014 (PTW-Freiburg, Freiburg, Germany). (From Gillin MT, Sahoo N, Bues M, et al. Commissioning of the discrete spot scanning proton beam delivery system at the University of Texas M.D. Anderson Cancer Center, Proton Therapy Center, Houston. *Med Phys.* 2010;37:154-163.)

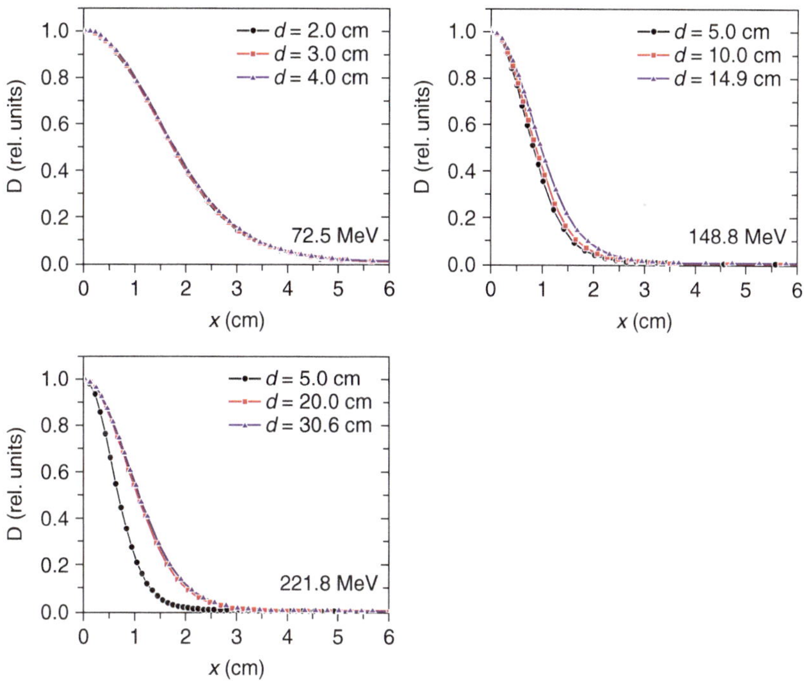

Fig. 3.12 In-plane half-lateral profile of single pencil beams measured in a water phantom for energies of 72.5 MeV, 148.8 MeV, and 221.8 MeV. The surface of the water was placed at the isocenter plane. (From Gillin MT, Sahoo N, Bues M, et al. Commissioning of the discrete spot scanning proton beam delivery system at the University of Texas M.D. Anderson Cancer Center, Proton Therapy Center, Houston. *Med Phys.* 2010;37:154-163.)

developed to consolidate the differences, but this should be done only as a last resort.[9] MD Anderson has developed such tools.

The end-to-end testing should include the entire process: "patient" setup, imaging guidance, and treatment delivery, with the treatment recorded by the EMR. Tests should include not only treatment delivery without issues but also treatments involving interruptions or failures of either the treatment delivery system or the EMR system, because the entire pencil beam pattern must be delivered as planned to treat the target with the prescribed dose.[9] Recovery from interruptions could be tested by deliberately causing failures in either or both the delivery system and the EMR.

After a failure, the number of delivered spots and MUs delivered should be verified, and this number must be consistent with the values defined in the treatment field. The number of remaining spots and MUs can then be determined, and the field can then be completely delivered. For example, one test involved sequential exposure of three films, with the first film being irradiated with a normal complete treatment and the second and third films being exposed together to the first part of treatment, followed by a beam abort. The second film was then removed while the third film remained in place. After recovery, the remainder of the treatment was then delivered to the third film. The films were then scanned and the dose distributions compared.[9]

Recovery from a treatment interruption may require going through the entire process again, from sending the treatment plan to the EMR and on to the treatment delivery system, including site setup and treatment fields. The image guidance may also need to be repeated to ensure the

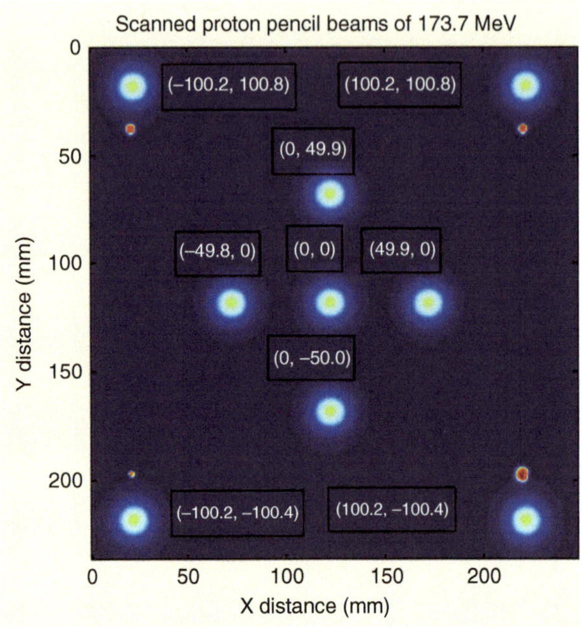

Fig. 3.13 Example of spot position measurements using radiochromic film. (From Gillin MT, Sahoo N, Bues M, et al. Commissioning of the discrete spot scanning proton beam delivery system at the University of Texas M.D. Anderson Cancer Center, Proton Therapy Center, Houston. *Med Phys.* 2010;37:154-163.)

correct setup of the patient to be treated. If imaging guidance is not necessary, then the couch coordinates must be verified as being correct, as described in Chapter 7 (Treatment Delivery Procedures).

Summary

Commissioning PBS systems for proton therapy can be daunting because it involves many tasks and processes unique to PBS and others that are similar to those for passive scattering proton beams and photons. The time required is measured in months. MD Anderson has used a phased approach in which intensity-modulated proton therapy is the most recent treatment modality to be offered. A diverse team is required for such an effort. At MD Anderson, irradiation of a large number of phantoms from the Imaging and Radiation Oncology Core, including head and neck and prostate, has provided independent validation of the entire system from imaging to planning to delivery. Other requirements beyond the scope of this chapter include the need for a comprehensive quality assurance program, with machine-specific and patient-specific components; a safety program that meets regulatory requirements; and an established set of operational procedures with which to train staff involved in treatment planning and delivery. Before attempting to treat disease at sites involving large inhomogeneities, the accuracy of the dose calculations for such sites should be verified by using inhomogeneity phantoms, and more advanced algorithms, such as those based on MC calculations, would need to be implemented. As an example, motion mitigation strategies would be needed to treat tumors at anatomic sites subject to substantial respiration-motion.[37]

References Available Online.

CHAPTER 4

Immobilization and Simulation

Archana S. Gautam ■ Richard Wu ■ X. Ronald Zhu ■ Falk Poenisch

Introduction

Intensity-modulated proton therapy (IMPT) using pencil beam scanning (PBS) technology is advancing rapidly for delivering precise and more conformal doses to target volumes while sparing surrounding normal and critical tissues. To fully use the advantages of IMPT, immobilization and simulation is a critical step, similar to intensity-modulated radiation therapy (IMRT) and volumetric-modulated therapy (VMAT) using photons. The goal is to have small intra- and interfraction variations for the patient setup and have the setup uncertainty be well understood. It does not matter how precisely the machine can deliver the treatment; if the setup is not reproducible and appropriate for the treatment site, a precise delivery is hard to achieve.[1] A well-designed immobilizing system can also reduce the time for daily patient setup. Devices such as headrests, Vaclock, body bags, and so on, are constructed to reduce external setup uncertainty and patient movement, whereas rectal balloons are used to reduce internal motion during treatment of prostate patients, and spacers are used to create more separation between the target volume and critical normal structures.

For radiation therapy, immobilization needs to not only immobilize the patient but also place them in a stable and reproducible position for each treatment.[1,2] Therefore, indexing of devices is very important: if there is only one device, it should be indexed to the treatment couch; if there is more than one device, each of them needs to be indexed relative to each other, and the system as a whole is indexed to the treatment couch. Accurately determining and maintaining the water-equivalent thickness (WET) along the beam path, including immobilization devices, is critically important in proton therapy. It helps to reduce the range uncertainty and the effect on proton beam penumbra. It should be pointed out that the setup uncertainty could result in a combined effect of range variations in inhomogeneous tissues of a patient, which can also alter the ranges of protons and influence dose distribution.[3] Therefore, a good immobilization system could effectively reduce range uncertainty as well.

In general, simulations for proton therapy are similar to IMRT and VMAT because they are done using computed tomography (CT) scanners to acquire volumetric images. Magnetic resonance imaging (MRI) and other imaging modalities are also used to facilitate target volume delineation. However, a proton beam has a finite range compared with the photon. Protons deposit much of their energy at the end of the range, also known as the Bragg peak. Proton range and interaction depend on tissue or material density in the beam path; hence, CT scanners for proton therapy simulation require special considerations for calibration to establish a relationship between Hounsfield unit (HU) values and proton stopping powers (see Chapter 3). The interactions between photons and media are functions of the x-ray spectrum; different kV will result in different spectra. For the same kV, different scanners may have different spectra because of the difference of x-ray tube housing construction, which can act as a filter for the x-ray spectrum. Therefore, when performing a CT simulation for proton therapy, the staff should only use the CT scan protocol that is calibrated for proton therapy. In addition, one should not apply a CT-stopping power calibration curve from one scanner to CT images from a different scanner, even if the kV is the same, unless it has been verified.

Immobilization Devices: General Considerations

Immobilization devices for radiation oncology should have the following general properties: (1) reproducible and comfortable for the patient, (2) ease of use and setup, (3) easy in making and cleaning, (4) maintaining the rigidity and shape throughout the course of treatment for patient-specific devices, and (5) indexing to the treatment table.

Additional considerations for immobilization devices for proton therapy have been discussed by Wore et al.[4,5] At MD Anderson, we include, but are not limited to, the following considerations when designing and selecting immobilization devices for proton therapy: (1) uniform, low-density if possible, material (i.e., minimal part-to-part variability) so that it would introduce minimal range perturbation in the beam path; (2) devices with gradual slope and no sharp edge; (3) devices producing minimal imaging artifacts; and (4) avoiding the field passing part of the frame and/or table edge during treatment planning.

Various external immobilization devices, including the headrest, mask, bit block, Vacloks, wing board and T-bar, and leg-knee device, are used, depending on the disease site being treated. For moving targets, some motion mitigation strategies may have to be used, including compression boards, breathhold, and gating.

The Hitachi treatment tabletops used at MD Anderson are rectangular slabs, as shown in Fig. 4.1, made of a foam core with a carbon fiber shell. These tabletops have the desirable properties of low density and of being homogeneous. They come in three lengths: long, medium, and short. The short one was originally intended for head and neck (HN) and brain patients. However, the rectangular shape would create large airgaps for lateral or lateral oblique fields often used for HN and brain patients. Large airgaps will enlarge the penumbra for passive scattering beam with aperture and the spot sizes with a range shifter for spot scanning beam for shallow targets. To minimize airgaps, HN couch tops specific for proton therapy were designed and manufactured. Shown in Fig. 4.2 is an example used at MD Anderson manufactured by CIVCO (Kalona, IA), in which the superior end of the couch top is contoured to have the shape of head and shoulder. Similarly, the BoS Headframe developed by Qfix (Avondale, PA) is used by some of the other institutions.

Although it has many advantages for radiation therapy, such as high mechanical strength and low specific density,[6] the carbon fiber couch top is conducting, which limits its compatibility with

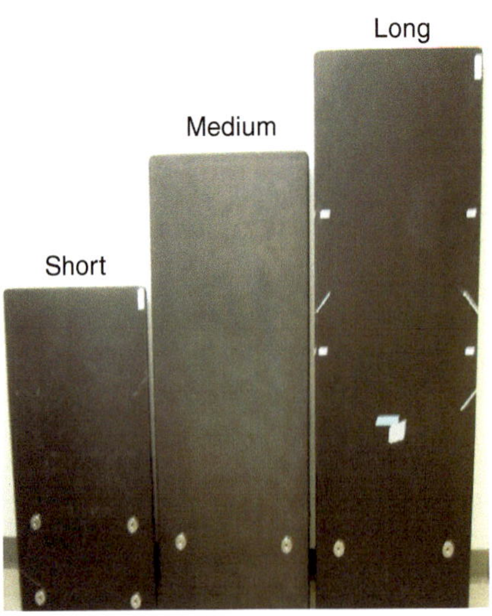

Fig. 4.1 The Hitachi treatment tabletops used at MD Anderson are three different lengths: short, medium, and long.

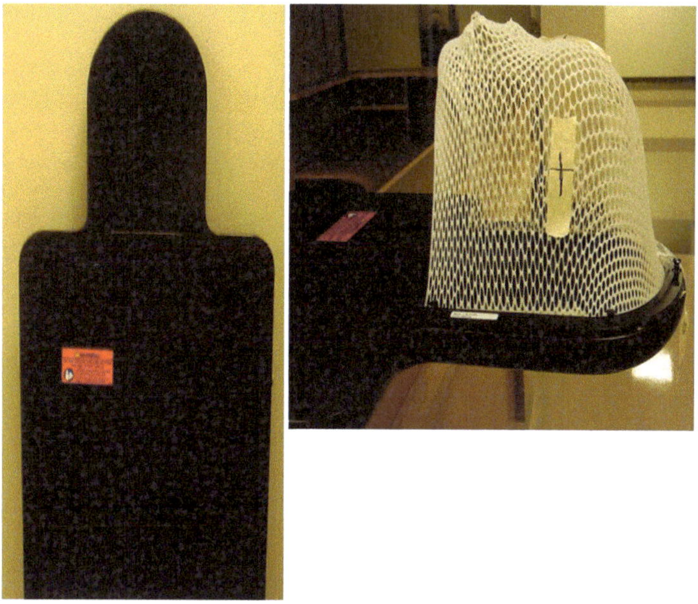

Fig. 4.2 Head and neck couch tops specific for proton therapy used at MD Anderson; the superior end of the couch top is contoured to have the shape of the head and shoulder.

MRI.[7] On the other hand, MRI has become an indispensable imaging modality in modern radiation therapy because of its superior soft tissue contrast and other advanced imaging applications, such as diffusion-weighted imaging and diffusion tensor imaging.[8] It is recommended to have MRI-compatible immobilization devices for proton therapy. Other materials, such as a composite of polypropylene and fiberglass,[7] have been developed as an MRI-compatible alternative to carbon fiber. Two approaches have been suggested[9]: (1) use the MRI-compatible couch top and immobilization devices with the same foam factor, shape, and size for imaging while the patient would be simulated and treated with the carbon fiber couch top; and (2) replace the carbon fiber all together using MRI-compatible materials for CT and MRI imaging and treatment. At MD Anderson, we currently use the first approach for all patient simulation and MRI imaging during the course of proton therapy.

Immobilization Devices and Modeling by the Treatment Planning System

The effects of the devices external to the patient receiving radiation therapy, including increased skin dose, reduced tumor dose, and altered dose distribution, were traditionally ignored as if the patient was suspended in air. Recently, this issue has been addressed by the Task Group Report 176 (TG176) of the American Association of Physicists in Medicine (AAPM).[6] Although the dosimetric effects on photon therapy should be incorporated in the planning process and they are nevertheless small, the range errors introduced by these devices could result in the dose changes up to 100% of a proton beam to a part of the target volumes and/or normal tissues. For proton therapy, the immobilization devices, including immobilization and treatment couch top, in the beam path act as range shifters. Anything in the beam path would contribute to the WET for the beam and should be correctly accounted for by the treatment planning system (TPS). Based on these considerations, TG176 recommends that, for proton therapy, TPS should be used to calculate the WET values of the devices, comparing the TPS calculated values with measurements to ensure the devices are properly modeled.[6]

To model the external devices in TPS, it is necessary to have the devices correctly represented in the planning CT images. A direct approach would be to include all devices used in treatment delivery during CT simulation. The treatment couch top is typically different from the CT simulator couch top. Several approaches have been used at MD Anderson to address this topic:

1. For patients to be treated with beams not passing any device and couch top, such as prostate patients using lateral fields only, no special consideration is needed in this regard.
2. For HN and brain patients, an identical couch top is placed on top of the CT simulator, and the patient is immobilized to the HN couch top. During CT simulation, special attention is paid to ensure the CT images include the entire couch top. A software tool was developed at MD Anderson to remove the CT scanner couch top. Fig. 4.3 shows a CT image for an HN patient with and without the CT couch top. The WET thickness of the HN couch top is 8 mm, which is within 1 mm of measured values.
3. For any patient to be treated with the posterior beam passing through the regular Hitachi couch top at MD Anderson, the CT couch top is replaced by a digital model of treatment couch using a different function of the same software tool mentioned in 2. Fig. 4.4 displays a CT image for a thoracic patient, with a CT scanner table and with the digital treatment couch top.

After the external devices are correctly represented in CT images, it is critical to verify the WET values predicted by TPS are within the established tolerance. Typically, TPS calculates the

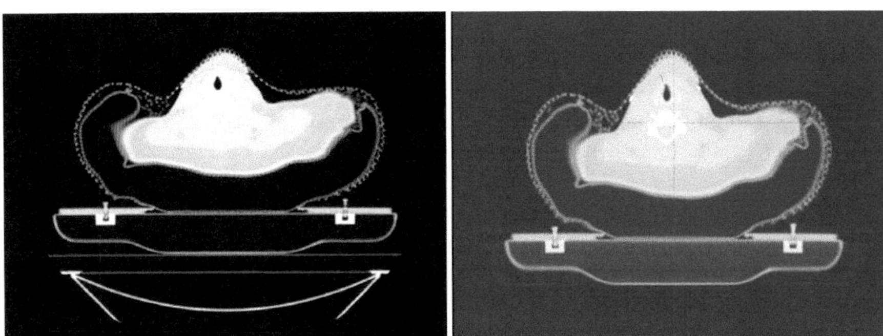

Fig. 4.3 A computed tomography (CT) image for a head and neck patient with and without a CT couch top.

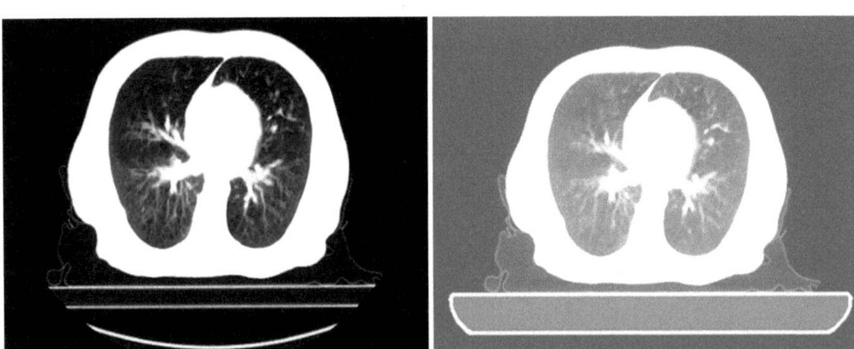

Fig. 4.4 A computed tomography (CT) image for a thoracic patient with the CT scanner couch top and with the digital treatment couch top.

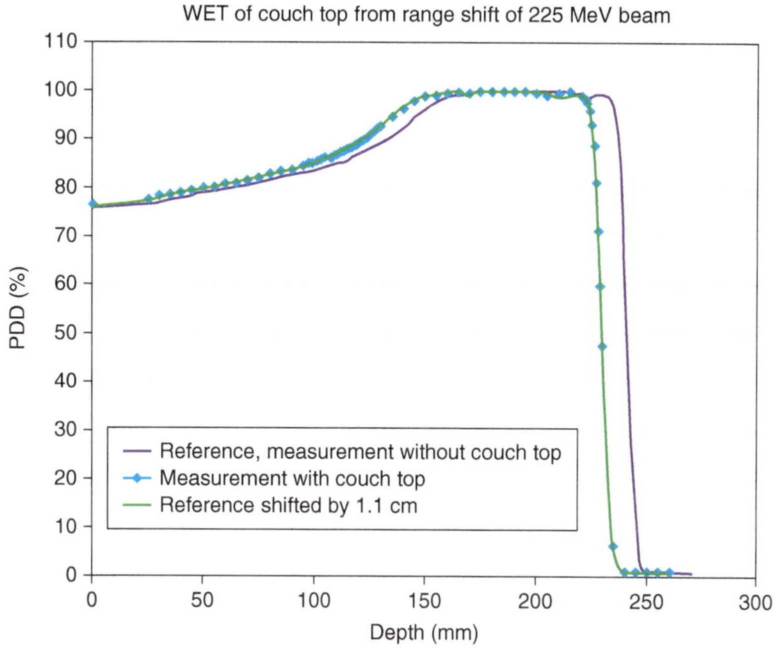

Fig. 4.5 An example of depth-dose curves with and without the Hitachi tabletop used at MD Anderson Cancer Center measured in a water tank. It was determined that the water-equivalent thickness *(WET)* of the tabletop was 1.10 ± 0.05 cm. *PDD*, Percent depth dose.

WET value based on the CT number of each voxel and the corresponding relative linear stopping power through the CT number and stopping power calibration curve accumulated over the beam path.

The WET value of a particular device can be determined by measuring the depth dose curve with and without the device. Depth dose curves for particle beams can be measured by scanning an ionization chamber in a water tank or a multilayer ionization chamber (MLIC).[10,11] Fig. 4.5 is an example of depth dose curves with and without the Hitachi tabletop used at MD Anderson Cancer Center measured in a water tank. It was determined that the WET of the tabletop was 1.10 ± 0.05 cm. In TPS, this tabletop has been confirmed to have the same value of WET. Wroe et al.[12] performed a WET analysis for various immobilization devices used in their clinic. It was found that multiple inserts of a commercial couch system had the WET values that were predicted by TPS within 1 mm. If the measured WET value could not be predicted by TPS, one would have to contour the device and override the HU or stopping power value such that the WET was within 1 mm of the measured value of WET of the device. In a recent study, Fellin et al. investigated the range errors introduced by modeling of WET in TPS and validation by measurements using MLIC.[11] They found the all the devices could be predicted by TPS except one.

Site-Specific Examples

HEAD AND NECK AND BRAIN PATIENTS

In general, one should minimize the potential variations in the patient setup when considering immobilization and simulation. For example, for brain and HN patients with long hair, the day-to-day variation of the amount of hair in the beam path, especially for a posterior-anterior (PA) beam, is a potential concern in the range perturbation. Thus special attention should be paid to patients with long hair to make sure the hair is consistently placed day-to-day between simulations and throughout the course of treatment. The variations in neck curvature, head rotation, and shoulder position in HN patients are potential setup concerns that may affect the dose coverages for the target volumes and normal tissue sparing.

HN and brain immobilization devices usually include a headrest and mask and bite block. Our technique for treating oropharynx and nasopharynx patients with bilateral node uses three fields, namely, PA and right and left superior-inferior oblique lateral fields.[13] There it is important in selecting the HN couch top with the proper length to allow the PA field as well as vertex field. For example, the original HN couch top was too short for the PA field when the isocenter was placed in the center of the total target volume in the middle of the neck. We had to work with the vendor to redesign and manufacture a new HN couch top, which is 12 cm longer, while keeping the contoured shape of the design. Over the years, various headrests have been tested and used, including a clear plastic headrest, colored foam headrests, Civco's Alpha cradle base products (CDRS system) such as Mayo Mold,[14] Klarity cushion (Klarity Medical Products USA, Heath, OH) without a headrest, and Klarity with a new design of headrest made of low-density foam, as shown in Fig. 4.6. Table 4.1 summarizes the pros and cons of each of the headrests. Thermal plastic masks are always used together with the headrests or molds or cushions. Generic

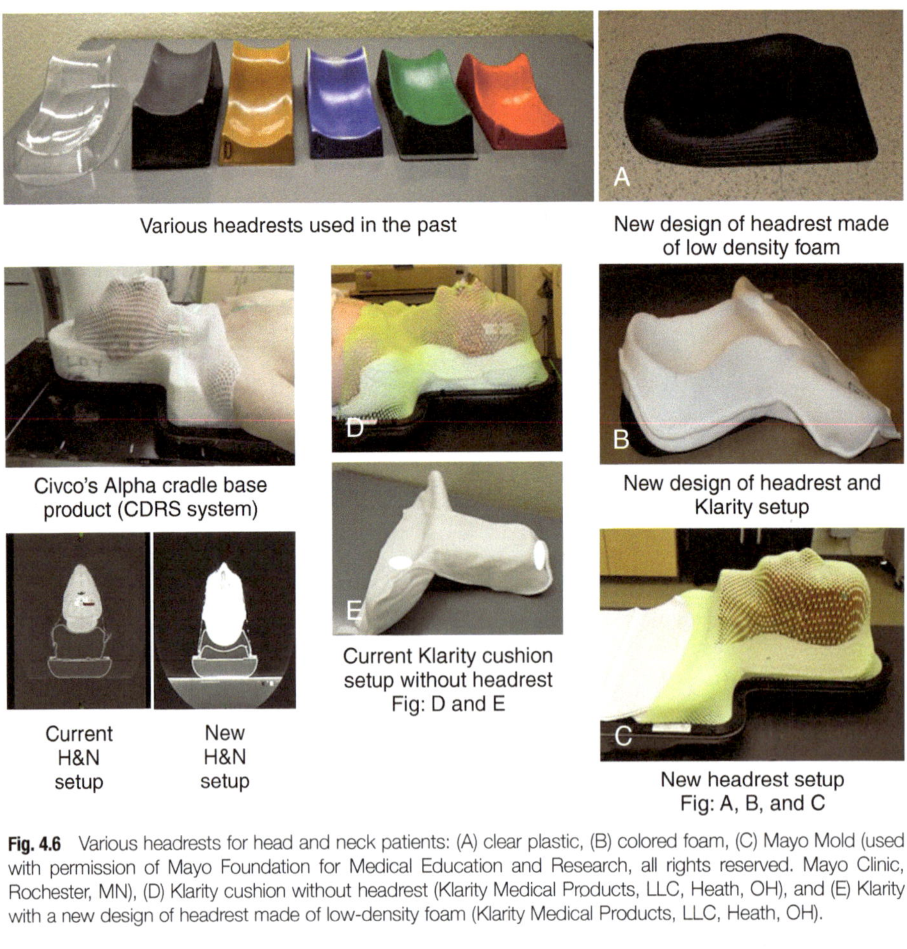

Fig. 4.6 Various headrests for head and neck patients: (A) clear plastic, (B) colored foam, (C) Mayo Mold (used with permission of Mayo Foundation for Medical Education and Research, all rights reserved. Mayo Clinic, Rochester, MN), (D) Klarity cushion without headrest (Klarity Medical Products, LLC, Heath, OH), and (E) Klarity with a new design of headrest made of low-density foam (Klarity Medical Products, LLC, Heath, OH).

TABLE 4.1 ■ **Comparison of Headrests**

Headrest	Pros	Cons
Clear plastic	Uniform and small WET inside	Sharp edge in the lateral sides
Colored foam	Uniform inside	Sharp edge in the lateral sides
Civco's Alpha cradle base product (CDRS system), such as Mayo Mold	Low density	Taking long time to simulate Shrinking over time
Klarity cushion without headrest	Very conformal to patient's neck Reduces the rotation and neck curve change	Difficult to indexing to couch top
Klarity cushion with low-density headrest	Very conformal to patient's neck Reduces the rotation and neck curve change Improves the indexing to the couch top	To be determined

WET, Water-equivalent thickness.

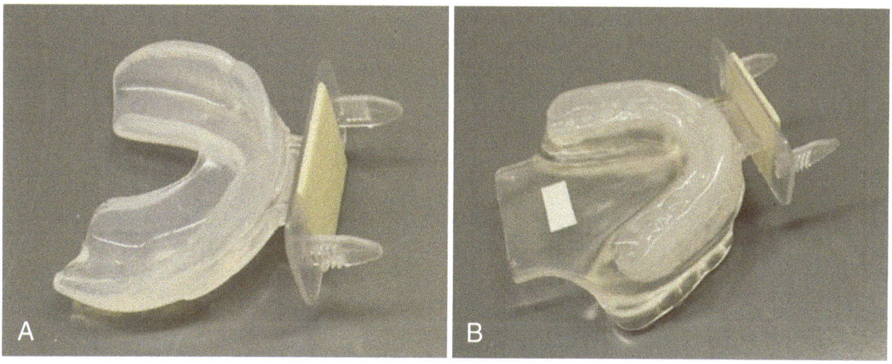

Fig. 4.7 (A) Generic bite block used for brain patients, and (B) custom bite block for head and neck patients.

bite blocks attached to the masks, as shown in Fig. 4.7A, are used for brain patients to minimize the head rotations. Patient-specific stents manufactured by the Dental Oncology Department at our institution are used for most of the HN patients, as shown in Fig. 4.7B. Shoulder position is often a concern for the consistent setup of HN patients. Attention should be paid to have the patient in a more relaxed and reproducible shoulder position. Recently, we have introduced a technique using clavicle bone position to assess if the shoulder is consistently set up through the course of treatment: the clavicle bony structure is contoured in the TPS and projected on setup digitally reconstructed radiographs, the clavicle bony contour is then passed onto the x-ray images during the daily imaging session before delivering the beams, and the consistency of the shoulder position is then determined by how good the matching is between the contour and clavicle bone on the daily x-ray images.

Thoracic and Abdomen

Thoracic and abdomen patients use similar immobilization devices, involving a large hemi-body vacuum bag (BlueBAG, Elekta Co., Atlanta, GA), a wing board, and a T-bar (Extended Wing Board; CIVCO, Kalona, IA), as shown in Fig. 4.8. The patient usually is in the arm-up position.

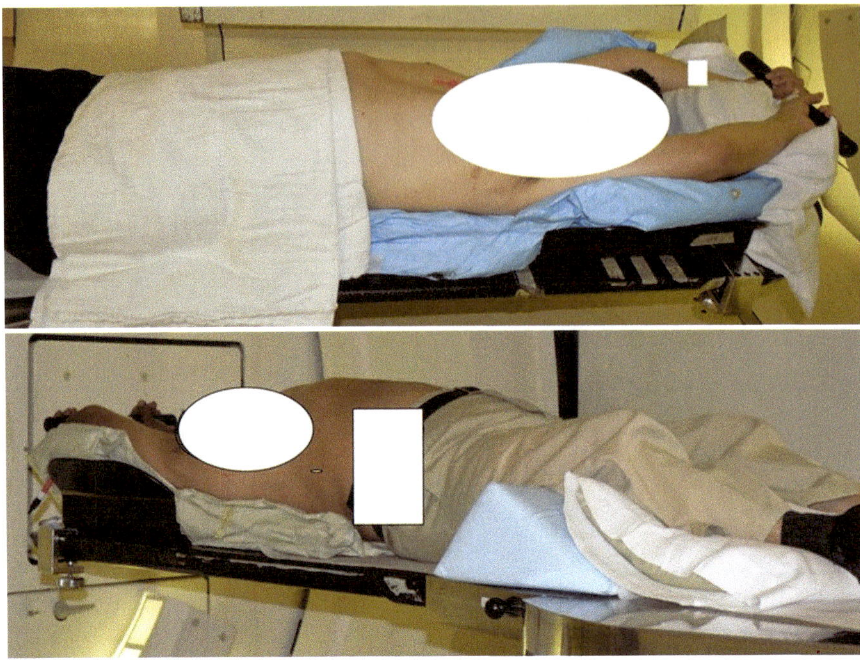

Fig. 4.8 Immobilization devices for thoracic and abdomen patients, involving a large hemi-body vacuum bag, a wing board, and a T-bar.

During the treatment planning, it is possible that one of the optimal fields is using a posterior oblique beam, which transverse across the couch top edge. The daily variation in the setup of the patient would translate into daily variation in the distal range of the proton beam in the patient, which could result in underdose of the target volume or overdose of the critical structures. Indexing the immobilization devices to treatment couch top would reduce this kind of daily variation. However, a study at MD Anderson showed that variations up to 1 cm were observed even with indexed devices.[15] Therefore one should use other beam angles that would not transverse across the couch top edge, if possible. An alternative method used at MD Anderson is to offset the immobilization device by 5 cm to the side where the beam is coming from, using an offset indexing bar. In this method, the patient is consistently offset to the side of the couch top such that the beam would not transverse the couch top edge with a margin. Potential edge issues may also exist for other disease sites.

Another important aspect of thoracic and abdomen patients is respiratory motion. Simulation, treatment planning, and treatment delivery strategies for moving targets in the thorax and abdomen include four-dimensional CT (4D CT),[16] abdominal compression, breathhold, layer and volumetric repainting, and gating.[17] Breathhold simulation is usually performed after 4D CT, assessing the magnitude of motion. Multiple (3–5) breathhold CT scans are normally performed to determine the reproducibility of the breathhold. Only one of the scans is used for treatment planning. Details of the breath-hold parameters are carried forward for the breathhold during treatment delivery.

Pelvis and Prostate

Although the soft tissues are dominant in the human body, the bony structures could contribute significantly to WET for a particular beam passing through it, such as a lateral field for the prostate. Therefore for pelvic and prostate patients, the position of femur heads and variation in prostate gland position relative to the bony structures in the pelvis are important factors to consider in selecting immobilization devices and simulation. A feet-knee fixation device is used to consistently position the femur heads (Klarity Medical Products USA, Newark, OH USA), as shown in Fig. 4.9. The separation of the feet and knee parts of the device and the device as a whole indexed to the couch top are customized to individual patients. To have a consistent setup, multiple CT imaging sessions are normally used. This allows the patient to sit up and walk around a little bit between the imaging sessions and finally settle into a more relaxed position, which is more reproducible during the course of treatment. To reduce intra- and interfraction position variations of the prostate gland, endorectal balloons (ERBs) are also used in prostate radiotherapy to immobilize the prostate and spare the rectal wall.[18,19] To account for the residual position variations of the prostate, two to three fiducial marks are placed in the prostate under transrectal ultrasound guidance.[20,21] The fiducials are used to align the prostate volume to the treatment field for image-guided proton therapy. The fiducial marks used at MD Anderson are made of carbon-coated zirconium dioxide, which has a smaller dose effect than higher Z materials such as gold.[22] A hydrogel spacer, SpaceOAR (Augmenix, Inc., Waltham, MA) has recently been used for proton therapy of prostate cancers.[23] The gel spacer is implanted between the prostate and anterior rectal wall to provide additional separation and therefore reduce the dose to the anterior rectal wall. However, the gel spacer does not reduce the intra- and interfraction prostate motion during prostate cancer radiotherapy.[24,25] Therefore the fiducials should be still used for patients with the gel spacer. Normally, the gel spacer is not used together with ERB.[23]

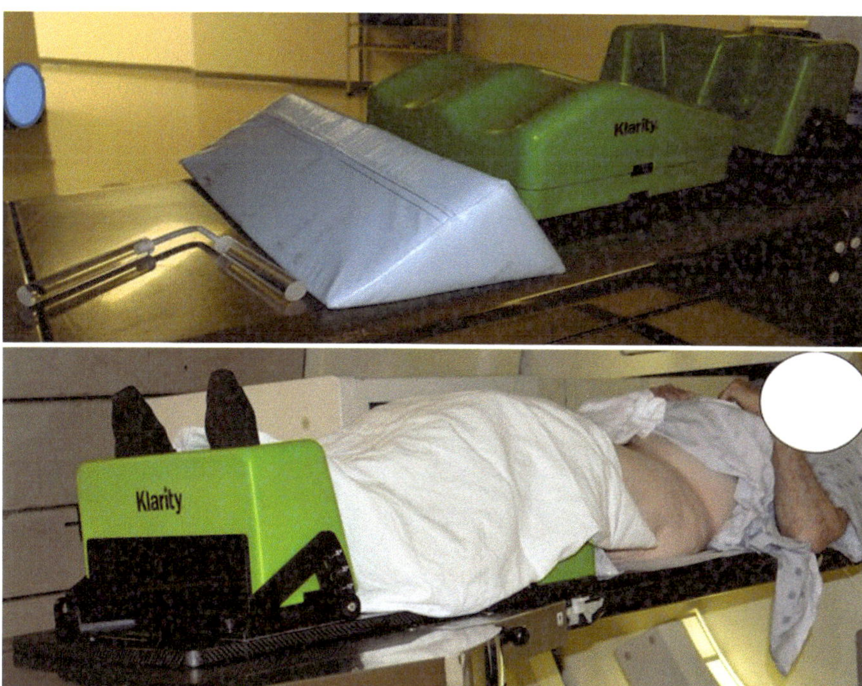

Fig. 4.9 A feet-knee fixation device is used for prostate patients (Klarity Medical Products, LLC, Heath, OH).

Craniospinal Irradiation

Craniospinal irradiation (CSI) is a radiation technique used for patients with central nervous system malignancies, such as medulloblastoma and primitive neuroectodermal tumors.[26] Immobilization devices for CSI patients treated in a supine position at MD Anderson include a headrest, head mask, and a large body vacuum bag (BlueBAG, Elekta Co., Atlanta, GA), as shown in Fig. 4.10. In addition, a Styrofoam slab is traditionally used to elevate the patient to allow the posterior oblique beams without transverse across the couch top edge, typically 15 degrees from the horizontal plane, for covering the cribriform plate yet sparing the lenses.[27] The entire central nervous system is normally longer than the maximum field size available and requires large fields with multiple isocenters.[28] For CSI using PBS, two neighboring fields from different isocenters should have a large overlap with low dose gradient through the IMPT optimization process. In this case, a match line change for the junction would not be required.[28–30]

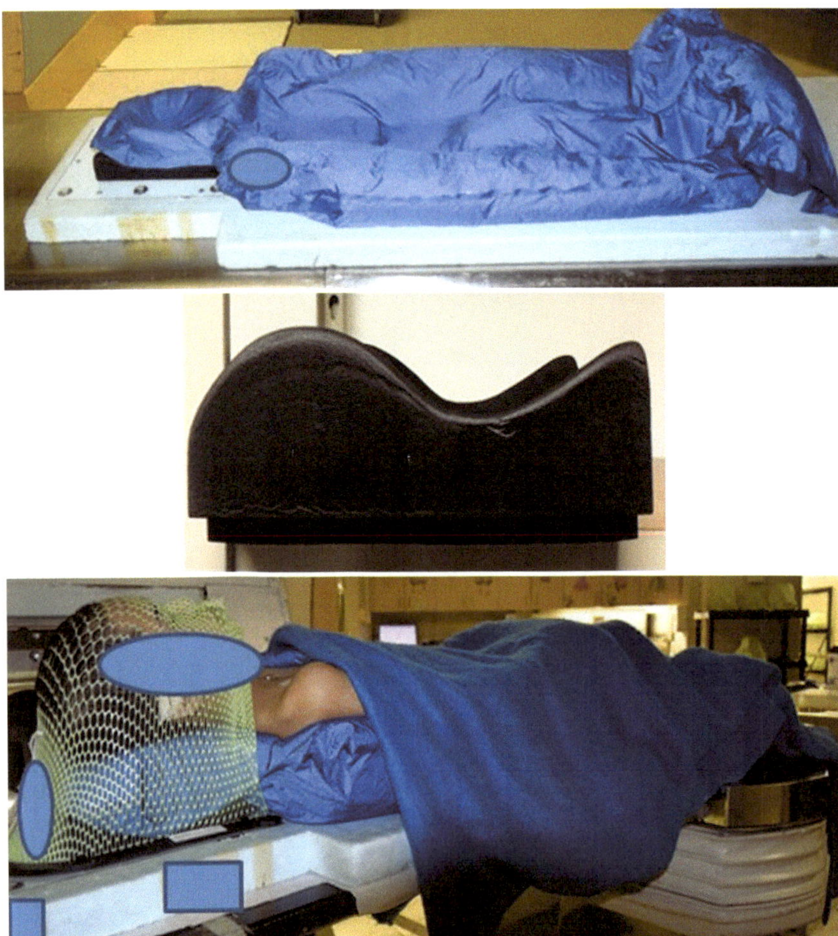

Fig. 4.10 An immobilization device for craniospinal irradiation patients treated in a supine position at MD Anderson includes a headrest, head mask, a large body vacuum bag.

Therefore it is important to index the Styrofoam slab and Vaclock bag to the treatment couch top to ensure that the patient's entire central nervous system is set up consistently. For pediatric patients, sedation is often applied to keep the patient in the treatment position. It is also important to position the head such that the airway is kept open.

Summary

Immobilization and simulation is one of the key processes for any successful radiation oncology practice. It is even more important for proton therapy and IMPT because of the finite range of the proton beam. Only the calibrated protocol should be used for CT imaging of the patients for proton therapy. Immobilization devices should create minimal range perturbation and avoid the sharp edge. The range shift effect should be accurately predicted by TPS.

References Available Online.

CHAPTER 5

Principles of Intensity-Modulated Proton Therapy Treatment Planning

Xiaodong Zhang ■ Yupeng Li ■ Heng Li ■ Richard Wu ■ Matthew Palmer

Intensity-Modulated Proton Therapy Is Effective for Complex Targets

Proton beam therapy (PBT), with its characteristic Bragg peak, holds the promise of further reducing toxicity. Several techniques exist for the administration of PBT, including passive scatter proton therapy (PSPT)[1–10] and intensity-modulated proton therapy (IMPT).[11–19] Although PSPT decreases dose distally, we also face a clinical challenge with dose-escalated radiotherapy using PSPT for tumors in very complicated anatomy. Because of a limited number of treatment fields, delivering ablative doses to targets with complicated shapes or locations, such as tumors curved around sensitive critical structures, is very difficult using PSPT. In IMPT, a pencil beam (spot or beamlet) can be magnetically scanned in two-dimensional directions perpendicular to the beam direction to form an irradiating field. By charging protons with different energies, pencil beams can be used to penetrate with different depths and "scan" the entire designated target volume. The delivery of the sum of all Bragg peaks individually modulated is thus sought to create highly conformal dose distributions to cover the three-dimensional (3D) tumor target. Mathematically, IMPT using scanning beam therapy can simultaneously optimize the intensities and the energies of all pencil beams using an objective function that takes into account targets as well as normal tissue constraints. Compared with PSPT, IMPT is more effective for designing treatment plans that deliver ablative doses to targets with complicated shapes or locations, such as tumors curved around sensitive critical structures. As shown in Fig. 5.1,[19] because of the close proximity of the spinal cord and planning target volume (PTV), the aperture has to be edited to meet the cord dose constraint. This aperture editing caused the underdose of the PTV, as shown in the enlarged image of the target region. Clinically, we have observed local recurrence in these underdosed regions for patients treated with PSPT technique at our center. Compared with intensity-modulated radiation therapy (IMRT)/volumetric-modulated arc therapy (VMAT) technology, IMPT treatment plan can be designed optimall to take advantage of the proton beam. The IMPT plan is able to significantly reduce the dose to the healthy organs while delivering a similar target dose. Fig. 5.2[11] shows a comparison of IMPT and VMAT plans for the first patient treated with multiple-field optimization (MFO) IMPT at our center. We can see that the mean lung dose for the IMPT plan is reduced by 4.4 Gy compared with the VMAT plan. Currently, patients with thoracic cancer are the most complex cases, for whom dose-volume constraints cannot be met by VMAT plans or because they need reirradiation.

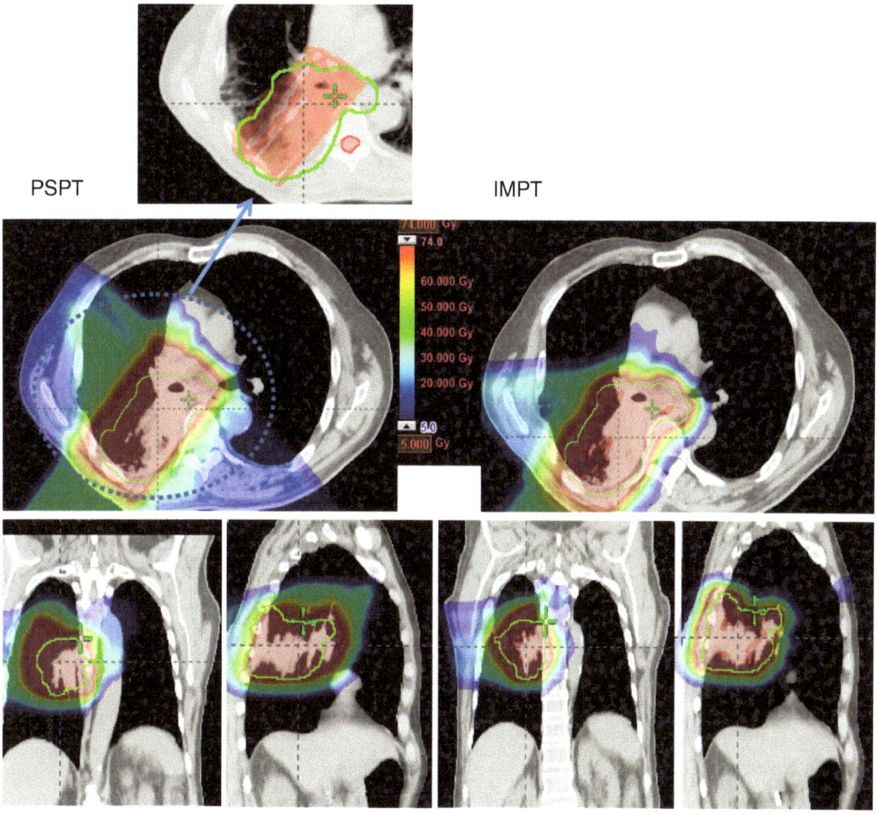

Fig. 5.1 Comparison between passive scatter proton therapy *(PSPT)* and intensity-modulated proton therapy *(IMPT)* for lung cancer. Dose distributions for the PSPT *(left)* and IMPT *(right)* plans are shown. Green lines delineate the PTV. An enlarged image of the target region for the PSPT is shown to indicate the inadequate dose coverage caused by aperture editing. (From Zhang X, Li Y, Pan X, et al. Intensity-modulated proton therapy reduces the dose to normal tissue compared with intensity-modulated radiation therapy or passive scattering proton therapy and enables individualized radical radiotherapy for extensive stage IIIB non-small-cell lung cancer: a virtual clinical study. *Int J Radiat Oncol Biol Phys*. 2010;77(2):357-366.)

Uncertainties

Because of the greater dosimetric advantage of IMPT compared with IMRT and PSPT, lately, newer proton centers have started adopting scanning beam–only delivery technology. Translational research on treatment planning centers on developing IMPT-specific planning technology. Among the most important planning technology developments is that of robust optimization for IMPT. There are several sources of nonrobustness of IMPT plans: (1) range uncertainty, (2) setup uncertainty, (3) motion/interplay uncertainties for moving anatomy, and (4) anatomical change uncertainties.

RANGE UNCERTAINTIES

The most important dose-sparing ability of the proton beam is that the proton can stop at roughly the end of the proton's range. However, because of approximation of tissues on computed

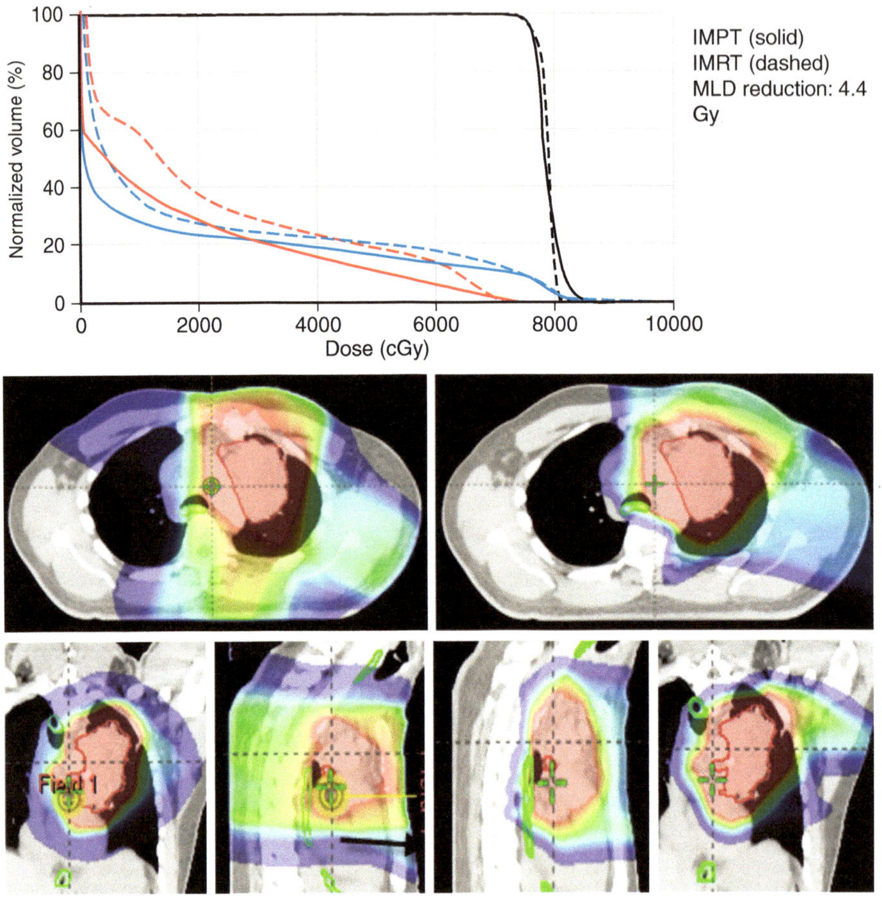

Fig. 5.2 The first patients treated using intensity-modulated proton therapy *(IMPT)* multiple-field optimization technology at MD Anderson Cancer Center. The comparison between the IMPT plan *(right)* and intensity-modulated radiation therapy *(IMRT)* plans *(left)*. *MLD*, Mean lung dose. (From Chang JY, Li H, Zhu XR, Liao Z, Zhao L, Liu A, et al. Clinical implementation of intensity modulated proton therapy for thoracic malignancies. *Int J Radiat Oncol Biol Phys.* 2014;90(4):809-818.)

tomography (CT) scans into Hounsfield units (HUs), there are systematic range uncertainties of about 3% in our understanding of where protons stop in patient tissues. Fig. 5.3[20] shows the dose distribution of an original plan and the dose distribution of a plan assuming a 3.5% range overshooting. The target dose is well covered by the prescription in the original plan, but the target is severely underdosed if the plan is 3.5% undershot. If a beam of a plan stops right before a critical organ, such as the spinal cord or brain stem on an original plan, the brain stem or spinal cord will actually receive much more dose than if the beam is overshot by 3.5%. Currently, one of the rules of thumb of selecting beams is still to not select beams stopping right before critical organs.

SETUP UNCERTAINTIES

All modalities of radiation therapy, regardless of whether they are proton or photon, suffer from setup uncertainties. Setup uncertainties are attributed to the misalignment of incident

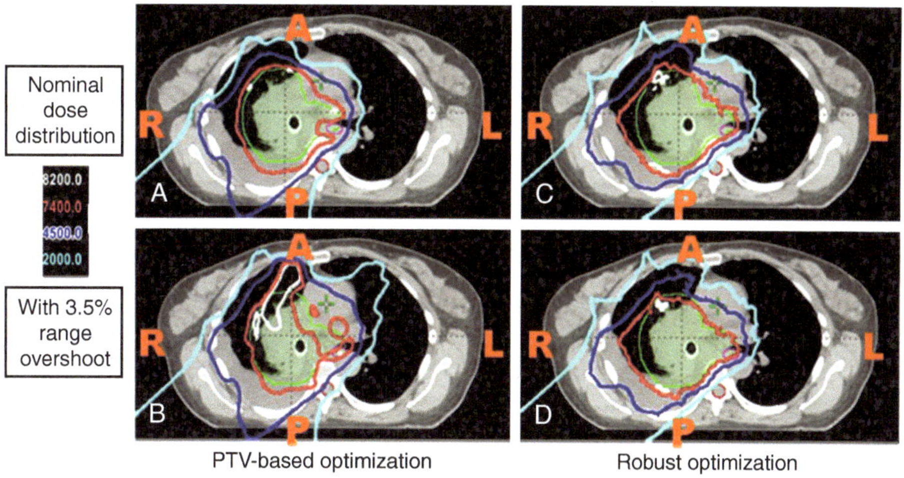

Fig. 5.3 Isodose contours of the dose distribution in the transverse plane of a lung cancer case: (A and B) planning target volume *(PTV)*–based plan; (C and D) robustly optimized plan; (A and C) with the nominal range; (B and D) with 3.5% higher than the nominal range. *Green color wash:* Clinical target volume (CTV); *purple color wash,* spinal cord. (From Liu W, Zhang X, Li Y, Mohan R. Robust optimization of intensity modulated proton therapy. *Med Phys.* 2012;39(2):1079-1091.)

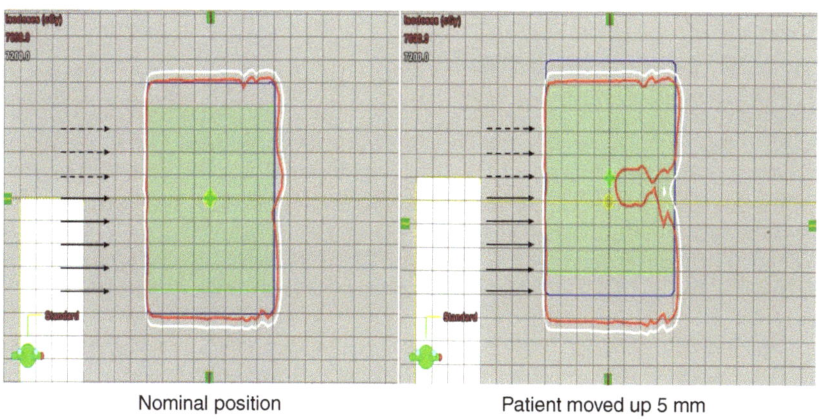

Fig. 5.4 Dose distribution symmetry broken under perturbation. (From Li H, Zhang X, Park P, et al. Robust optimization in intensity-modulated proton therapy to account for anatomy changes in lung cancer patients. *Radiother Oncol.* 2015;114(3):367-372.)

beams and the patient anatomy and the realignment of internal heterogeneities among themselves and with respect to the target volume. For photon therapy, setup uncertainties are mitigated by the use of expansion margins from the clinical target volume (CTV) to the PTV. The margin approach works well for photon therapy and is based on a nice property of the photon: the spatial nature of photon dose distributions is minimally perturbed by uncertainties. In other words, a photon dose distribution is relatively robust in the face of uncertainties. Unkelbach et al.[21] have used the term *static dose cloud* to describe a photon dose distribution. However, the margin approach does not work well for proton therapy. Distal and proximal to the beam direction, the margins for proton therapy should be determined by the range uncertainties. In the lateral direction, the static dose cloud will be broken under the lateral setup uncertainties. As shown in Fig. 5.4, the symmetry of the dose cloud, shown as the red isodose line that covers

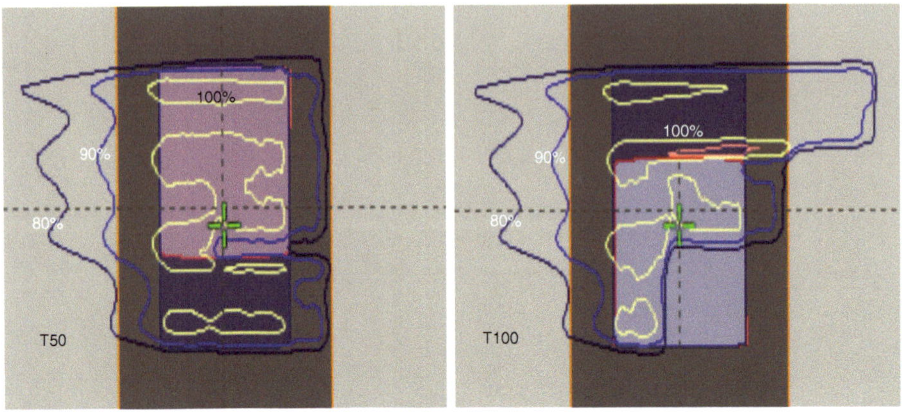

Fig. 5.5 Uncertainty caused by breathing motion: *left,* plan designed on the T50 phase of the computed tomography (CT) scan; *right,* same plan recalculated on the T0 phase of CT.

the target (blue shaded region), is broken if the patient moved up by 5 mm. The target is still covered in the up direction but is underdosed in the middle. The underdose shown in Fig. 5.4 cannot be mitigated by the margin.

MOTION/INTERPLAY UNCERTAINTIES

Protons are sensitive to variations in tissue density in the beam path.[5,22–26] This is particularly important when the tissue moves, as in the case of tumors in the lung. The sensitivity of protons to moving anatomy can be seen by calculating dose distributions on different phases of four-dimensional CT (4D CT). Fig. 5.5 shows uncertainties caused by breathing motion imitated with a phantom. In this extreme case, we can see that the dose in the T0 phase is drastically different than in the T50 phase if the plan is designed using only the T50 phase.

Both PSPT and IMPT techniques have uncertainties in dose distribution in the different phases of CT. However, for the IMPT plan, there is an extra uncertainty. For the IMPT technique, a magnetically deflected particle beam scans the tumor volume laterally by sequentially delivering a series of scanning spots and longitudinally, layer by layer, by altering proton energy. If the target moves at the same time as the scanning beam is delivered, the motion of the pencil beam might interfere with the delivery of the intended dose distribution, causing deviations from the planned dose distributions. This interference usually results in local regions of underdoses and overdoses, referred to as interplay effects. As shown in Fig. 5.6, if the tumor motion and dynamic delivery are synchronized unfavorably, we might have a complete miss of the target in extreme cases.

ANATOMICAL CHANGE UNCERTAINTIES

Anatomical changes during radiation therapy are sometimes a consequence of radiation therapy. Because radiation is used to eradicate tumors, the tumors will shrink during the course of treatment. This can be seen in Fig. 5.7[27]; the tumor/gross tumor volume (GTV) at simulation is different from the tumor/GTV shown on the day 50 CT scan. Also, patients often lose weight during the course of treatment, especially those with head and neck (HN) cancer. The anatomical

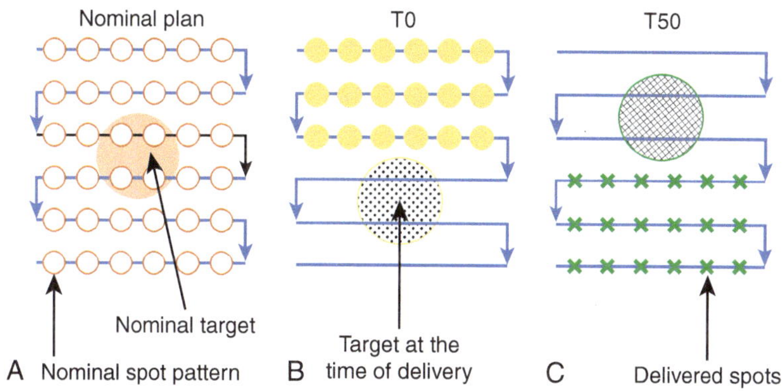

Fig. 5.6 Interplay uncertainties because of dynamic motion and moving target: (A) nominal plan designed at free-breathing phase; (B) when delivering the yellow spots, target on T0 phase does not see any spots; and (C) when delivering green spots, target on T50 phase does not see any spots.

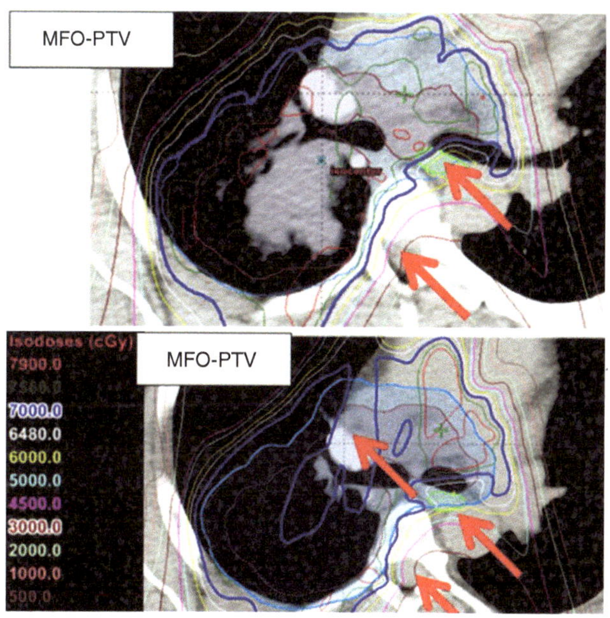

Fig. 5.7 Anatomical change uncertainties: target miss caused by target shrinkage by radiation therapy. At the top is the dose distribution of the plan generated at the time of simulation, and the blue line is the prescription line (70 Gy). At the time of day 50 shown at the bottom, the target (gross target volume [GTV]) shrinks, leading to the underdose. *MFO,* Multiple-field optimization; *PTV,* planning target volume. (From Li H, Zhang X, Park P, et al. Robust optimization in intensity-modulated proton therapy to account for anatomy changes in lung cancer patients. *Radiother Oncol.* 2015;114(3):367-372.)

change during the course of the treatment affects proton much more than photon therapy. Because of the larger perturbation of the IMPT plan attributed to anatomical change, we propose that plan adaption is mandatory for lung cancer IMPT plans to ensure target coverage.[28] At our center, more 30% of lung IMPT plans need adaptation during the course of treatment to compensate for the uncertainties caused by anatomical change.[29]

Robust Evaluations

PLANNING TARGET VOLUME AND CLINICAL TARGET VOLUME CONCEPT

As a result of the various uncertainties discussed previously, the major challenge facing the proton therapy community is how to evaluate the robustness of the treatment plan. In the photon world, the major tool for evaluating robustness is the concept of PTV and planning risk volume (PRV). The PTV is usually defined as the CTV plus a margin. One formula for margins is $2.5\ \Sigma + 0.7\ \sigma$, where Σ is the systematic error, and σ is the random error. Based on the famous work of Van Herk,[30,31] if the PTV margin is set based on $2.5\ \Sigma + 0.7\ \sigma$, the CTV treated based on the facility's systematic and random error, the chance that the CTV will receive 95% of the prescription dose is 95%. The margin formula has been widely adopted as the guideline for evaluating the robustness of photon therapy. However, using PTV as a means to evaluate the robustness of a proton plan was increasingly realized to be ineffective for IMPT plans. Fig. 5.8 shows the dose-volume histograms (DVHs) of two plans; the PTV coverage of plan A represented by the solid line is worse than that of plan B represented by the dashed line. However, the range of DVH variation of CTV under different uncertainty scenarios (shown by the shaded DVHs for plan A) is much narrower than that for plan B. For this plot, we used the same uncertainty scenarios for both plan A and plan B; apparently, plan A is more robust than plan B. Thus Fig. 5.8 indicates that better PTV coverage for the proton plan does not necessarily lead to more robustness of the plan. In other words, PTV is not a good way to evaluate the robustness of proton plans.

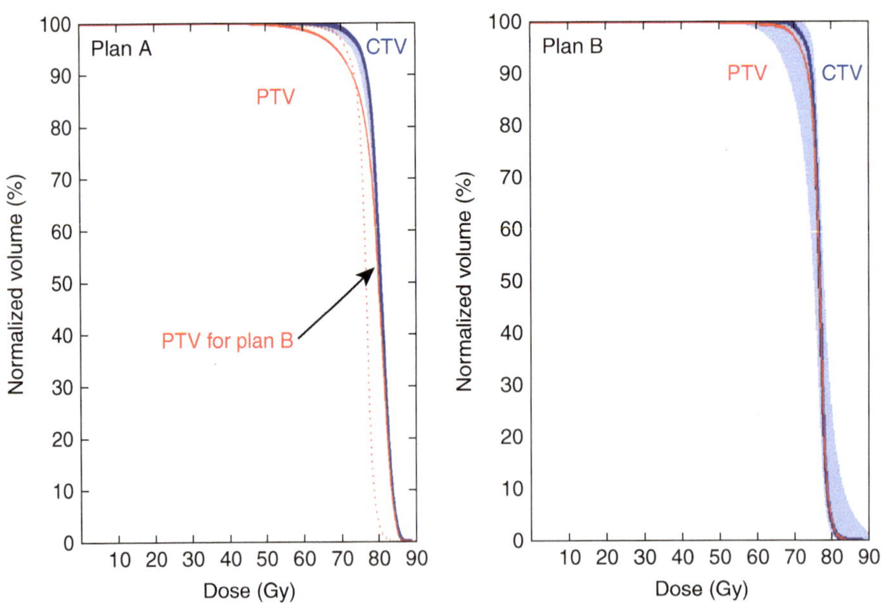

Fig. 5.8 The dose-volume histogram for plan A and plan B for the same patient. Plan A has worse planning target volume *(PTV)* coverage *(solid line)* on the left than plan B *(dashed line on left panel)*. But the clinical target volume *(CTV)* variation *(shaded area)* on left for plan A is much narrower than that *(shaded area on right)* for plan B with the same range of uncertainties.

WORST-CASE ROBUST EVALUATION

Currently, worst-case dose distribution and worst-case DVH are increasingly being adopted as the major tools for evaluating the robustness of proton plans. Worst-case dose distribution was first proposed by Lomax et al.[32] After a treatment plan was designed, it was recalculated with different uncertainty scenarios. Each uncertainty scenario essentially leads to a new plan. Because it is not convenient to evaluate so many new plans, Lomax et al. proposed to use a "worst-case" dose distribution to represent many plans with different uncertainty scenarios. The worst-case dose distribution introduced by Lomax et al.[32] is a method of combining multiple dose distributions (e.g., dose distributions calculated for different ranges of the Bragg peaks) into a single one. For a voxel inside the target volume, the minimum dose of this voxel in all dose distributions is stored in the worst-case dose distribution. For a voxel outside the target volume, the maximum is taken. The worst-case dose distribution evaluation is not actually adopted in commercial treatment planning systems (TPSs). In practice, the commercial Eclipse TPS used at our center released a tool, termed a *range uncertainties tool,* to facilitate calculation of many new perturbation plans. It can also plot DVHs from many uncertainty plans. The DVHs of a particular organ of interest from many plans are essentially combined to form a band of DVHs. We can gauge the robustness of the plan by the "band" of DVHs. Trofimov et al.[33] even proposed redrawing those band DVHs as shaded DVHs and using them as a standard approach to evaluate the robustness of IMPT plans.

Although the concept of worst-case dose distribution and worst-case DVHs seems to be a valid approach to evaluate the robustness of IMPT plans, two unanswered questions remain: (1) how many uncertainty scenarios should be used? and (2) what is the criterion to say that a plan is robust or not robust?

Much work has been done to address the first question. One approach is to use statistical uncertainties.[34] However, in our practice, we adopted only eight different scenarios and plotted the banded DVH with nine scenarios (eight perturbations plus the original one.) The eight scenarios are calculated by shifting the isocenter of the original plan by $+-$dx, $+-$dy, $+-$dz, and over/undershooting range by $+-$dr, where dx, dy, dz are the systematic uncertainties in x, y, and z directions, and dr is the range uncertainty, normally chosen to be 3.5%. We were tempted to use 95% coverage of the worst-case CTV to be equivalent to 95% coverage of the PTV as in the photon plan. But this concept has not been valid. Moreover, the nine-scenarios approach is only an approximation. The assumptions of this method may not be solid for the following reasons: (1) it is not always appropriate to assume that only cold spots have negative effects in treating the target; (2) the error on a perturbation dimension, say dx, cannot be +3 mm and −3 mm at the same time; (3) worst-case analysis (WCA) examines the shift in x, y, and z directions and beam range uncertainties separately, but shift always happens in all directions simultaneously with range uncertainties. It is therefore not clear whether WCA would over- or underestimate the plan sensitivity to uncertainties. It is necessary to validate the WCA method in a comprehensive way. We used a Monte Carlo–like approach to examine a large number of possible treatment plan–related scenarios with different perturbations. In our study, a series of perturbations to modify proton beam range and to shift the isocenter was sampled 500 times with the Ziggurat rejection sampling algorithm to derive the probability distribution of possible plan qualities for a prostate case and an HN case. The magnitude of the perturbation was assigned randomly following a Gaussian distribution with specified standard deviations in each perturbation dimension. The perturbed dose was calculated for each sampling, and DVHs were obtained. Dose-volume indices, including dose that was received by 95% of the target volume (D95) of CTV, volume of rectum and bladder exposed to at least 70 Gy (V70), V25 of femoral heads (V50 and V45 were all zero in the studied case), maximum dose to brain stem and spinal cord, and mean dose to brain and right parotid, are inspected here for demonstration purposes. The results were compared with the ones derived by WCA. The probabilities by which the dose volume indices of a perturbed dose are superior to the ones from

WCA are shown in Fig. 5.9. For CTV, 97.6% in the prostate case and 97% in the HN case of perturbed doses show a D95 value higher than the value given by WCA. For normal tissues, at least 96.4% of perturbed doses show lower dose-volume indices than the ones by WCA. As shown in Fig. 5.10, the DVHs of 500 perturbed doses spread over narrow or broad bands, and the DVH curves from WA lie within those bands and near the "worst" edges. This suggests that WCA may reasonably evaluate the IMPT plan's sensitivity to setup and range uncertainties. On the other hand, the observation that the perturbed dose could be worse than the WCA results with low but finite probabilities suggests that the plans' sensitivities were not overestimated by WCA.

Regarding the second unanswered question about the uncertainty criterions, no research has been done to date on this question. We believe that to fully address this question, one must correlate clinical outcomes with the IMPT plan to determine the robust evaluation criterion. When this chapter was written, this was an active focus of our research.

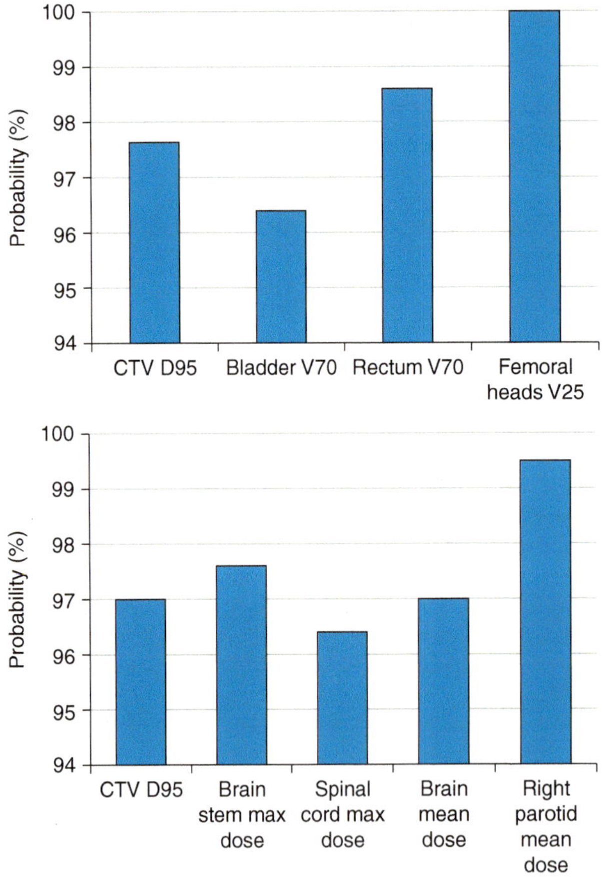

Fig. 5.9 Probabilities by which a perturbed dose is within the worst-case estimation under selected dose-volume indices. For the prostate case *(top)*, 97.6% of clinical target volume *(CTV)* D95, 96.4% bladder V70, 98.6% of rectum V70, and 100% femoral heads V25 values are within the estimated boundary values by the worst-case analysis. For the head/neck case *(bottom)*, 97% of CTV D95, 97.6% of brain stem maximum dose, 96.4% of spinal cord maximum dose, 97% of brain mean dose, and 98% right parotid mean dose values are within the worst-case estimations.

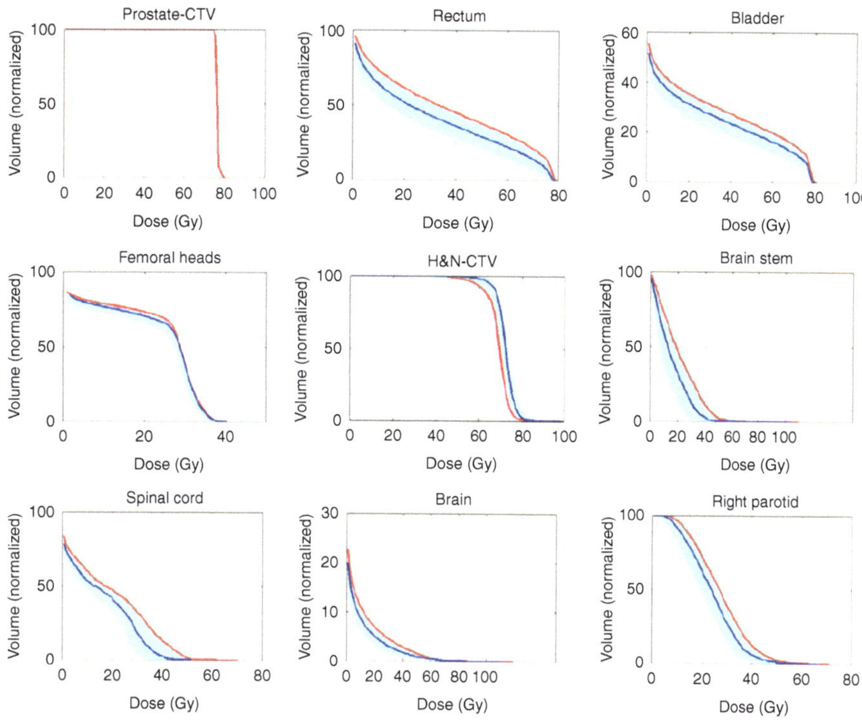

Fig. 5.10 Dose-volume histograms of all 500 possible dose distributions are plotted together, respectively, for the prostate and the head/neck case *(congregated curves in cyan)* with the dose-volume histogram of the worst-case doses *(red solid line)*. The nominal doses without any perturbation are plotted in blue solid lines. In all cases, the worst-case lines located near the "worst" edge of the bands covered by all 500 sampled perturbations, indicating that the worst-case analysis is likely to provide reasonable estimates of the negative impact of perturbations. *CTV,* Clinical target volume.

ROBUST EVALUATION CONSIDERING MOTION

The worst-case dose distribution considered only setup and range uncertainties. However, for lung and liver tumors, tumor and normal tissue organ motion can be very large. The effect of that motion on proton plans poses another challenge for evaluating the robustness of proton plans. As seen in Fig. 5.5, the same plan may produce very different dose distributions on different breathing phases. At MD Anderson Cancer Center MD Anderson strongly discourages the use of this (or other) initialisms; it prefers to be spelled out as "MD Anderson Cancer Center" at first mention and simply "MD Anderson" elsewhere., regardless of whether the plan is PSPT or IMPT, the dose must always be calculated on both the T0 and T50 phases as a robust evaluation strategy for thoracic cancer. To evaluate the interplay effect of the dynamic delivery and mobile tumor or anatomy, we developed a dynamic dose simulator. The 4D dynamic dose simulator calculates dose on the basis of the treatment planning procedures and beam delivery system details at our institution. With this 4D dynamic dose simulator, we defined a metric that represents the target coverage of a single-fraction 4D dynamic dose without considering rescanning, denoted as the 1FX dynamic dose.[23] The target coverage of the 1FX dynamic dose, calculated with the use of our 4D dynamic dose simulator, has become our clinical standard for evaluating the magnitude of interplay effects.

Robust Optimization

After we understood the various sources of uncertainties, different strategies were proposed to make the plan robust against those uncertainties. To compensate for the range uncertainties that were not seen in photon planning, a concept termed beam-specific PTV (bsPTV)[35] was proposed. The beam-specific target is the CTV/GTV, expanded laterally using the margins similar to CTV to PTV margins but expanded distally and proximally using the distal margins and proximal margins determined by the range uncertainties. One drawback of the bsPTV approach is that this approach can work only for single-field optimization (SFO).

Since the mid-2010s, robust optimization by incorporating errors directly into the optimization algorithm has evolved from early exploratory research[21,36,37] into clinical practice.[20,38–41] Robust optimization can be done in several ways: the probabilistic approach and worst-case optimization. The probabilistic approach[21,37] assumes prior knowledge of the probability distribution of the uncertainty; in most cases, the distribution was assumed to be normal. The worst-case optimization optimized the worst case that could have occurred. After Pflugfelder et al.[36] implemented the first version of the worst-case optimization in their in-house TPS for particle therapy (KonRad, Heidelberg, Germany), the worst-case dose optimization or its slight variations have now become the standard method implemented at MD Anderson or commercially.[39,40] The worst-case optimizations were first formulated as[20]:

$$\begin{aligned}\text{Min } F_{\text{Robust}} = & \sum_{i\in T} w_{T,\min}\left(D_{i,\min} - D_{p,T}\right)^2 \\ & + \sum_{i\in T} w_{T,\max}\left(D_{i,\max} - D_{p,T}\right)^2 \\ & + \sum_{i\in OAR} w_{OAR}\left(D_{i,\max} - D_{p,OAR}\right)_+^2 \end{aligned} \quad [5.1]$$

The terms $D_{i,\min} = \min_m\left(D_i^m\right)$ and $D_{i,\max} = \max_m\left(D_i^m\right)$ indicate the minimum and maximum dose among m possible doses D_i^m in voxel i, which are calculated using $D_i^m = \sum_j k_{i,j}^m w_j^2$ in each iteration. The mth influence matrix $k_{i,j}^m$, , incorporating either range or setup uncertainties, is precalculated before the optimization and stored in memory. Notably, the optimization target is the CTV rather than the PTV in Eq. (5.1). Also, each dose was forced to use either minimum or maximum doses among m possible doses. We refer to this kind of objective as a robust objective. In practical clinical scenarios, it may be necessary to compute selected objectives by using only the nominal dose distribution in robust optimization; such objectives may be referred to as nominal objectives. We call this the robust planning approach, in which robust objectives and nominal objectives are selectively applied on different planning structures to yield selective robust optimization. The selective robust optimization was implemented into the Eclipse TPS through collaboration. Worst case–based robust optimization was originally designed to apply objectives directly to the CTV, in contrast to conventional PTV-based optimization. Naturally, without considering PTV in the optimization process, PTV coverage cannot be guaranteed and will likely be undesirable according to conventional standards. Before the reliability of the plan robustness evaluation using the aforementioned worst-case dose can be thoroughly established and widely accepted through further studies, PTV evaluation may remain a necessary part of clinical practice.

The standard worst-case optimization considered only the setup and range uncertainties, for example, the nine-perturbation scenarios introduced before. However, for disease sites involving anatomical motion, 4D CT is now becoming the standard for treatment planning and simulation. When 4D CT is available, we also implemented a simple version of 4D robustness optimization.[18] We added two extra scenarios in Eq. (5.1): dose to the maximum inhale phase and exhale phase in the nominal dose distribution. We validated this approach for IMPT planning for esophageal cancer. We demonstrated that the 4D robustness-optimized IMPT plans notably reduced the overall dose deviation of multiple fractions and the dose deviation caused by the interplay effect in a single fraction.

INTENSITY-MODULATED PROTON THERAPY PLAN DESIGN

Similar to IMRT-type photon technology, the IMPT plan design process is essentially painting complex targets and a target-avoidance shape by using the directions and physical properties of each beam. The parameters of the IMPT beams include beam directions, number of beams, energy layers of each beam, spot spacing, and intensity of each spot. For nearly all commercial TPSs providing proton planning capabilities, the planner needs to specify manually or preconfigure the beam directions, number of beams, energy layer spacing, number of energies of each beam, and spot spacing of each energy layer. The TPS provides an inverse planning module so that the planner can define dose-volume or equivalent uniform dose (EUD)–type objectives. The DVH parameters, EUD parameters, and weights are user-adjustable parameters. The planner's main job is to adjust those parameters through trial and error to achieve the best target coverage while maximally sparing the normal tissues. The following is a breakdown of our research and understanding of parameter selection and the inverse planning process.

BEAM ANGLE

Because IMPT allows modulation of beams in the depth directions, it needs fewer beams to design complex plans for most sites. At the Proton Therapy Center-Houston, we use only two lateral opposed beams for prostate cancer and three beams for most other disease types. For prostate cancer, we[42,43] used beam angle optimization (BAO) and found that the three-beam plan outperformed the two-beam plan, but use of more than three provided no increased benefit. We also provided a three-beam class solution for prostate cancer.

Similar to prostate cancer cases, we have begun to generate a class solution for some other disease sites with relatively invariant tumor shapes among different patients. For example, for a bilateral HN case, we use the following three-beam class solution: a posterior-anterior (PA) beam and two lateral anterior beams with couch kick. Notably, the three-beam class solution is from our experience; at other institutions, a two-beam posterior-oblique beam is used for bilateral HN cancers.

Besides the two class solutions for prostate and bilateral HN cases, we also have a three-beam class solution for esophageal cancer at the gastroesophageal junction. The consideration in this three-beam class solution is that the three posterior beams provide adequate target coverage and minimal exposure of the normal tissue to the proton beam, and, more importantly, the effects of motion are the smallest.

Currently, to our knowledge, arc delivery technology has not yet been developed for proton therapy. However, some research is beginning to explore using arc delivery for proton therapy.

ENERGY SPACING

To "scan" the target volume, the proton beam is controlled by varying its energy to penetrate the patient's body to different depths. Although scanning proton beamlets or spots with the same energy can take as little as 10 to 20 m/s, changing from one proton energy to another requires approximately 2 additional seconds. The total IMPT delivery time thus depends mainly on the number of proton energies used in treatment. Current TPSs typically use all proton energies that are required for the proton beam to penetrate in a range from the distal edge to the proximal edge of the target. To address the optimal selection of proton energie, we developed an iterative mixed-integer programming optimization method to select a subset of all available proton energies while satisfying dosimetric criteria.[44] We applied our method to six patient data sets: four cases of prostate cancer, one case of lung cancer, and one case of mesothelioma. The numbers of energies were reduced by 14.3% to 18.9% for the prostate cancer cases, 11.0% for the lung cancer cases, and 26.5% for the mesothelioma case. These results indicate that the number of proton energies used in conventionally designed IMPT plans can be reduced without degrading dosimetric performance. The IMPT efficiency of delivery could be improved by energy layer optimization, leading to increased throughput for a busy proton center in which a delivery system with a slow energy switch is used.

SPOT SPACING

In the current TPS (Eclipse, Varian Medical Systems, Palo Alto, CA) at MD Anderson, the arrangement of spatial positions of spots is predetermined to cover the target volume. In all energy layers, a set of discrete spots is located with a defined spot spacing between one spot and the next.

The default setting of Eclipse assigns the value of spot spacing for each field as a fraction of the spot size for the highest energy used for the field. The spot spacing can range from approximately 6 mm (spot size is approximately 13 mm) for the 221.8-MeV energy to approximately 16 mm (spot size is approximately 35 mm) for the 72.5-MeV energy. Based on the arranged spots, an optimization process is performed to optimize the intensity of each spot from each treatment field.

Studies have shown that smaller spot spacing can increase target dose homogeneity and reduce dose to organs at risk (OARs), but results in many low-intensity spots and reduces plan optimality. There are minimum monitor unit (MU) constraints for delivering each pencil beam (spot) for the scanning spot system. An MU is defined by a fixed number of output pulses from the main dose monitor ion chamber in the scanning nozzle. Hence, an MU value is used to represent spot intensity. The minimum MU (0.005 at MD Anderson) must be set to ensure accurate delivery. However, deliverable minimum MU constraints are not considered in the current TPS. Instead, postprocessing is used to satisfy those constraints. MU values over 0.0025 are rounded up to 0.005, and ones below 0.0025 are rounded down to 0. Rounding errors in postprocessing can result in significant distortion from optimized dose distributions to the delivered ones.[49] The distortion becomes worse if there are more spots with small MU values that can be caused by small spot spacing. Therefore, a threshold value for spot spacing needs to be set to resolve the tradeoff between dosimetric advantage and delivery constraints when designing a treatment plan. Using spot spacings less than the threshold value is hence avoided in designing IMPT plans because of the dose distribution deterioration from the rounding errors.

We developed a two-stage optimization approach to optimize spot intensities and incorporate minimum deliverable MU constraints simultaneously in IMPT treatment planning. [45] Compared with current commercial TPSs, this approach allows treatment planners to use small spot spacing to improve dosimetric performance of IMPT plans without diminishing delivery robustness. Our results demonstrated that more dosimetric benefit in both target dose uniformity and normal sparing could be achieved when the smaller spot spacings were used for IMPT plans for four prostate cancer cases. The proposed approach avoids the troublesome postprocessing routine required by the current IMPT TPS. More importantly, the trial-and-error step for selecting an appropriate spot spacing can be eliminated. In addition, the deliverable spot intensity optimization can automatically create a nonuniform spot arrangement by using only a small fraction of candidate scanning spots. Therefore, deliverable scanning spots are selected within the optimization process without adding a postprocessing step.

Planning Parameters for Inverse Planning

The inverse planning process for IMPT is similar to that for IMRT. The planner needs to interactively adjust the planning parameters and go through many rounds of trial and error to design a plan that can be approved by the physician. Thus, the goal of the planner is to design an approved plan but not necessarily the most optimal plan. This is not the desired goal, but the optimal plan is not known; the trial-and-error process of the treatment plan design, means that the quality of the treatment is often determined by the experience of the treatment planner. Actually, it could happen that an IMRT/VMAT plan designed by a very experienced planner could be better than an IMPT plan designed by an in experienced planner. Recently, the knowledge-based or automatic planning for IMRT/VMAT has seen rapid progress.[46–48] The automatic planning tries to eliminate or reduce the differences among different planners and also improve the planning efficiency by eliminating or reducing the trial-and-error process. We developed an MD Anderson AutoPlan system that can essentially achieve IMRT/VMAT plans without manual intervention that are better (or at least or no worse) than those created by very experienced planners. This automatic planning technique is ready to be implemented into the Eclipse TPS once the Eclipse research application programming interface (API) is fully available. But before the automatic planning technology can be made available to planners through a research API, we will implement an intermediate automatic planning process that can ensure that our IMPT plans are better (or no worse) than VMAT/IMRT plans. To design a new IMPT plan, a VMAT plan is first generated either by an experienced planner or by an in-house-developed automatic planning system. An in-house-developed tool is used to generate the dose-volume constraints for the IMPT plan as a plan template for the Eclipse TPS. The beam angles for the IMPT plan are selected based on the preferred angles in the VMAT plan. The IMPT plan is designed by importing the plan objectives generated from the VMAT plan. As an example, we selected a thoracic IMPT plan under the Radiation Therapy Oncology Group (RTOG) 1308 protocol to demonstrate the effectiveness and efficiency of this approach. The PTV D95, lung V20, mean lung dose, mean heart dose, esophagus D1, and cord D1 are 70 Gy, 31%, 17.8 Gy, 25.5 Gy, 73 Gy, and 45 Gy, respectively, for the IMPT plan and 65.3 Gy, 34%, 21.6 Gy, 35 Gy, 74 Gy, and 48 Gy, respectively, for the VMAT plan. For most cases, the high-dose region of the normal tissue that is near the PTV is comparable between IMPT and VMAT plans. The low-dose region of the IMPT plan is significantly better than the VMAT plan. Using the knowledge gained in VMAT plan design can help efficiently and effectively design a high-quality IMPT plan. The quality of the IMPT plan can be controlled to ensure the superiority of IMPT plan compared with the VMAT/IMRT plan.

Site-Specific Treatment Planning Design

TREATMENT PLANNING FOR PROSTATE CANCER

At MD Anderson, IMPT plans for prostate cancers currently use two parallel-opposed right and left lateral fields for a prescribed dose of 78 cobalt Gray equivalent (CGE) in 39 fractions and are designed using the SFO method.[49] The CTV includes the entire prostate gland and the proximal seminal vesicles (typically the first centimeter). An optimization volume for scanning proton beam treatment planning, called the *scanning target volume (STV)*, was defined for each prostate cancer patient by using the distal margin for the lateral anatomic expansion, 0.6 cm for the posterior expansion, and 0.8 cm for the expansion from the CTV to everywhere else. The STV is essentially a bsPTV with 3.5% range uncertainties in the beam direction. Expansions in lateral directions are based on our experience with setup uncertainties, which are similar to the margins used for x-ray–based IMRT and passive scattering proton therapy for

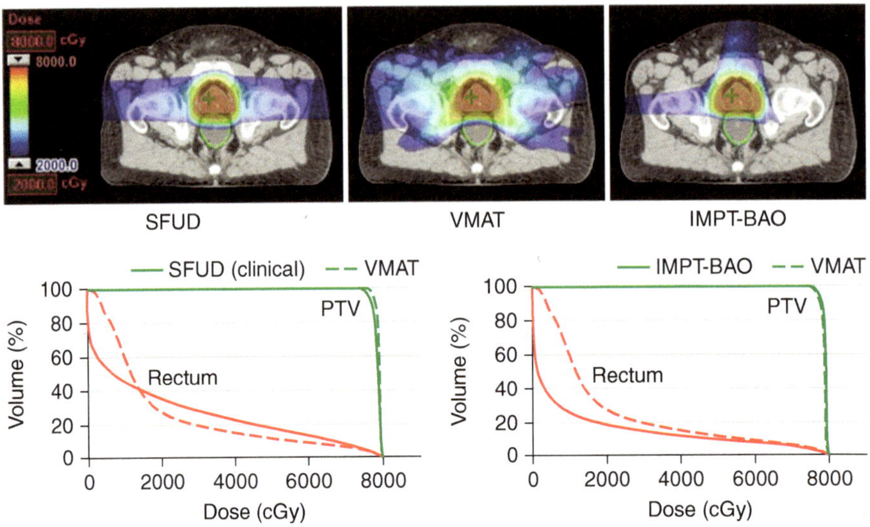

Fig. 5.11 Comparison of single-field uniform dose distribution *(SFUD)*, volumetric modulated arc therapy *(VMAT)*, and intensity-modulated proton therapy *(IMPT)* treatment plans for one prostate cancer patient. Here, SFUD represents a two-beam IMPT single-field uniform dose distribution plan. This plan is used to treat patients at MD Anderson. *VMAT* represents a photon volumetric modulated arch therapy plan. *IMPT-BAO* represents a class three-angle IMPT plan, where *BAO* represents beam angle optimization. (From Cao W, Lim GJ, Li Y, et al. Improved beam angle arrangement in intensity modulated proton therapy treatment planning for localized prostate cancer. *Cancers.* 2015;7(2):574-584.)

prostate cancer. The field lateral margin in the beam's-eye view was set to be equal to the spot spacing; that is, we allowed one spot to be outside the STV. The prescription-isodose line was fixed for each patient at 97% or 97.5%.

Fig. 5.11[43] compares a two-beam SFO IMPT plan with a VMAT plan. The target coverage is similar. The rectum sparing is better in the low-dose region but worse in the higher-dose region for the two-beam SFO plan. Fig. 5.11 also compares a three-beam IMPT plan with a VMAT plan. The IMPT plan is superior to VMAT plan in terms of rectum sparing at all dose levels with similar target coverage. The three-beam IMPT plan was designed by using robust optimization, and the rectum sparing does not change, even though there might be a 3.5% range overshoot.

TREATMENT PLANNING FOR PROSTATE CANCER INVOLVING PELVIC LYMPH NODES

For patients with prostate cancer and with pelvic lymph node involvement, treatment involves a primary treatment that covers the pelvic lymph nodes with proper margins followed by one or more boost treatments. The primary treatment involves a three-field beam arrangement including a PA field and two lateral parallel-opposed fields. Fig. 5.12 shows the GTV, CTV, and PTV for a prostate case involving pelvic lymph nodes in transverse, coronal, and sagittal views and three-beam arrangements. Fig. 5.12D also illustrates the anatomy and beam arrangements in 3D view. Unlike the SFO technique, all fields are optimized together to achieve optimal sparing of OARs. Fig. 5.12 shows the contribution of each field for a three-beam prostate plan and composite dose from the three beams. Critical organs such as the rectum, bladder, and sigmoid colon are located between bilateral pelvic lymph nodes and can be protected by splitting the

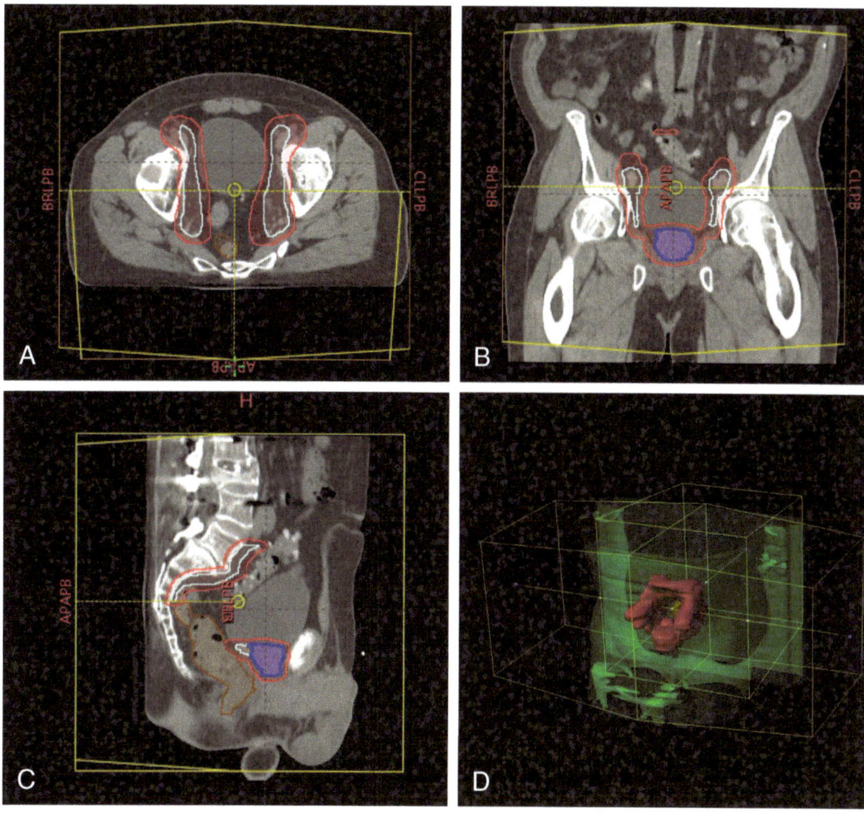

Fig. 5.12 The gross target volume (GTV), clinical target volume (CTV), and planning target volume (PTV) for a prostate case involving pelvic lymph nodes in transverse (A), frontal (B), and sagittal (C) views and three-beam arrangements. (D) The anatomy and beam arrangements in three-dimensional view. *Blue,* GTV; *cyan,* CTV; *red*, PTV; *brown*, rectum.

target into right and left lateral subtargets. Each lateral field covers only the subtarget on the same side, without passing across the midbody line. The PA field is designed to cover the entire target. This way, any part of the target is covered by at least two fields. For the plan shown in Fig. 5.12, the PA beam contains 57 energy layers with 8100 spots, the right lateral beam contains 63 energy layers with 4964 spots, and the left lateral beam contains 64 energy layers with 5473 spots. Notably, the Hitachi machine at MD Anderson cannot deliver more than 64 energy layers for one beam. The treatment plan was designed to satisfy that constraint by deleting some energy layers in the planning process. Because of the use of the PA field, the patient support device needs to be digitally replaced with the one that is consistent with the daily treatment setup in the TPS.

We use robust optimization that incorporates setup and range perturbations in the planning process. For the plan shown in Figs. 5.11 and 5.12, we used 0.5-mm setup uncertainties and 3.5% range uncertainty for the robust optimization. We applied only the robust objectives for the CTV and rectum by using the selective robust optimization strategy.[40] In Fig. 5.13, we show the final dose distributions and the DVH for the above plan. The DVH plot includes the DVH with eight possible uncertainty scenarios, and it was used as our robust analysis method (Fig. 5.14). We can see

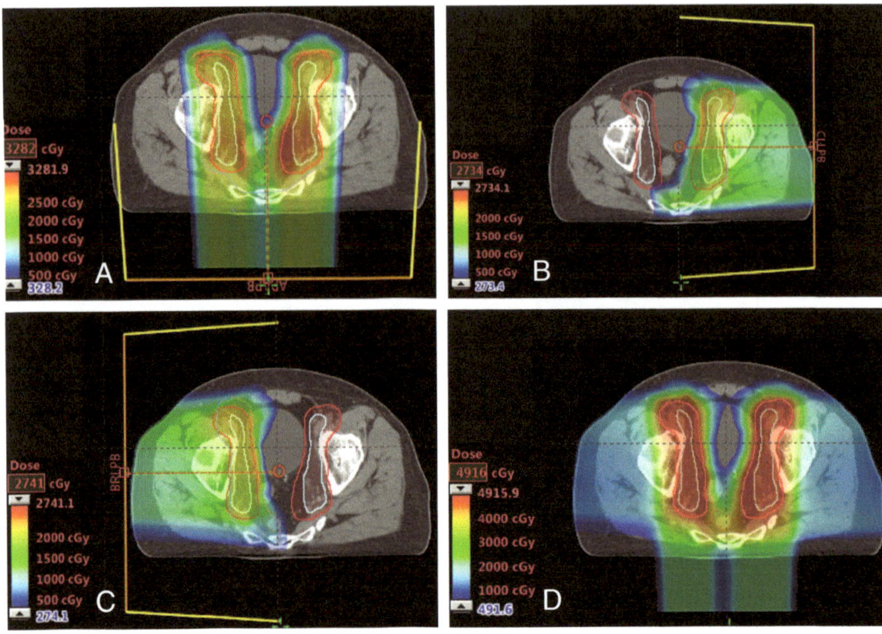

Fig. 5.13 The contribution of each field for a three-beam prostate plan. Field dose contributed from posterior-anterior beam (A), left lateral beam (B), and right-lateral beam (C) and composites dose from the three beams (D).

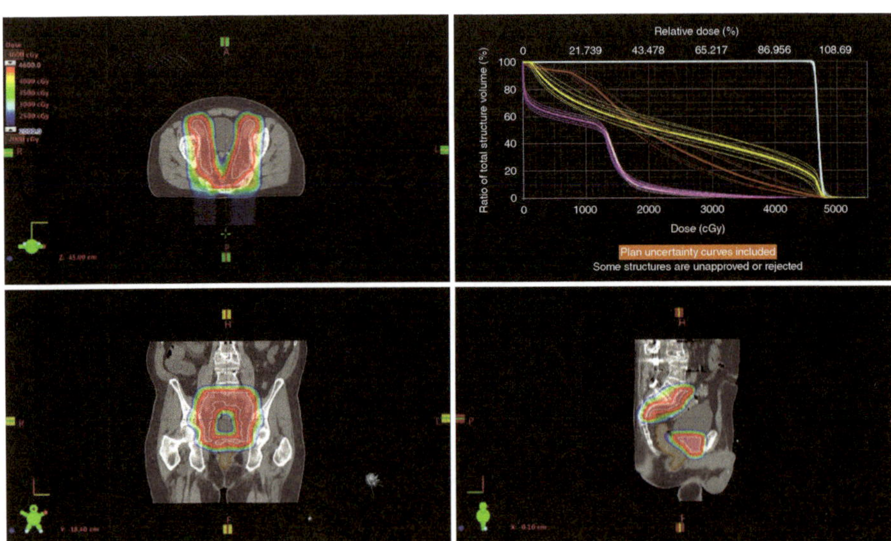

Fig. 5.14 The dose distributions and dose-volume histogram (DVH) for a prostate case with pelvic lymph nodes involvement. The DVH also includes the DVH with eight possible uncertainty scenarios, which was used as our robust analysis method.

that the CTV was quite stable under 4 mm and 3.5% range uncertainty perturbation, but the rectum and bladder had relatively larger variations. However, those variations were considered clinically acceptable because they resulted from geometrical misalignment, which can be explained by the PRV of the bladder.

TREATMENT PLANNING FOR LUNG CANCER

In addition to range and setup uncertainties, the major challenge for designing lung IMPT plans is the management of respiratory motion. A consensus guideline for implementing pencil beam scanning beam proton therapy for thoracic malignancies on behalf of the Particle Therapy Co-Operative Group (PTCOG) was proposed with a major contribution from MD Anderson.[50] The MD Anderson effort on the clinical implementation of lung treatment planning and motion management is described elsewhere.[4,11,23,50–54] For lung cancer, all patients should undergo 4D CT-based treatment simulation to determine the magnitude of tumor motion. For patients who can be treated while "free breathing," an internal GTV (IGTV) should be generated by using either a union of GTVs on all respiratory phases or an outline of the GTV on the maximum-intensity projection CT scan and verified through different breathing phases. For patients to be treated with breathhold (BH), multiple BH CT scans should be acquired, and the IGTV should be generated by using a union of all GTVs defined on each different BH scan. For patients to be treated with respiratory gating, the IGTV should be defined based on the gating window. The internal CTV (ICTV) is defined as a 5- to 10-mm isotropic expansion of the IGTV that is edited clinically based on the pattern of tumor spread and anatomic boundaries (vertebral body, chest wall, esophagus, heart, and great vessels, among others). The PTV, defined as an expansion of the ICTV, typically by 5 mm, should be used for reporting and evaluation purposes. Fig. 5.15 from Chang et al.[50] shows a typical workflow implemented at MD Anderson for lung cancer planning. That article also provides a good summary of treatment planning for lung cancer, as paraphrased here:

1. Perform basic measurements with a moving phantom to establish a threshold of the motion amplitude where the interplay effect is small.
2. Evaluate tumor motion using 4D CT-based evaluation and/or management to allow better selection of beam angles.
3. Perform motion analysis. Compare single-fraction four-dimensional dynamic accumulated dose (1FX4DDD) and single-fraction four-dimensional accumulated dose (1FX4DD) to determine whether motion mitigation is necessary or sufficient.
4. Use dose distributions calculated on T0 and T50 scans to quantify the extremes of systematic dose degradation caused by respiratory motion.
5. Use rescanning (either layered or volumetric) to reduce interplay effects, bearing in mind that the use of SFO plans with multiple fields is effectively equivalent to volumetric rescanning, and fractionated treatment delivery also provides effective rescanning. Use BH or gating as needed based on motion evaluation or a combination of any of these techniques with rescanning.
6. Use an optimized delivery sequence, including scanning direction, to minimize interplay effects.
7. Use 3D robust optimization to minimize the impact of organ motion. Use 4D robust optimization to further improve the robustness to intrafractional motion for large organ motion or in short fractionation schemes.
8. Use verification 4D CT often, such as on a weekly basis, to determine whether adaptive replanning is needed to maintain plan robustness.

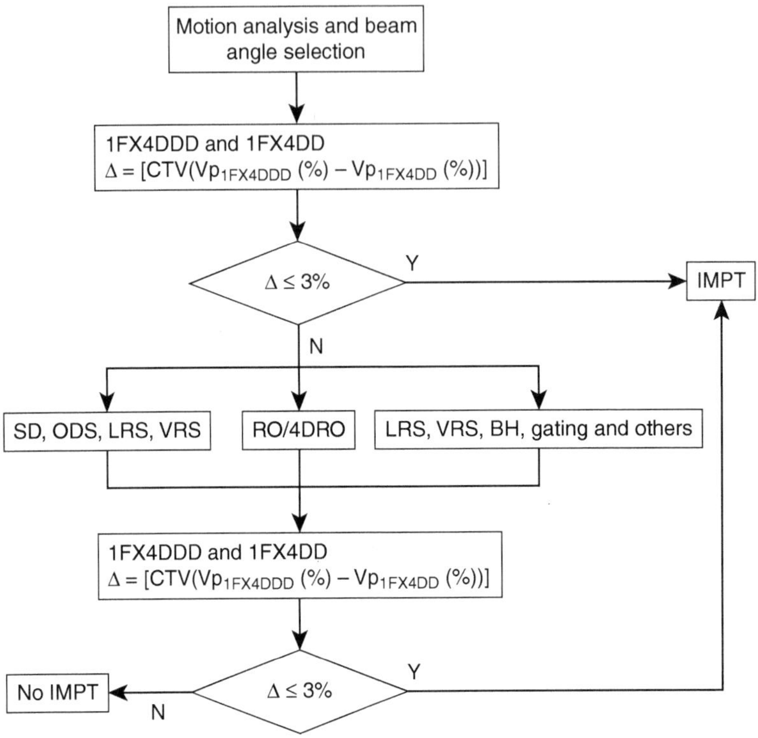

Fig. 5.15 Example of a clinical workflow based on using the difference between single-fraction four-dimensional dynamic accumulated dose *(1FX4DDD)* and single-fraction four-dimensional accumulated dose *(1FX4DD)* to evaluate the target volume to be covered by the prescribed dose, with various motion mitigation strategies to be used if needed. *BH,* Breathhold; *CTV,* clinical target volume; *IMPT,* intensity-modulated proton therapy; *LRS,* layered rescanning; *N,* no; *ODS,* optimized delivery sequence; *RO,* robust optimization; *SD,* scanning direction; *Vp,* volume of CTV that receives at least prescribed dose; *VRS,* volumetric rescanning; *Y,* yes; *4DRO,* four-dimensional robust optimization. (From Chang JY, Zhang X, Knopf A, et al. Consensus guidelines for implementing pencil-beam scanning proton therapy for thoracic malignancies on behalf of the PTCOG thoracic and lymphoma subcommittee. *Int J Radiat Oncol Biol Phys.* 2017;99(1):41-50.)

TREATMENT PLANNING FOR HEAD AND NECK CANCER

Proton therapy for cancers of the HN is considered one of the most complex types of treatment delivery. HN cancer scenarios can be considered in two categories of treatment delivery: Scanning beam delivery is indicated when multiple dose tiers are required and bilateral nodal beds that extend into the low neck are to be treated; passive scatter delivery can be indicated for one dose level is used and the nodal bed is limited to one side, generally not extending into the low neck. Examples of scanning beam scenarios may include cancers of the nasopharynx, tonsil, base of the tongue, gingivobuccal sulcus, and submandibular glands. The scanning beam delivery technique is discussed here. Treatment planning starts with the acquisition of planning CT images. The physician then draws the target volumes, which include a built-in setup margin. Normal tissue structures are also drawn based on the site of treatment. An HN prescription and dose-limiting document is then produced by the radiation oncologist and is loaded into the documents section within the MOSAIQ environment for planning reference. Special structures that serve the purpose of helping to conform the prescription isodose line are then drawn by the dosimetrist. Treatment field geometry is determined, and optimization parameters are entered into the TPS. The type of optimization (SFO or MFO) is determined. Typically, patients are treated with definitive chemoradiation with IMPT to the primary disease site (the GTV) to a dose of 70 GyE (relative biological equivalence [RBE]), typically in 33 fractions overall at 2.12 Gy (RBE)/fraction. The CTVs (CTV1, CTV2, and CTV3) were designed accordingly based on the clinical evaluation of the anatomic areas at risk of gross and/or microscopic involvement, including nodal regions. In our practice, the Eclipse TPS (Varian Medical System, Palo Alto, CA) is used. All plans are calculated using the TPS to deliver proton therapy with discrete spot beam scanning.[55] The delivery of the actual IMPT plan is done by the use of a synchrotron and the Hitachi PROBEAT PBT system (Hitachi, Ltd., Tokyo, Japan). A standard three-field beam arrangement is used, with right anterior oblique, left anterior oblique, and PA direction beams that were noncoplanar, with robustness consideration (Fig. 5.16).[15,56] The Eclipse proton-based IMPT inverse planning techniques are used, with overall target margins of 0 cm distally and proximally and 1 cm laterally. The spot spacing is determined by the TPS according to maximum energy for each individual field ($s = \alpha$ times FWHM [full width at half maximum], $\alpha \leq 0.65$).[49] The planning goals for all CTVs are V100% greater than 95% (i.e., at least 95% of prescription doses cover 100% of the corresponding CTV volumes), V95% greater than 99%, V105% less than 10%, and maximum dose (Dmax) less than 120%. The spot scanning system has a total number of 94 energies ranging from 72.5 to 221.8 MeV. The depth of penetration (range) of the proton beam is proportional to the energy. The range for the minimum energy of 72.5 MeV is 4 cm. This presents a problem when the target volume is located at a depth of less than 4 cm. To accomplish dose coverage for these shallow depths, a block of plastic (67 mm thick) is inserted into the beam path. The thickness of the plastic reduces the range that the

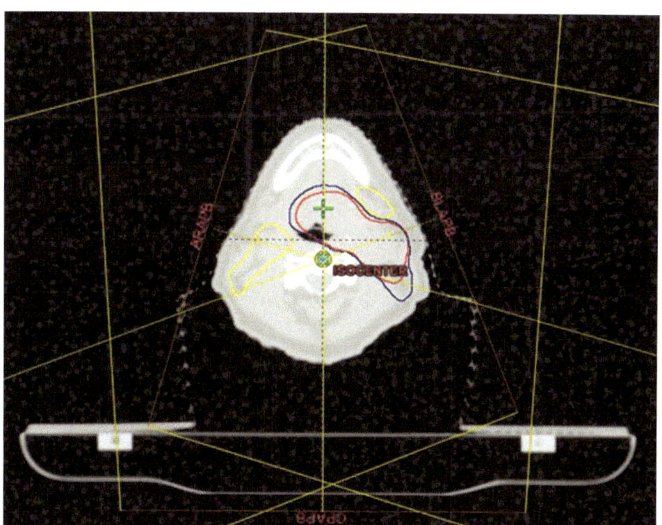

Fig. 5.16 A noncoplanar beam arrangement in a typical dosimetric planning case for a patient with oropharyngeal cancer, using intensity-modulated proton therapy techniques. (Data from Quan EM, Liu W, Wu R, et al. Preliminary evaluation of multifield and single-field optimization for the treatment planning of spot-scanning proton therapy of head and neck cancer. *Med Phys.* 2013;40(8):081709, and Liu W, Frank SJ, Li X, et al. Effectiveness of robust optimization in intensity-modulated proton therapy planning for head and neck cancers. *Med Phys.* 2013;40(5):051711.)

proton travels into the patient. This allows the dose to be deposited at superficial depths or in the shallow area of the HN regions near the skin.

Verification and Adaptive Planning Strategies

Our retrospective study[57] showed that verification and adaptive planning are required during the course of proton therapy for patients to ensure that adequate dose is delivered to the planned CTVs while maintaining safe doses to OARs. In this section, we discuss our current verification and adaptive planning strategy, illustrating potential dose differences to CTVs and OAR volumes between the original and adaptive plans, as well as between the adaptive and verification plans, to simulate doses that would have been delivered if the adaptive plans had not been used.

Typically, patients received radiation to the bilateral neck volumes and had verification CT scans before treatment and also at 4 weeks (±1 business day) after radiation therapy began. A previous internal study indicated that weight loss led to deviation in body contours starting at about 4 weeks after radiation therapy had begun.[58] In our practice, almost 100% of patients had verification plans, and more than 90% of patients had adaptive plans. Some adaptive plans were done earlier than 4 weeks, which in most cases was attributed to poor initial setup. Some patients (<10%) may not require adaptive planning (as determined by the radiation oncologist). The criterion to implement an adaptive plan for patient treatment was to maintain the CTV1 D95% greater than or equal to 100% (i.e., dose to 95% of CTV1 volume ≥100% prescription dose), and also respecting OAR dosages according to RTOG guidelines.

Body contours changed significantly, usually at about 3 to 4 weeks into the treatment course (Fig. 5.17). CTV and OAR locations inside the patient's contours also changed, which ultimately could affect the actual dose distribution (Fig. 5.18); indeed, the CTV coverage was shown to change between the original and verification CT scans.

Verification CT scans were acquired before the first treatment and then weekly depending on the disease characteristics and physician's preference and definitely during the fourth week.

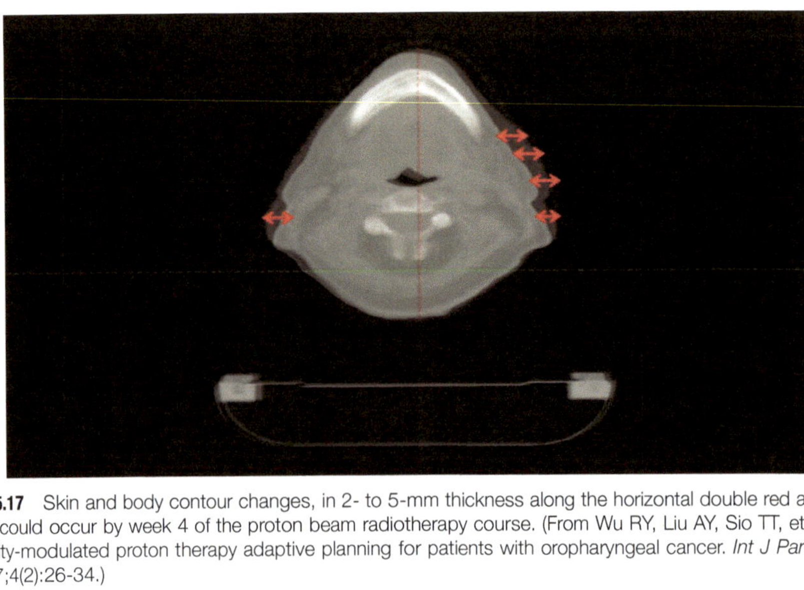

Fig. 5.17 Skin and body contour changes, in 2- to 5-mm thickness along the horizontal double red arrows, that could occur by week 4 of the proton beam radiotherapy course. (From Wu RY, Liu AY, Sio TT, et al. Intensity-modulated proton therapy adaptive planning for patients with oropharyngeal cancer. *Int J Part Ther.* 2017;4(2):26-34.)

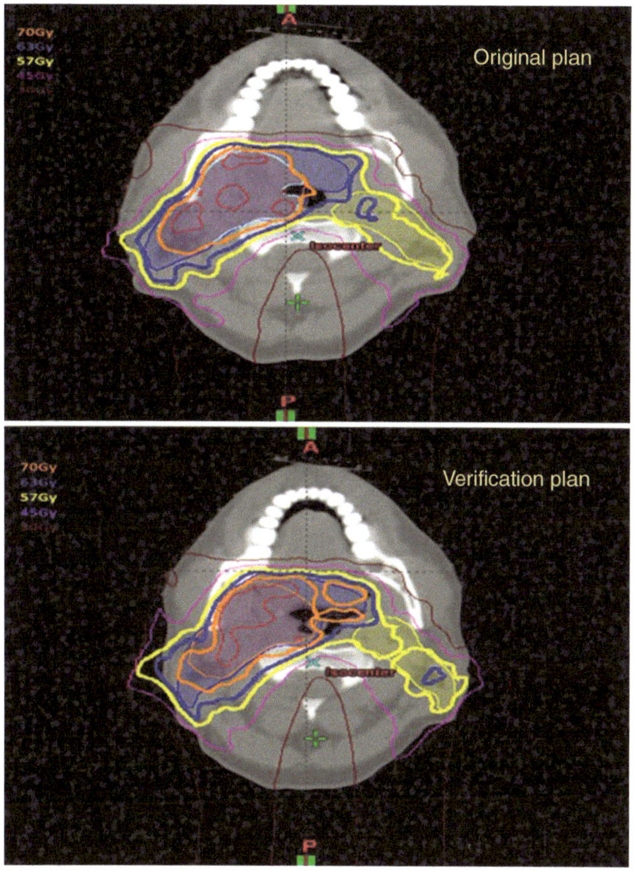

Fig. 5.18 Example of a patient's plan with carcinoma at the tongue base. The top image represents the original plan, and the bottom image is the verification plan. The dose distribution changes can be seen because of slight changes in the tongue position and also weight loss that the patient experienced during the course of treatment; adaptive planning was certainly indicated in this case. (From Wu RY, Liu AY, Sio TT, et al. Intensity-modulated proton therapy adaptive planning for patients with oropharyngeal cancer. *Int J Part Ther.* 2017;4(2):26-34.)

To compare, the verification CT images were registered with the original planning CT images by using the Eclipse rigid registration tool simulating the daily patient treatment alignment process.

Deformable image registration (DIR) was done between the two CT image sets by using commercial deformable registration software (Velocity Medical, Varian Medical Systems, Palo Alto, CA). The accuracy of the DIR algorithms was previously evaluated by Kirby et al.[59,60] Our systems were also validated according to Mohamed et al.[61] The treatment targets had three CTVs (CTV1, CTV2, and CTV3) corresponding to intended dose levels of 70, 63, and 57 Gy(RBE), respectively. Major OARs were parotids, oral cavity, spinal cord, and brain stem. Both CTVs and OARs were deformed and transferred from the original CT images to the verification CT image data set. All deformed contours were reviewed by a staff radiation oncologist before the adaptive plan was generated. The beam configuration and intensity distribution profile from the original treatment plan were then copied to the verification CT image set to create a verification plan for the calculation of the updated radiation dose levels reflecting the most recent anatomic changes.

Based on the dosimetric results, the radiation oncologist would then evaluate, compare, and determine whether the adaptive treatment plans should be created. These plans were highly individualized and depended on several other clinical characteristics. We then compared the accumulated dose to CTVs and OARs between the original and adaptive plans, and also looked at the difference between the adaptive verification plans to simulate the doses that would have been delivered if the adaptive plans had not been used.

For adaptive plans, there should not be any significant dosimetric differences between the original and adaptive plans (Fig. 5.19). This was expected because the replanning process should

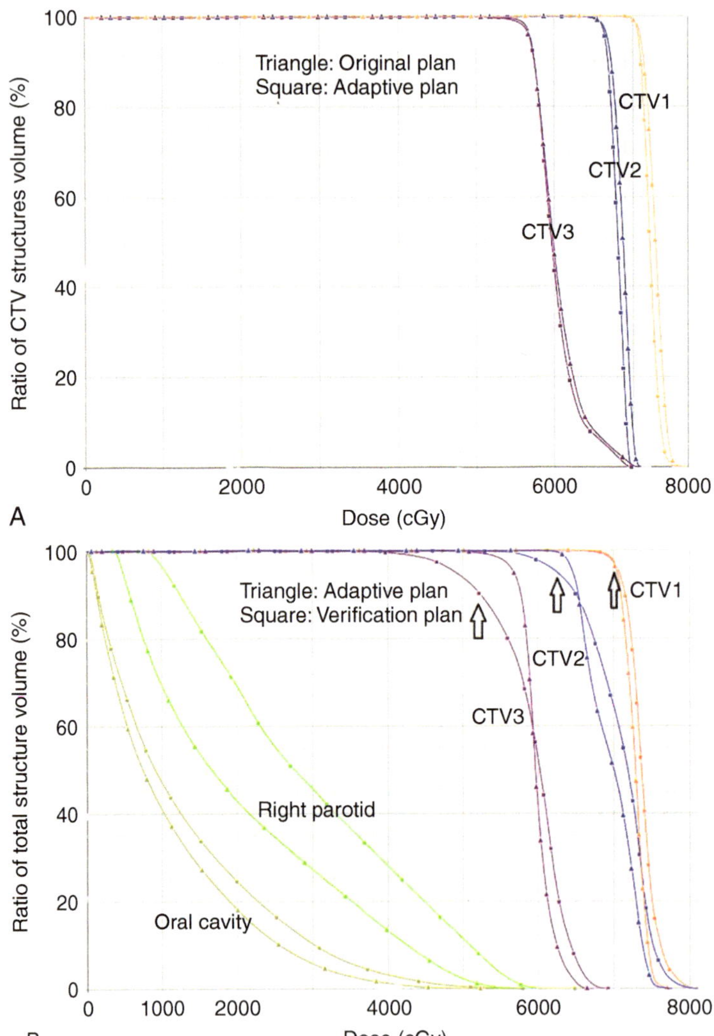

Fig. 5.19 (A) The generated dose-volume histograms (DVHs) were used for clinical target volume *(CTV)* comparisons (all shown in 33 fractions), which were derived from the original *(square lines)* and adaptive *(triangles)* plans. (B) These DVHs were generated for CTV and organs-at-risk comparisons based on the verification *(square lines)* and adaptive *(triangle lines)* plans. In this case, there were no significant differences for CTV coverage. However, a significant difference between the verification and adaptive plans was seen.

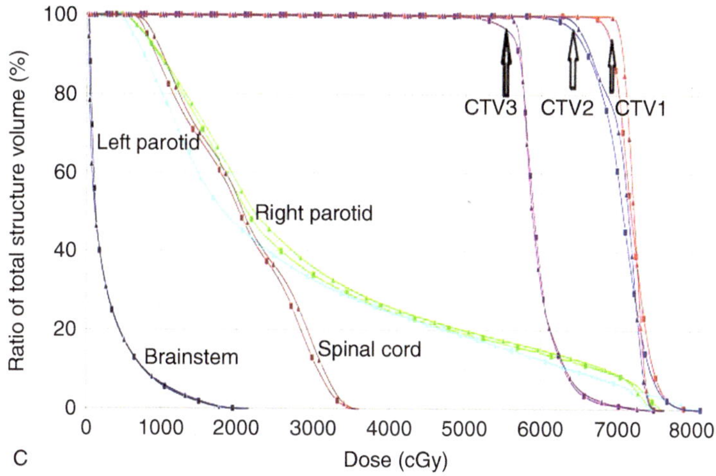

Fig. 5.19, cont'd **(C)** In this DVH, D95 was noted to be less than the prescription dose for CTV1. As a result, an adaptive plan was required even though other organs at risk had no significant changes. *CTV,* Clinical target volume; *DVH,* dose-volume histogram; *D95,* dose that was received by 95% of the target volume. (From Wu RY, Liu AY, Sio TT, et al. Intensity-modulated proton therapy adaptive planning for patients with oropharyngeal cancer. *Int J Part Ther.* 2017;4(2):26-34.)

mimic and reproduce the same planning goals that were originally set with the specified dose constraints as closely as possible based on the verification CT. However, significant dosimetric differences were found between the adaptive and verification plans, as illustrated in Fig. 5.19. On the verification DVH plan, 95% of the CTV1 volume was covered by the prescription dose (70 GyE); however, the dose homogeneity and conformity were degraded. The decrease in both dose homogeneity and conformity became more significant for CTV2 and CTV 3; also, doses to the right parotid and oral cavity increased.

Our retrospective study demonstrated the importance of using verification CT imaging and the need for developing a systematic workflow for adaptive planning during the course of IMPT for patients with HN cancer undergoing radiotherapeutic treatments. Wang et al.[62] found that anatomical structure changes could occur during radiotherapy for HN cancer owing to shrinkage of the tumor or lymph nodes or body weight loss, and GTVs can be reduced by as much as 70%.[63] Therefore, it is important during proton therapy to evaluate the dosimetric effect over the complete duration of the treatment course. Our results were consistent with those stated in previous studies,[62,63] for which several authors concluded that CTV and parotid volumes consistently decreased after radiation treatment (in our case, after 3 weeks). The dosimetry outcomes reported here are consistent with those findings.[64,65] DIR can reduce the workload of physicians in recontouring all structures in the new CT image data set, which can be time-consuming during a busy clinical practice in both academic and community settings; however, DI certainly represents an important step for ensuring the basis and accuracy of the adaptive treatment plan design and evaluation. The new contours review or modification process on the new CT data set cannot be completely eliminated and replaced with DIR[61]; this is a subject of ongoing research at MD Anderson.

References Available Online.

CHAPTER 6

Physics Quality Assurance

Falk Poenisch ■ Narayan Sahoo ■ Heng Li ■ Yoshifumi Hojo

Introduction

This chapter describes the physics quality assurance (QA) program for the proton pencil beam scanning (PBS) gantry of the Hitachi ProBeat machine (Hitachi America, Ltd., Tarrytown, NY) at the Proton Therapy Center University of Texas MD Anderson Cancer Center (UT MDACC PTC), which has been in clinical use since May 2008. This QA program has two components, namely machine QA and patient treatment field–specific QA. The machine QA program is designed to test the functionality of the various components of the delivery system so as to ensure that safe and accurate delivery of the dose to all the patients treated with the machine. The patient treatment field–specific QA is designed to assure that the delivered dose and planned dose distributions for the specific treatment plan for the patient and fields in that plan are in agreement within acceptable tolerance limits. These QA programs were designed by using the recommendations from the International Commission on Radiation Units and Measurements Report 78[1] and American Association of Physicists in Medicine TG-40 report[2] on the comprehensive QA program for radiation oncology and with the consideration of practicality and effectiveness of the QA checks to assure safe and accurate treatment delivery. The objective of the QA program for the PBS proton beam is to assure the accuracy or constancy of the following delivery system components:

1. dose monitor calibration
2. energy or range of the individual spots
3. spot depth dose distribution
4. spot lateral fluence and dose profiles
5. spot positioning
6. gantry and couch isocentricity
7. x-ray and radiation isocenter coincidence
8. couch translation
9. x-ray imaging system functionality
10. patient treatment field dose distribution

Items 1 through 9 constitute the machine QA program, and item 10 is the patient treatment field–specific QA program. Various tasks in the QA program for the scanning proton pencil beam gantry at UT MDACC PTC are summarized in Table 6.1 and are described in detail in the following sections. The QA programs at other centers are described briefly using the information available in the published literature.

Machine Quality Assurance

The machine-focused QA program at PTC has daily, weekly, monthly, and annual components. The original QA program at PTC was derived from our passive scattering proton beam QA program described in a paper by Arjomandy et al.[3] as well as from the original commissioning of

TABLE 6.1 ■ **Quality Assurance Tasks for the PTC Scanning Proton Pencil Beam Gantry**

Quality Assurance Check	Frequency	Tolerance (±)
X-ray, laser, and couch alignment	Daily, monthly, annually	1 mm
Proton pencil beam range constancy	Daily, annually	1 mm
Spot position accuracy	Daily, annually	1 mm
Spot size constancy	Daily, annually	1 mm or 10%
Volumetric dose constancy	Daily, monthly, annually	3% for daily, 2% for monthly and annual
Couch rotation isocentricity	Weekly, monthly, annually	1 mm
Couch translation	Monthly, annually	1 mm
Snout translation	Monthly, annually	1 mm
Gantry isocentricity	Monthly, annually	1 mm
Proton field and x-ray field coincidence	Monthly, annually	2 mm
Patient imaging and analysis system shift calculation accuracy	Monthly	1 mm
Radiation vs. mechanical isocenter coincidence check	Monthly, annually	1 mm
Output as a function of gantry	Monthly, annually	2%
Dose monitor calibration using IAEA TRS 398 protocol	Annually	2%
Daily and monthly QA dosimetry system baseline verification	Annually	2%
Dose and MU linearity and Dynamic MU delivery constancy	Annually	2%
Validation of inverse-square factor	Annually	2%
Integral depth dose constancy	Annually	2%
X-ray imaging system: kVp accuracy	Biennial (once in every 2 years)	10%
X-ray imaging system: HVL	Biennial	>2.3 mm @ 80 kV
X-ray imaging system: timer accuracy	Biennial	5%
X-ray imaging system exposure reproducibility	Biennial	Coefficient <0.005
X-ray imaging system: mA linearity	Biennial	<10%
X-ray imaging system: output constancy	Biennial	20%
X-ray imaging system: field light vs. x-ray alignment	Biennial	2% of Source to Image Distance
X-ray imaging system: image quality	Biennial	Consistency with baseline
X-ray imaging system: safety, dead man switch, 5 minute time, radiation warning sign, and door interlock	Biennial	Functional

Continued on following page

TABLE 6.1 ■ **Quality Assurance Tasks for the PTC Scanning Proton Pencil Beam Gantry** (Continued)

Quality Assurance Check	Frequency	Tolerance (±)
Delivery system safety interlocks: beam pause, in-room beam stops, facility beam stop, beam delivery indicator light, radiation monitors, door interlock, audiovisual monitoring, gantry rotation sensor, room clearance push button, room motion sensor	Annually	Functional
Patient treatment field–specific dose distribution: agreement between plan and measurement	Before start of treatment	Gamma pass rate for 3% dose and 3-mm distance agreement >90%
Patient treatment field–specific spot positions: agreement between planned and delivered spot positions and spot monitor units	Before start of treatment and after each field delivery	1 mm for mean deviation in spot position and 1% for mean deviation in spot MU

HVL, Half-value layer; *kVp*, kilovoltage peak; *MU*, monitor units, *PTC*, University of Texas MD Anderson Cancer Center Proton Therapy Center in Houston.

the spot scanning beamline described in a paper by Gillin et al.[4] However, over the years, we have adapted this program, especially the daily QA and monthly QA, based on our initial experience. Therefore, more emphasis is put on those two subjects.

The daily QA is performed once a day before treatment and takes about half an hour. The monthly QA is done within one calendar month. The annual QA is performed within 365 days and is the most comprehensive among the three.

DAILY QUALITY ASSURANCE

The goal of the daily QA is to verify: (1) the dosimetric characteristics of the proton pencil beam; (2) proper functioning of the dose monitor chambers; (3) proper functioning of the spot position monitor; (4) proper functioning of the imaging system used for patient setup; (5) seamless communication between the electronic medical record (EMR), Patient Positioning Image and Analysis System (PIAS), and treatment delivery system; and (6) proper functioning of all mechanical and safety aspects of the treatment machine before patient treatment. Our scanning beamline is capable of delivering 94 different energies. Because it is nearly impossible to check the dosimetry features of proton PBS for all these energies daily, a smart QA program had to be developed. The dosimetric checks have three parts: range check, spot position check, and volume-dose check. The dosimetric checks are performed using the Keithley Tracker detector (Fluke Biomedical, Cleveland, OH). It consists of an array of five single parallel-plate ion chambers (∅ = 2.5 cm × 0.8 cm), which are separated by 10 cm and are arranged as a cross. The tracker is snapped into a jig placed tightly on the Hitachi tabletop, as shown in Fig. 6.1.

All daily QA tasks are performed through our EMR and verify system MOSAIQ using a QA patient, thus providing the same data flow as treating a patient. When running the QA checks through MOSAIQ, the Hitachi Treatment Control System, Zenkei, is switched to treatment mode, providing the same conditions as real patient treatment.

X-Ray, Laser, and Couch Alignment Check

There are two objectives for this test: testing communication and data flow as well as checking the functionality of the x-ray imaging system. In this procedure, a stored plan in MOSAIQ is sent to

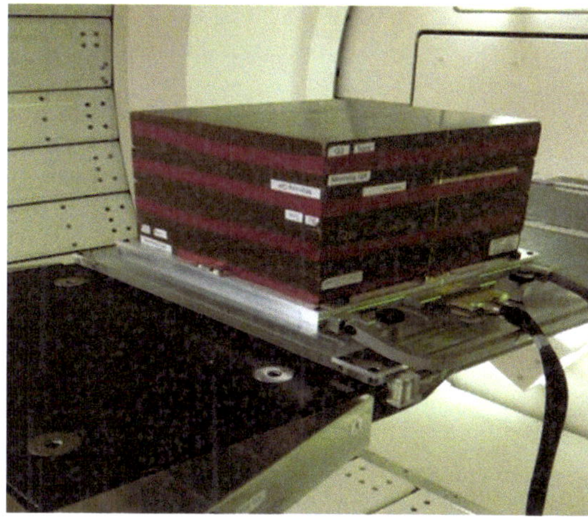

Fig. 6.1 Measurement setup with the tracker detector between buildup and the jig.

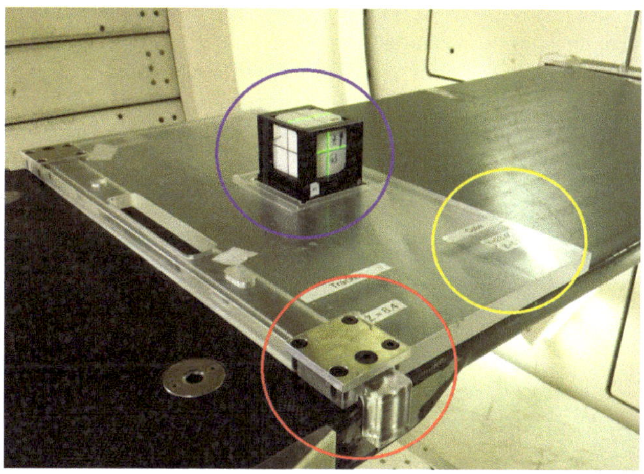

Fig. 6.2 Setup to determine the correct couch position as well as proper functioning of the x-ray. A custom-made jig is placed on the treatment table and indexed using the knobs on the table together with a ball bearing at the jig *(red circle)*. A Varian OBI cube (dimensions of the white plastic: 5 × 5 × 5 cm^3) is sunken into the acrylic board *(purple circle)* so that there is no play between the cube, the board, and the table. The Varian cube contains a 2-mm-diameter radiopaque metal sphere at the center of the white plastic. The metal sphere is positioned to the center of the mechanical isocenter using couch coordinates written on the jig *(yellow circle)*.

the Hitachi HMI (Hitachi machine interface) computer. This will initiate the MOSAIQ site setup task, which sends the two-dimensional (2D) orthogonal reference images from MOSAIQ to the Hitachi imaging system, which is called PIAS (Patient Positioning Image and Analysis System). In the case of actual patient treatment, the reference images are compared with a set of two setup verification x-ray images. In the case of the QA patient, the purpose of sending the reference image from MOSAIQ to PIAS is to ensure that two systems are communicating as expected. Fig. 6.2 shows the x-ray setup consisting of an acrylic jig and a Varian On-Board Imaging (OBI) cube that has a 2-mm metal sphere in its center. The imaging cube is tightly secured to the jig, which is also tightly snapped onto the treatment couch using a ball-and-bearing screw system. This setup ensures reproducible placement of submillimeter accuracy of the center of the x-ray imaging cube. The couch is then moved to its expected calibrated coordinates (*x*, *y*, and *z*) using the Hitachi couch control pendant. This brings the metal sphere into the gantry isocenter, and the room lasers should be aligned to the crosshair in the cube if no change has taken place in the couch calibration and laser alignment. If a misalignment outside the 1-mm tolerance is observed, the cause of the misalignment is investigated, and corrective actions have to be taken before the patient treatment can start. A major reason for misalignment has been found to be a collision between the treatment head and the couch that affects the couch positioning calibration.

During routine daily QA, the location of the center of the imaging cube is compared with the center of the x-ray system using two orthogonal x-rays. The daily tolerance level for this test is 1 mm, which is the radius of the sphere. The PIAS system has a pixel size of 0.3 mm, but it allows shifts in increments of 0.1 mm (therefore, some shifts do not move the image). If the tolerance is exceeded, but within 2 mm, the covering medical physicist will be notified, and further tests will be required at a later time. If those tests confirm the deviation, a Hitachi engineer will have to recalibrate the couch coordinates. As a side note: the absolute couch coordinates are actually more important for correct QA setup to get accurate dose readings (see subparagraphs later) because if the table origin has shifted, the setup of the ionization chamber will not be correct. For patient setup, however, this is will not be a problem because the patient's daily position is shifted according to the result of the x-ray and is not based on absolute couch coordinates. The daily shifts are recorded, and the two orthogonal images are sent from the PIAS system via couch pendant back to MOSAIQ. The correct data transfer of those images is part of the daily QA check. In addition, safety tests are performed every day. This includes the check of the audio system, video-TV system, the room search audio warning signal, the radiation monitor (inside/outside), the beam pause button, as well as the door interlock.

Proton Pencil Beam Range Check

The way the range check is performed has changed over time, but it can be divided into two periods: before 2016 and after 2016. The measurement devices and the idea behind the measurement remained the same: A different energy spot pattern has been used on each weekday. The corresponding proton pencil beam ranges vary from 28.8 to 5.1 cm. The amount of buildup (Solid Water, Gammex, RMI) is fixed for a particular weekday for the proton beam checked on that day.

Range Check Before 2016

The original range check was a convolution of positioning as well as dose output. Thus dose readings were obtained, but not actual ranges. This test consisted of that monoenergetic spots that are centered to the positions of the ion chamber. Their energies were selected in such a way that dose values at a depth close to the Bragg peak and at two more depths, one proximal to the Bragg peak and other distal to Bragg peak, were measured. The proximal dose and D_{max} were an average of two chamber readings, whereas the distal one was only from one ion chamber. The method was able to detect output changes, setup shifts, and range changes (see the green symbols in Fig. 6.3 from February 2014 to December 2015).

Range Check Since 2016

Similar to the procedure used before 2016, each weekday, a different set of energies and a different amount of buildup are used. However, the revised range check now uses five different energies daily compared with three energies before. In addition, the spots are not delivered on a single point over the ion chamber as was done before 2016, but instead on a 3×3 cm^2 square using optimized weights in such a way that the dose within this square is uniform. Thus this new pattern makes the dose reading not sensitive to any phantom setup variation. The five monoenergetic

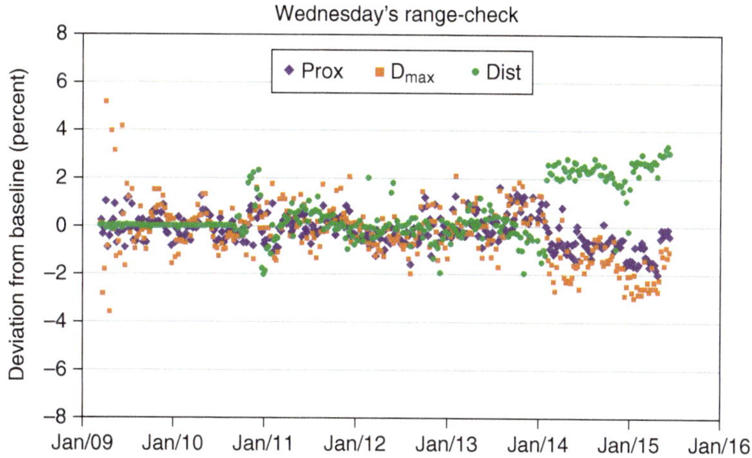

Fig. 6.3 Range check deviation compared with baseline data as an example of the Wednesday readings between 2009 and 2015.

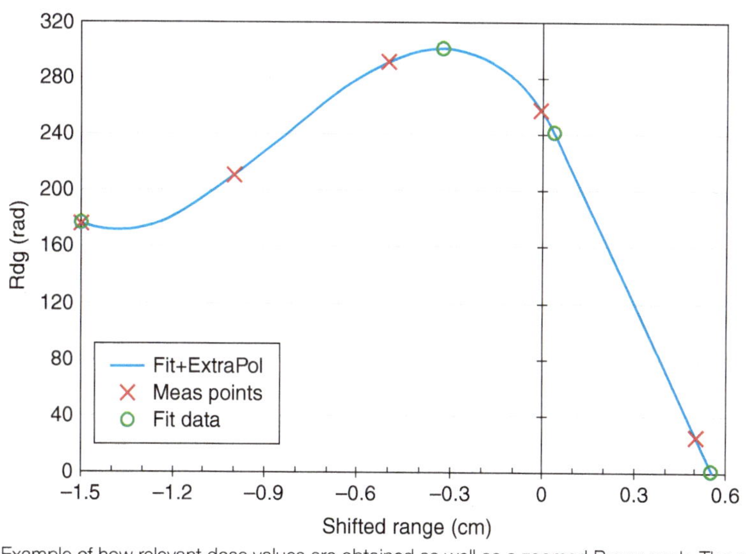

Fig. 6.4 Example of how relevant dose values are obtained as well as a zoomed Bragg peak. The measured doses are shown as red crosses. The *x*-axis is shifted so that the four-dose value is $x = 0$. The green circles are four derived points from inter- and extrapolation. The blue line connects those green point circles.

energies resulting in different dose readings since the buildup remain constant for each 3×3 cm^2 square delivery, and the measurement depth is always close to the Bragg peak. An example of this test is shown in Fig. 6.4. The first derived data point is used as a verification of the output check. The tolerance for this is 3%. Then, from the first four dose readings, a third-order polynomial fit is performed, connecting all four measured points with a line. This polynomial fit creates a maximum value that can be used to derive its position (second green circle) as well as the maximum dose value. From the dose maximum, the 80% dose value (third green circle)

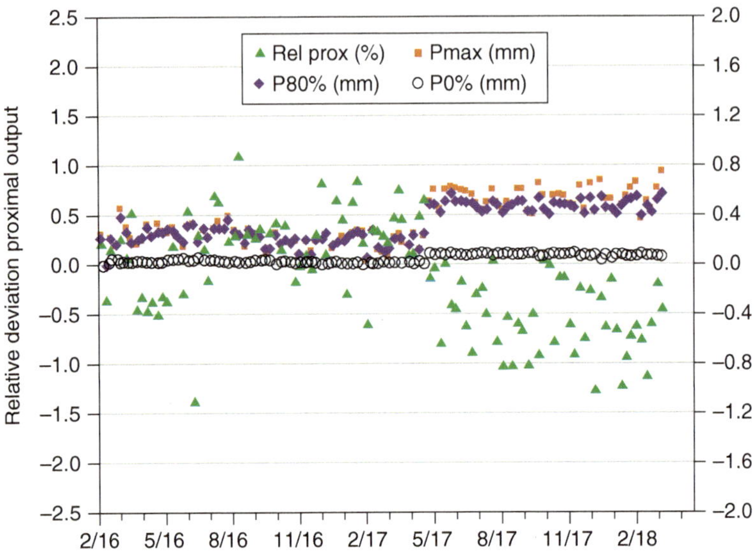

Fig. 6.5 New range check of output and range differences compared with baseline data as an example of the Wednesday readings between 2016 and 2018, where P80% is the position in which the dose drops to 80% and P0% is the position where dose is null.

and the 0% dose values (fourth green circle) are estimated by interpolation between the fourth and fifth measured dose values.

The new method allows measuring the ranges indirectly by deriving them from charge readings. The trend of those measurements is shown in Fig. 6.5. The output has been within 1% over more time shown. The changes in the positions Pmax, P80%, and P0% have remained constant over the last 2 years, being within 0.6 mm of the baseline values. However, in May 2017, a noticeable jump in the trend was observed. This was caused by the installation of a new primary dose monitor whose water-equivalent thickness differed from the one it replaced by 0.2 mm. Because the change was rather small, the baseline data were not changed.

Spot Position Accuracy Check

For this test, five monoenergetic spots are delivered at the central axis and at ±10 cm along the *x*-axis and along the *y*-axis. The highest available energy of 221.8 MeV is used because it provides the smallest spot size available for our scanning proton pencil beam. This spot size, however, is increased by 15% because of the use of a 20-cm solid water buildup, which is used to increase the dose reading by more than 50% to about 112 cGy. The spot position check has been performed since 2008 on every treatment day, and its baseline value was not changed until May 2017. The change was necessary because of the replacement of the primary dose monitor, which was built using thinner copper foils and thus resulted in a reduced spot size of about 10%. This change in spot shape increased the dose reading by 7% after replacement of the hardware. This system is capable of detecting both spot size changes as well as spot position change, as shown in Fig. 6.6 and Table 6.2. Although the overall deviations in Fig. 6.6 are fairly constant, there are, however, some jumps, for example, October 2010, February 2011, August 2012, August 2013, March 2015, and February 2016. Most of those deviations are attributed to misalignment of the absolute couch coordinates after a collision between nozzle and couch pedestal, resulting in a drop of dose value because the detector is not anymore located at the maximum dose value. This is corrected by recalibrating the couch by the Hitachi engineer.

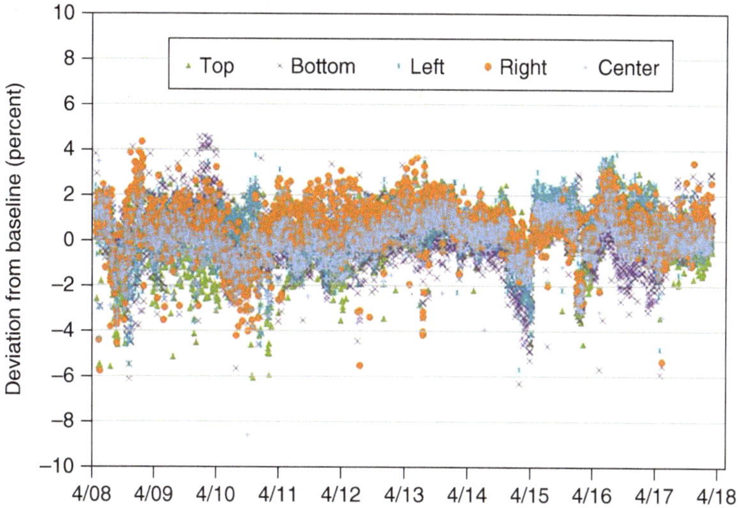

Fig. 6.6 Deviation from the baseline for daily spot position check over the last 10 years.

TABLE 6.2 ■ **Average Relative Deviations of Five Chambers and Their Standard Deviations**

	Chamber Position				
	Top	Bottom	Left	Right	Center
Average	0.1%	0.0%	0.3%	0.5%	0.0%
STD	1.3%	1.4%	1.2%	1.2%	1.1%
Max	3.5%	4.6%	3.8%	4.3%	3.6%
Min	−6.1%	−6.3%	−5.7%	−5.8%	−8.6%

Max, Maximum; *Min,* minimum; *STD, standard* deviation.

Volumetric Dose Check

The volumetric dose check was initially done as part of the weekly dose output check using a cube-like water tank. However, because this required an additional setup, we decided in 2012 to use the same tracker detector (see previous paragraphs) for this test as well. We used three different volumetric spot scan patterns (all using a field size of about 10 × 10 cm^2 and a spread-out Bragg peak [SOBP] of 10 cm) with maximum ranges of 30.6, 20.0, and 14 cm. The first pattern is our standard calibration file that delivers 1 cGy/monitor unit (MU) as described in the paper by Gillin et al.[4] Other files are derived from different versions of the Eclipse treatment planning system (TPS). Every day, one volumetric spot pattern file is used for the volumetric dose check, and over the course of the week, each pattern is delivered at least once. Fig. 6.7 below shows the deviation in the daily volumetric dose check results. All data points are within ±2%. However, there were some outliers in August and December 2013, when the dose monitor cable was changed. In addition, there were two dose monitor exchanges, one in January 2016 and one in May 2017. The first change resulted in a different energy response, especially for the R30 file

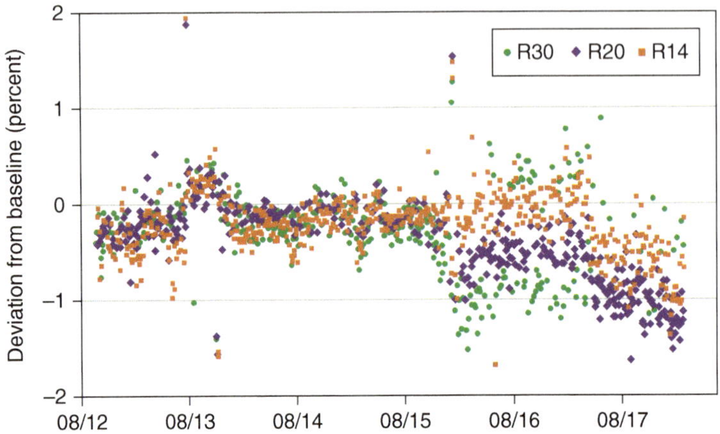

Fig. 6.7 Volumetric output check: relative deviation from baseline.

(purple symbols) that now exhibits a larger fluctuation, as well as an offset to the R20 file (yellow symbol). Again, the baseline data were not changed over the 5-year period.

WEEKLY MACHINE QUALITY ASSURANCE CHECKS

As part of the weekly machine QA check program, all measurements from daily QA are reviewed by a board-certified medical physicist. In addition, a couch rotation isocentricity check is also performed once a week as described below.

The Hitachi couch rotation axis is located away from the gantry rotation plane. An isocentric couch is emulated by translating in two axes (x and y) and rotation of the couch head. This requires a fine interplay of all three rotations (and their motors) to achieve an isocentric rotation. Any collision between the gantry head and the couch can result in a failing isocentric rotation. Because this is a sensitive parameter, this test is performed weekly. The test requires the gantry to be at 0 degrees and the OBI cube (see Fig. 6.2) to be aligned at the x-ray isocenter. Then the couch is rotated to 90 and 270 degrees, and an x-ray image is taken. The deviations in the x and y directions of the cube's radiopaque steel ball called BeeBee (BB) with the couch are recorded. The tolerance for deviation is ± 1 mm.

MONTHLY QUALITY ASSURANCE

The goal of the monthly QA is the same as the daily QA, namely, to verify constancy of dosimetric data, x-ray imaging system alignments, and safety checks. Unlike the daily QA, the monthly QA is performed by a board-certified physicist, and it uses different detector systems: IBA Matrixx 2D ion chamber array and EBT3 film to complement the daily QA checks. The original monthly QA program was derived from the program for the passive scattering proton beamlines at the PTC that went into operation 2 years before the scanning proton beam gantry became clinical. The monthly QA program consists of mechanical checks, gantry isocentricity and couch isocentricity checks using an x-ray imaging system, together with the PIAS system, as well as x-ray versus radiation isocenter check and dose output as a function of gantry angle.

Mechanical Quality Assurance Checks

The couch translation is checked by moving it to predefined positions (−10, −3, 0, +3, +10 cm) in *x*, *y*, and *z* directions. The position of the laser is measured using a ruler, and the deviations from the expected shift are recorded. The tolerance is less than 1 mm, which was always the case during the time of operation of the scanning beam gantry. The movable snout of the PTC is checked similarly using a ruler and laser. The snout position is set to 38, 23, and 8 cm, and the actual position is recorded. The deviation was always within 1 mm of the expected value. In addition to the gantry angle, the six-dimensional couch, as well as the snout rotation, is measured using a spirit level.

Gantry Isocentricity Check With X-Ray Imaging System

For this check, the jig shown in Fig. 6.2 is used to set up the Varian OBI cube. The table is moved to the expected reference coordinates. Then a pair of orthogonal x-rays are taken at the reference gantry angle used for patient setup of 0 degrees. There should be no additional couch shift required unless a collision between gantry and table occurred or work was performed on the x-ray imaging system. The couch location is recorded; the gantry is rotated to 90, 180, and 270 degrees; and x-ray images are repeated after the table mechanical couch adjustment was applied. The mechanical isocenter adjustment was implemented by Hitachi in the design phase of the PTC to meet the requirement of mechanical isocenter being within 0.5 mm. This could only be achieved by making software corrections to the couch called mechanical couch adjustments. The tolerance of the deviation of the isocenter position with the gantry angle is ±1 mm.

Couch Rotation Isocentricity Check

This test is also carried out as part of the monthly QA following the same procedure described in "Weekly Machine Quality Assurance Checks" in this chapter. This is an independent check of the same check done once in a week.

Patient Position Image Analysis System Shift Calculation Accuracy Check

The PIAS software allows a couch shift of up to 3 cm determined from the analysis of the acquired x-ray images by the software. This test is to verify whether an intended shift of 3 cm is actually mechanically performed by the couch movement control system as well as whether the calibration of the PIAS system has not changed. After the BB in the Varian OBI cube is aligned with the PIAS crosshair, the couch is shifted in all three directions by a specific distance under 3 cm, and an orthogonal x-ray image set is acquired. The shift to bring the BB back to the center of the PIAS crosshair is determined and compared with the applied couch shift. The obtained shift is always about 1 mm more compared with the expected shift because the image acquisition of the x-ray panel is 2D, but the shift of the BB is done in 3D, and the cube is shifted away, thus resulting in an increased value.

Radiation Versus Mechanical Isocenter Coincidence Check

To check the coincidence between radiation isocenter and x-ray imaging system isocenter, a spot pattern is delivered to the isocenter location into the aligned Varian OBI QA cube described in "Gantry Isocentricity Check with X-Ray Imaging System" in this chapter. Thus the metal BB of the Varian cube is located at the x-ray isocenter, and the spot penetrates the cube and leaves a dose variation on the radiographic EBT3 film (see Fig. 6.8). The test is repeated for all cardinal angles. The films are scanned using a flatbed scanner Epson Expression 10000XL, and films are analyzed using IBA OmniPro software. The BB should be within 1 mm of the radiation isocenter. However, one should remember that the spot delivery is performed by deflecting the beam using magnet fields; thus, the actual spot position can change from each spill. To determine the actual location of the delivery, we use the spot analysis tool, which is described in papers by Li et al.[5] and Mackin et al.,[6] in our QA software called HPlusQA to determine the deviation of the delivered spot position from the planned spot positions, as shown in Fig. 6.9. A comparison of the actual delivered spot positions with the film data provides a more meaningful comparison of whether the difference of radiation and x-ray imaging system isocenter locations is within tolerance.

Fig. 6.8 Image of the EBT3 film with BeeBee at the center of the spot.

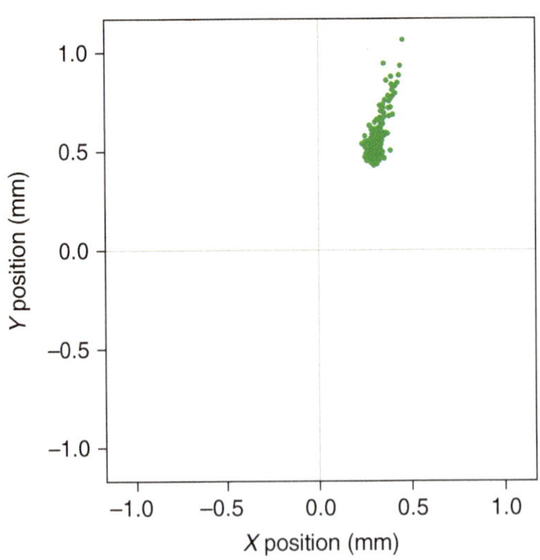

Fig. 6.9 Spot position record of a quality assurance (QA) field used for monthly QA. A total of 15 monitor units (MUs) are delivered with 0.04 MU per spot; thus, there are 375 spots total. The green dots represent the individual spot locations recorded by the multiwire spot position monitor. In this delivery, the average spot deviation in x and y was 0.31 and 0.54 mm, respectively.

Output as a Function of Gantry

Output as a function of gantry angle (0, 90, 180, and 270 degrees) is obtained by using the IBA MatriXX EVO, a 2D ion chamber array, with an in-house manufactured nozzle attachment that has a fixed water-equivalent acrylic buildup of 5 cm. The MatriXX readings are compared with a baseline and thus provide an independent output check. The results are summarized during the annual QA report and agree very well with the maximum deviation being less than 0.3% for all gantry angles.

ANNUAL QUALITY ASSURANCE CHECKS

The annual QA measurements are designed to check the constancy of a subset of machine parameters and data acquired during the commissioning of the beamline for clinical use. The details of our beam commissioning data are described in a paper by Gillin et al.[4] The list of annual QA checks carried out at our center are given in Table 6.1 and are described later.

Mechanical Quality Assurance Checks

The annual mechanical QA consists of the following tests:

1. Gantry rotation mechanical isocenter location using mechanical pointers to determine mechanical isocenter; this isocenter position is then used as a reference in the subsequent tests described below.
2. Couch mechanical rotation isocentricity using a 2-mm ball pointer.
3. Coincidence of gantry and x-ray imaging system rotation isocenters x-ray using a ball pointer that was positioned at mechanical isocenter.
4. Coincidence of laser marker with mechanical isocenter.
5. Coincidence of proton radiation isocenter with mechanical isocenter using radiographic film and custom jig.

The tolerances for those tests are generally all 1 mm. More details can be found in the publication by Arjomandy et al.[3]

X-Ray Imaging System Performance Quality Checks

These checks are designed to ensure that the two x-ray tubes and digital panels are functioning within the diagnostic imaging required parameter. The tests for the x-ray imaging system are performed by a board-certified diagnostic imaging medical physicist, and emphasis is put on safety and imaging dose during operation of the x-ray equipment. The following tests are performed for the x-ray imaging system annually. The procedure and tolerance for these tests are described in the literature.[7]

1. kilovoltage peak (kVp), half-value layer, and timer accuracies
2. exposure reproducibility
3. mA linearity
4. output (exposure as a function of kVp)
5. image quality (high and low contrast resolution)
6. safety

Dosimetric Quality Assurance checks

Formal Calibration of the Dose Monitors

This is a mandatory annual QA check to ensure that dose monitor calibration by using the International Atomic Energy Agency (IAEA) Technical Report Series (TRS) 398[8] protocol under a reference condition has not changed beyond the acceptable tolerance. Our reference condition to define MU at the main dose monitor is that for a spot pattern with a range of 30.6 cm (called the

R30 pattern) and delivering a uniform dose to $10 \times 10 \times 10\ cm^3$ volume. The delivered MU of 217.13 equals the expected dose of 217.13 cGy. As per the requirements of the IAEA TRS-398 protocol,[8] we use a water tank, a Farmer-type ion chamber with a valid dose-to-water calibration factor for the Co-60 beam from an accredited dose calibration laboratory, and a calibrated electrometer. The ion chamber is positioned at the center of irradiated volume and at the gantry isocenter to perform the calibration. We use worksheets provided by the IAEA TRS protocol to record and calculate the dose per MU. In addition, as mentioned in paragraph 2.1.4, we use two more volumetric reference spot delivery patterns (R20 and R14) for which the dose/MU are also verified during annual dosimetric calibration. If any deviation is noticed from the required tolerance for dose/MU values, the pulses per MU are adjusted to bring the dose/MU to the required values after diligent investigation of the cause of deviation and second independent check of the dose/MU values measured during the annual calibration. Our calibration is also checked with two different ion chambers to ensure proper functioning of the ion chambers. We also perform annual thermoluminescent dosimeter (TLD) irradiations under the same condition using the R30 and R20 patterns. The TLDs are provided by the US National Cancer Institute–funded IROC (Imaging and Radiation Oncology Center) QA center, and the results have been always within 3% of expected values. The monitor chamber calibration has been very stable over the past 10 years, and changes required in the number of pulses per MU have been minimal. Such changes occurred when there was either a cable replacement or ion chamber replacement in the nozzle.

Daily Quality Assurance Dosimetry System Baseline Verification

We check our daily QA dosimetry check baseline standards during the annual QA checks after the IAEA TRS 398 calibration is completed to ensure that there is no change in the baseline standard values. If needed, the baseline values are reestablished after diligent investigation of the cause of the change above the tolerance limits of ±2%.

Dose and Monitor Unit Linearity Test and Dynamic Monitor Unit Delivery Check

The linear increase in dose with MU is measured using a PTW Bragg peak chamber. The measured charge is compared with the requested MUs (starting from 0.5 to 25 MU) both for the spots with the lowest and highest energies (72.5 and 221.8 MeV). Then the charge readings are extrapolated to a dose of "0 MU," which is the end effect dose and is typically very small: 12 pC corresponding to 0.002 MU. This is a constancy check to ensure that no significant change has taken place since the commissioning of the beam in the dose monitor end effect.

The maximum number of MUs for our discrete spot scanning beam is 0.04, whereas the minimum is 0.005. The dynamic MU check was studied using the Bragg peak chamber at a depth of 2 cm in a plastic water phantom for both the lowest energy beam and the highest energy beam. The same number of MUs (10) was delivered using 0.005 MU/spot (2000 spots), 0.01 MU/spot (1000 spots), and 0.04 MU per spot (250 spots). The results are normalized to the average of the three readings. We see often a trend that the 0.04 MU/spot delivery gives slightly higher readings of 0.3% and 0.6% for 221.8 and 72.5 MeV, respectively. This is again a constancy check to ensure that no significant change has taken place since the commissioning of the beam in the delivery of spots with MUs both at their highest and lowest values.

Validation of Inverse Square Factor for Change in Dose With Source-to-Detector Distance

The inverse-square factor (ISF), representing the variation of dose with source-to-detector distance (SCD), is an important dosimetry parameter used in our Eclipse TPS. Therefore, its validity is reestablished during the annual QA check. The ISF measurements are performed using the spot pattern with a range of 20 cm and are designed to deliver uniform dose to 1 L of water. A Farmer-type ion chamber is used in a water tank to determine the dose as a function of SCD. This chamber is positioned at different distances from the isocenter by moving the water tank.

The measured charge readings are compared with an expected value calculated using the ISF with 253 cm as the reference SCD. This parameter has remained within 1% of their expected values over the past 10 years.

Spot Size in Air

The spot size, which is determined from the spot profiles, is an important input for the configuration of in scanning pencil beamline in the TPS. It also affects the deviation of the delivered dose compared with the planned dose. Therefore, a constancy check of the spot sizes is carried out during the annual QA checks. The spot profiles at isocenter in air are measured using the IBA MatriXX ion chamber array as well as a PTW 3D scanning tank using a small ion chamber. The MatriXX raw data are smoothed and interpolated using the IBA OmniPro software using a cubic spline interpolation. The full width of half maximum and the 80/20 dose falloff are compared with reference data acquired during commissioning as well as reference data from previous years. It has been found that for lower energies (<150 MeV), the MatriXX data agree very well with the pinpoint-ion chamber data; however, the MatriXX data are systematically found to be too high for higher energies because of the interpolation artifact. Therefore, for high energies, the ion chamber measured data are used to check the constancy of the spot profiles and sizes. The tolerance for the spot size variation from the initial commissioning data is 1%. There have been no instances where the spots sizes were found to have exceeded these tolerance values from the baseline over the past 10 years during the annual QA checks. As described in "Spot Position Accuracy Check" in this chapter, the spot sizes were impacted when a new dose monitor was installed in 2017, leading to reestablishment of the baseline values.

Output as a Function of Gantry Angle

The output (dose/MU) as a function of gantry angle is checked to ensure that the dose monitor response is not affected by the gantry position. This check is carried out during monthly QA using the MatriXX detector. However, the MatriXX detector does not have absolute calibration but instead is cross calibrated. Thus, this cross calibration needs to be checked once a year to ensure the constancy of the MatriXX chamber response and baseline data for monthly QA. The absolute output as a function of gantry angle is measured using a Farmer-type chamber placed in a water-filled acrylic cube that can be rotated so that the buildup is always the same at all gantry angles. The agreement has been within 0.5% over the past 10 years.

Proton Pencil Beam Range Test

Proton pencil beam range is a critical parameter in the beam configuration in the TPS as well as in the accuracy of the delivered dose to the patients. Therefore, it is verified during the annual QA check. To verify the range of the proton pencil beams precisely and to compare with baseline data, we use the PTW scanning system together with a PTW Bragg peak chamber. The chamber was set such that the front face of the chamber was set at the water surface. The gantry was at 0 degrees. The purpose of these scans was to establish the range, not to measure the entire pristine spot dose distribution. Our range was defined at the distal 90% dose and is measured over the entire span of all energies. Fig. 6.10 shows the deviation from the measured to the nominal range. From this illustration, one can see that with increasing range, the deviation becomes larger. At 306 mm, the deviation was about 1.4 mm.

Spot Position Test

The spot position test of the delivery system is necessary, as any deviation from the planned positions will affect the accuracy of the delivered dose. It was previously discussed in the section Radiation Versus Mechanical Isocenter Coincidence Check that we can perform log file analysis of the recorded spot position if the delivery is performed through MOSAIQ treatment mode. For

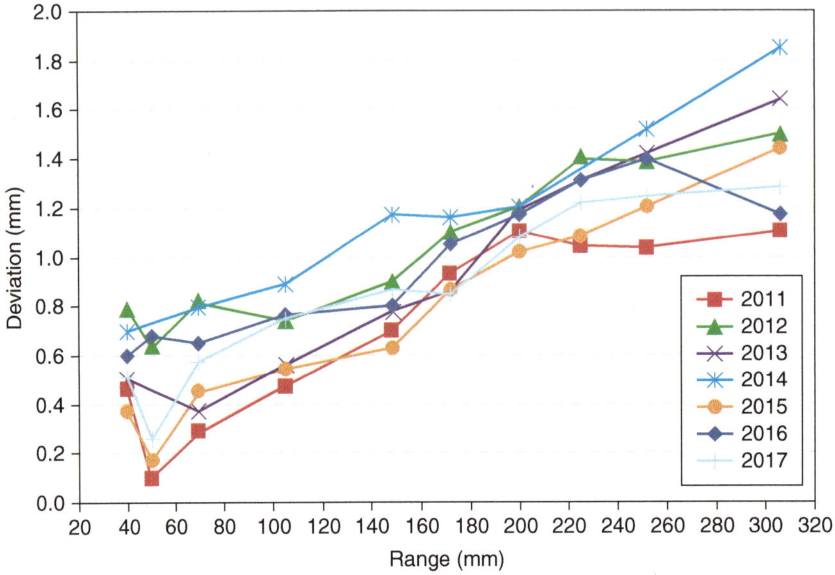

Fig. 6.10 Deviation between nominal ranges to measured ranges as a function of energy. Results are shown for the last seven annual quality assurance checks.

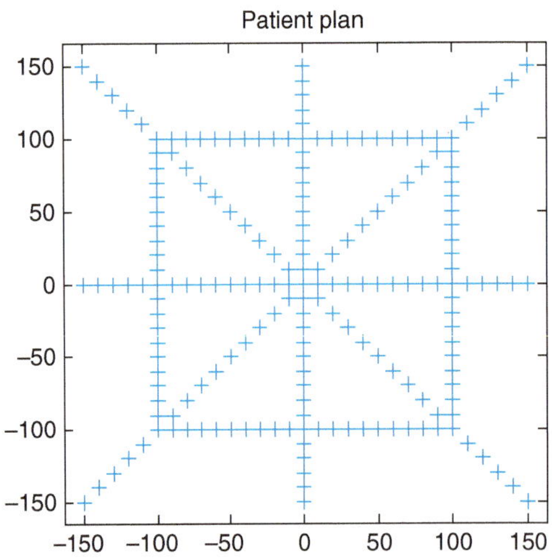

Fig. 6.11 Shape of the irradiated cross pattern delivered through MOSAIQ control. Dimensions are given in millimeters.

the annual QA check, we combine the log file analysis with MatriXX ion chamber array measurements and then compare both data. A monoenergetic cross/rectangular pattern (Fig. 6.11) is used for pencil beam spots with energies of 96.9, 148.8, and 221 MeV. There are two sets of patterns, the "planned" and the "intentionally modified" ones. The latter pattern has a distinct offsets of −0.05, +0.1, −0.2, and 0.3 cm. Although the detector array grid size is rather course with 0.76 cm, the method is capable of detecting submillimeter deviations accurately. The results in Tables 6.3 and 6.4 show that both methods can precisely determine shifts by a fraction of a millimeter and that the requested positions are precisely delivered with deviations within 1% or 1 mm.

TABLE 6.3 ■ **MatriXX Results for Annual Quality Assurance**

Location Cm E (MeV)	Planned Pattern 96.9	148.8	221.8	Intentional Modified 96.9	148.8	221.8	Offset (cm)	Differences (cm) 96.9	148.8	221.8
9.7 ^{+}x	10.1	1.04	10.12	9.68	9.64	9.64	−0.30	−0.33	−0.40	−0.48
−10.5 ^{-}x	−10.2	−10.09	−10.13	−10.08	−10.15	10.18	−0.05	−0.06	−0.06	−0.05
10.1 ^{+}y	10.07	10.10	10.14	10.17	10.19	10.22	0.10	−0.10	0.09	−0.08
−10.2 *y*	−9.95	−9.99	−10.06	−10.17	−10.21	−10.25	−0.20	−0.22	−0.22	−0.19

TABLE 6.4 ■ **Spot Scanning Beam Log File**

Location Cm E	Planned Pattern 96.9	148.8	221.8	Intentional Modified 96.9	148.8	221.8	Offset (cm)	Differences (cm) 96.9	148.8	221.8
9.7 ^{+}x	10.6	10.05	10.02	9.76	9.75	9.74	−0.30	−0.30	−0.30	−0.28
−10.5 ^{-}x	−10.6	−10.07	−10.09	−10.12	−10.11	−10.14	−0.05	−0.06	−0.04	−0.05
10.1 ^{+}y	10.01	9.99	10.00	10.10	10.10	10.13	0.10	−0.09	0.11	−0.13
−10.2 *y*	−9.99	−9.98	−10.00	−10.19	−10.19	−10.21	−0.20	−0.20	−0.21	−0.21

Bragg Peak Chamber Measurements of Dose at a Depth of 2 cm

The beam configuration in our TPS requires the integral depth dose of the proton pencil beam spots. The constancy of this parameter is checked during annual QA using the PTW Bragg peak chamber at a depth of 1.8 cm (0.4 cm intrinsic and 1.4 cm additional plastic water buildup). Five monitor units are delivered in physics mode on the central axis, and the charge is measured. As shown in Fig. 6.12, the reading has been stable over the last 6 years for all energies measured with deviations being below the 2% tolerance limit.

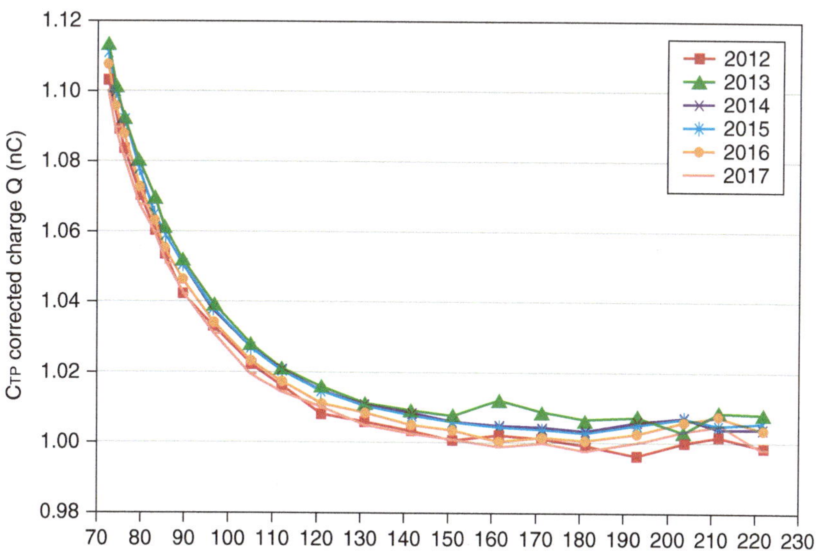

Fig. 6.12 CTP (temperature and pressure)-corrected charge of the Bragg peak parallel plate ion chamber as a function of energy. The charge was normalized to the five highest energy readings.

MACHINE QUALITY ASSURANCE PROGRAMS FOR SCANNING PROTON PENCIL BEAMS AT OTHER INSTITUTIONS

There are only a small number of published reports regarding the machine QA programs for the scanning proton pencil beams at other institutions. We will briefly summarize some of these reports. The daily QA checks for scanning proton pencil beams at other institutions are carried out using different devices and procedures as described in the published literature. The underlying objectives of the QA programs at different institutions are the same: namely, constancy checks of the following dosimetry parameters: (1) dose output, (2) beam range check, and (3) spot position accuracy check and proper functioning of the safety interlocks of the delivery system.

The daily QA program for the scanning proton pencil beamline at the Center for Proton Therapy of the Paul Scherrer Institute (PSI) in Villigen, Switzerland, is described in a paper by Actis et al.[9] A specialized daily QA phantom consisting of a multilayer ionization chamber, strip detectors, a dosimetry phantom made of a acrylic block with two embedded ionization chambers and a temperature sensor, and scintillating screens are used to check the spot position, beamwidth, and range of the proton pencil beams and dose at the SOBP region and 50% distal falloff region. Additionally, laser alignment and safety interlock functionality tests are carried out daily. The use of QA software tools to record and analyze the results of QA measurements, optimized workflow, and all-in-one phantom has led to an efficient in terms of time savings and a comprehensive daily QA program at PSI.

The Mayo Clinic[10] uses a Sun Nuclear daily QA 3 device and a custom-made acrylic block that allows simultaneous measurements of beam ranges of low- and high-energy proton beams using a single nonuniform field. The efficiency of their device and procedure is illustrated in terms of the time savings and the ability of the system to measure the deviations from the baseline values under tighter tolerance limits, namely, 1% for output, 0.5 mm for range, and 1.5 mm for spot position.

The QA program at the Italian National Centre for Oncological Hadrontherapy consists of daily, half-yearly, and yearly checks.[11] EBT films, all-in-one phantom, strip chambers, ion chambers, and the PTW Peakfinder device are used to measure the spot position, spot size, beam calibration constancy, dose homogeneity in 2D fields, energy constancy, beam contamination, dose distribution in inhomogeneous phantoms and CT-range calibration constancy, and are checked as part of the QA program.

Patient Treatment Plan–Specific Quality Assurance Checks

MATERIALS AND METHODS

The patient treatment plan–specific QA (PSQA) has two parts. The first part involves the plan review by a physicist to ensure that appropriate beam arrangements and beam parameters are being used to design the best possible plan. The setup digitally reconstructed radiographs (DRRs) and treatment field DRRs are also reviewed to ensure that they are correctly generated. The transferred fields in the record-and-verify system or EMR are also checked to confirm that all the necessary information is being correctly transferred from the TPS. Field-specific apertures, if used in the treatment plan, also undergo a physics QA check after they are fabricated. For this purpose, the outline of the planned aperture is overlaid on the aperture to check for any deviations. The second part involves the comparison of the planned dose distribution of every treatment field with the measured dose distribution in a water-equivalent phantom. Measurement of treatment field dose distribution is necessary because the machine QA program described in previous sections only checks dosimetric features of a subset of available of proton pencil beam energies and a very limited number of spot positions to ensure that the critical delivery system interlocks are functioning as expected. Certain important beam parameters such as spot profiles or Bragg peak shapes are not measured frequently, and QA measurements for all beam options are not performed. Additionally, the broad beams used for patient treatment are unique for specific patients. Therefore, a comparison of delivered dose distribution with the planned dose distribution is important to ensure that any deviations are within acceptable tolerance limits. Additionally, the measurements of patient-specific treatment field dose distributions also serve as indirect machine QA of the delivery system. Any failure in meeting the tolerance standards for treatment field dose distribution would indicate either failure of the delivery system components and/or the beam configuration in the TPS. The dosimetric QA program for patient-specific scanning proton pencil beam plans is based on the same philosophy used for the QA program for intensity-modulated photon radiation therapy. The details of the patient treatment field-specific dosimetric QA program at PTC are described in the following sections.

There are two different types of measurements: (1) measurement of dose distribution at one depth by delivering the beam through the record and verify system, MOSAIQ, termed as *Mosaiq QA*; and (2) measurements at additional depths by delivering the beam without the use of MOSAIQ, termed as *additional depth QA*. In the Mosaiq-QA session, the scanning beam is delivered with the scanning beam accelerator control system (ACS) put in the treatment mode. The beam parameters and spot pattern are sent to the ACS through our MOSAIQ Medical Oncology Management (IMPAC Medical Systems, Sunnyvale, CA) running in "QA mode." During this delivery, as described in the paper by Zhu et al.,[23] the following items are verified: (1) data transfer integrity from the TPS to the ACS by end-to-end testing, and (2) proper functioning of the beam steering magnets by measuring the dose distribution of treatment fields being delivered at the treatment gantry angles and comparing them with the predicted dose by the TPS. Additionally, the bending magnet field strengths, which were not provided by the TPS, are acquired and stored in the treatment field definition in MOSAIQ for use as a change check parameter during patient treatment with these fields.[4] Furthermore, Mosaiq QA enables the transfer of the spot position log files from the ACS to MOSAIQ, allowing further analysis. Additional depth QA measurements are performed with Hitachi ACS in the physics mode and at a fixed gantry angle of 270 degrees for all treatment fields to be more time-efficient. For this purpose, the Digital Imaging and Communications in Medicine (DICOM) RT plan file from Eclipse is used to create the control point and spot position files that are needed by the ACS to deliver the spots in the treatment field of interest.

The first step in the preparation for the QA process is to create a verification plan in the TPS. The verification plan computes the dose distribution for the treatment fields in a digitally created water phantom using the pencil beam convolution superposition algorithm of the Eclipse TPS. The treatment plan is uploaded to MOSAIQ to make the treatment fields available for QA measurements.

Our first 249 patients treated in proton scanning pencil beam had prostate cancer. They were treated using the single-field uniform dose (SFUD) delivery technique[12] using two parallel-opposed lateral fields. A characteristic of SFUD is that the entire target volume receives the prescription dose. Therefore, SFUD is less sensitive to proton range uncertainties than intensity-modulated proton therapy (IMPT).[13] Because the target dose is uniform over a rather large volume (>50 cm^3), the QA dose measurements are much easier, and simpler tools were used.

To measure the dose distribution of treatment fields for prostate cancer patients, an oval-shaped water phantom together with a small volume ion chamber CC04 (IBA Scanditronix Wellhoffer, Barlett, TN) were used as shown in Fig. 6.13. Using this phantom, it becomes feasible to measure the dose at the center of the phantom for the two lateral fields at gantry angles of 90 and 270 degrees without shifting the phantom.

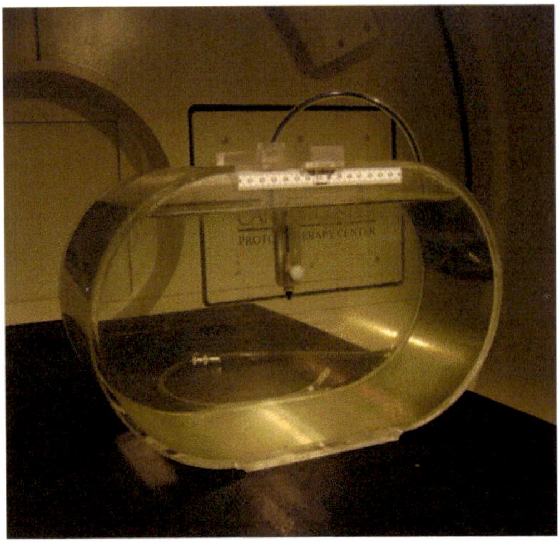

Fig. 6.13 "Fishbowl" phantom for patient-specific quality assurance for prostate patients used between 2008 and 2011. In the center of the phantom, a small volume ion chamber was placed. (From Zhu XR, Poenisch F, Song X, et al. 2011: patient-specific quality assurance for prostate cancer patients receiving spot scanning proton therapy using single-field uniform dose. *Int J Radiat Oncol Biol Phys*. 2011;81(2):552-559.)

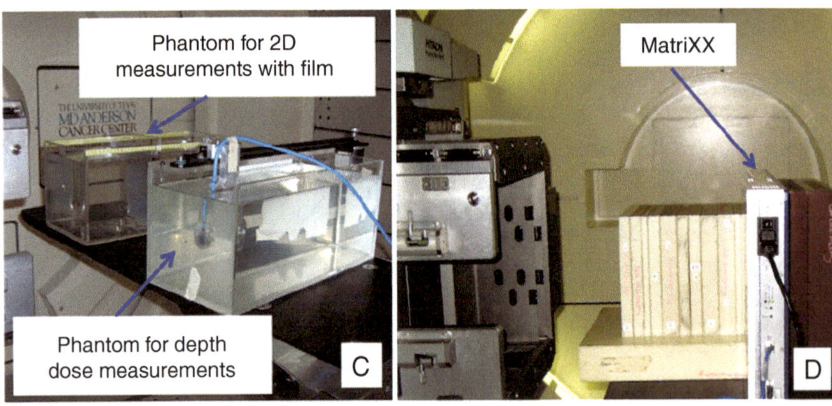

Fig. 6.14 Experimental setup for patient quality assurance. *(Left)* Two-dimensional (2D) film measurements and 1D depth dose measurements. *(Right)* 2D depth dose measurement using MatriXX 2D ion chamber array with plastic water as buildup. (From Zhu XR, Poenisch F, Song X, et al. 2011: patient-specific quality assurance for prostate cancer patients receiving spot scanning proton therapy using single-field uniform dose. *Int J Radiat Oncol Biol Phys*. 2011;81(2):552-559.)

The point dose measurements were supplemented by depth dose measurements and relative 2D dose distribution measurements. For a central axis dose depth dose measurement, a 1D scanning tank and a parallel plate ion chamber (type 34045; PTW, Freiburg, Germany) were used, as shown in Fig. 6.14. The 2D dose measurements were done initially using Gafchromic EBT film inside a water tank, as shown in Fig. 6.14. Later, we replaced the film measurements using a 2D ion chamber array detector MatriXX (Scanditronix Wellhofer, Schwarzenbruck, Germany) and plastic water (CIRS Inc., Norfolk, VA) for buildup.[3,12] For the first 5 years, we analyzed the 2D dose distribution using the IBA OmniPro software. The results of our dosimetric QA for treatment fields for prostate cancer patients are described in a paper by Zhu et al.[12] Results of comparison of depth dose curves and isodose lines from measurements and TPS calculations are shown in Figs. 6.15 and 6.16 as examples.

The QA program was changed after the scanning proton pencil beam was used to treat sites other than the prostate using IMPT plans with energy absorber. The Mosaiq QA is now

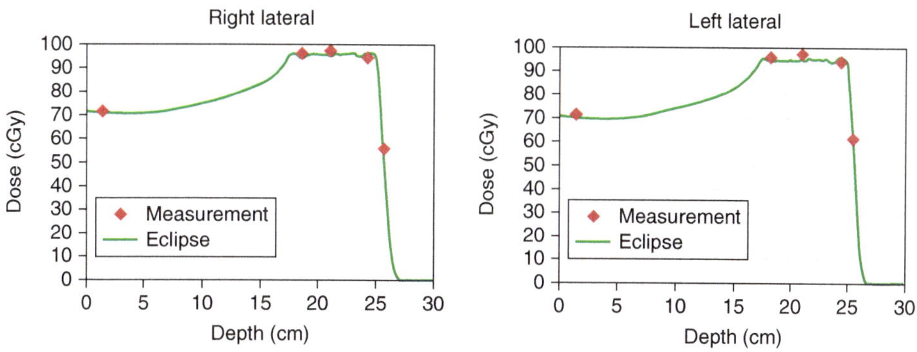

Fig. 6.15 Central axis depth doses for two lateral fields used to treat cancer in the prostate. Points are from measurements; lines are from the calculation by the treatment planning system.

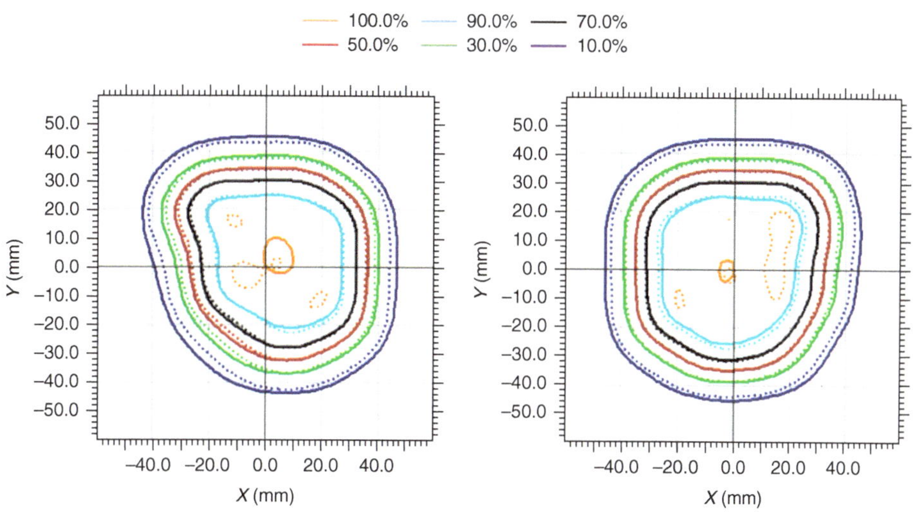

Fig. 6.16 Isodose comparison of right lateral *(left)* and left lateral *(right)* fields used to treat cancer in the prostate with proton pencil scanning beams. Solid lines are from measurement, and dashed lines are from treatment planning system (TPS) calculation.

performed using the MatriXX 2D ion chamber array together with an in-house designed table attachment, which is shown in Fig. 6.17.

The MatriXX detector exhibits an angular dependence,[14] and it is necessary to position the MatriXX surface perpendicular to the beam axis. Therefore, we have built an attachment that allows the MatriXX detector to rotate around the mechanical isocenter so that the detector plane remains perpendicular to the beam axis during the dose measurement for any gantry angle. This design also allows the movable snout to be positioned at the same location as in the treatment plan, providing similar air gaps as for patient treatment. There is a provision to attach a piece of buildup material to the MatriXX attached to the rotating platform. Currently, this choice is limited to 2 , 5, or 20 cm in addition to the 0.4 cm of inherent buildup depth of the MatriXX, which are found to work well for plans for targets in every anatomical site treated at PTC with scanning

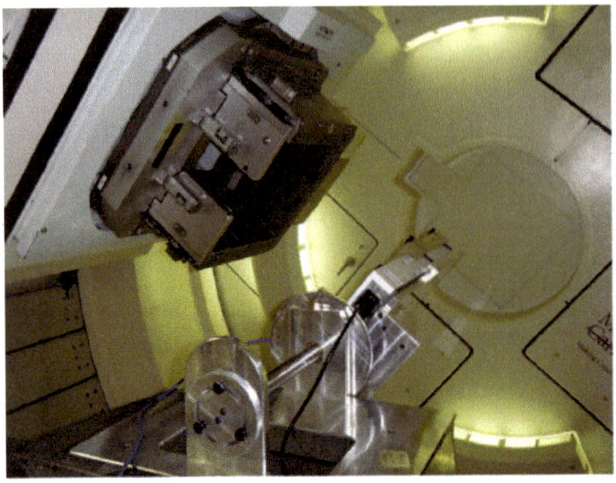

Fig. 6.17 Measurement setup for Mosaiq QA: the MatriXX is bolted onto the custom tabletop attachment. (From Mackin D, Li Y, Taylor MB, et al. Improving spot-scanning proton therapy patient specific quality assurance with HPlusQA, a second-check dose calculation engine. *Med Phys*. 2013;40(12):121708.)

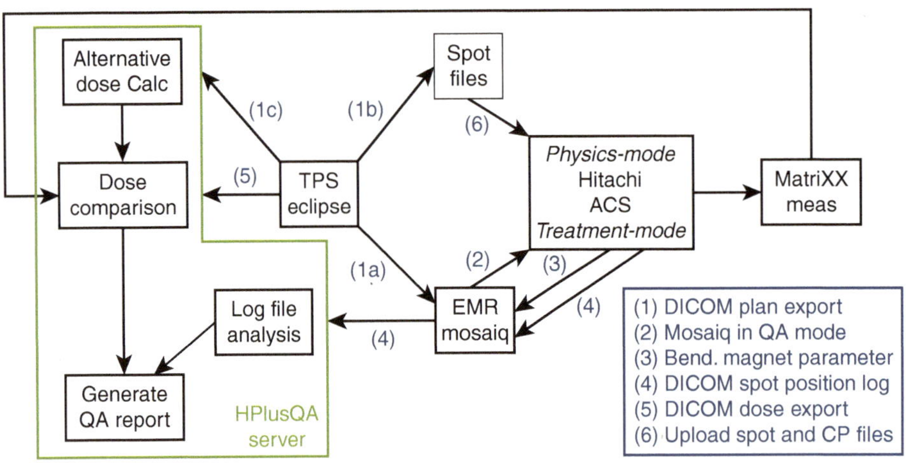

Fig. 6.18 Patient-specific workflows for scanning beam quality assurance *(QA)*. Green lines indicate calculation performed on the HPlusQA server. *ACS,* Accelerator control system; *EMR,* electronic medical record; *TPS,* treatment planning system. (Modified from Zhu XR, Li Y, Mackin D, et al. Towards effective and efficient patient-specific quality assurance for spot scanning proton therapy. *Cancers (Basel)*. 2015;7:631-647.)

proton pencil beams. The additional depth QA measurements are performed at a fixed gantry angle of 270 degrees using the MatriXX and plastic water phantom (CIRS Inc., Norfolk, VA) instead of using an ion chamber in a water phantom, as described earlier. These measurements are done at a fixed SSD setup to match with the setup used in the verification plan in the TPS. We typically measure no more than 3 depths per field, namely, proximal, center, and distal with regard to the SOBP. However, this categorization is subjective if multifield optimized IMPT plans are measured. The measured dose distributions are now compared with the dose calculated by TPS using our in-house developed HPlusQA software.[6] The efficiency of the QA program was improved by using this automated analysis software. HPlusQA also performs independent dose calculations in the water phantom using the proton PBS fields of the treatment plans.[23] It also provides the results of a comparison of three dose distributions, namely, HPlusQA calculated, Eclipse calculated, and measured dose distributions. Details of the HPlusQA dose calculation and implementation are described in papers by Li et al.[14] and Mackin et al.[6] Our current patient treatment field–specific dosimetric QA workflow is shown in Fig. 6.18.

After the creation of the verification plan in TPS for the treatment plan to be checked by the PSQA process, the following additional tasks are performed to complete the PSQA process: (1a) transfer of the plan to MOSAIQ, (1b) creation of control point files and spot position files, (1c) transfer of plan information from TPS to HPlusQA for independent dose calculation, (2) Mosaiq QA measurements in treatment mode, (3) recording of the bending magnet values in EMR MOSAIQ after beam delivery, (4) transfer of DICOM files containing the spot position log to HPlusQA after beam delivery, (5) transfer of the DICOM file containing the verification plan dose to HPlusQA, and (6) additional depth QA measurements in physics mode using the Control Point (CP) and spot files and transfer of all the measured dose distributions to HPlusQA for analysis. The results of intercomparison of dose distributions are provided in terms of comparative depth dose curves and 2D gamma indices using both 2%/2 mm and 3%/3 mm dose/distance agreement criteria, as shown in Fig. 6.19. Additionally, the HPlusQA software displays two selected dose distributions, a 2D gamma map, a histogram of gamma pass rate, as well as a plot of isodose lines, as shown in Fig. 6.20.

In addition to the dose comparison, the spot log analysis is performed in HplusQA. The map of planned and delivered positions, results of statistical analysis of the deviations in delivered spot positions, and MUs from the planned spot positions and measured MUs are displayed[16] as shown in Fig. 6.21 for one of the five fields of an IMPT plan used to treat a target in the head and neck. The summary of the deviations for the five fields for this plan is given in Table 6.5 as an example of the information available from the spot log file analysis by the HPlusQA software.

After the independent dose calculation, dose distribution intercomparison analysis, and spot log file analysis are complete, a complete QA report is generated using the HPlusQA software in an MS Word–compatible file format. This report includes the description of the patient's treatment course as well as other details such as dose, number of fractions, beam parameters such as number of spots and MUs for each field in the plan, the gamma pass rates for every field at different depths, and average deviation of the spot positions and spot MUs from their planned

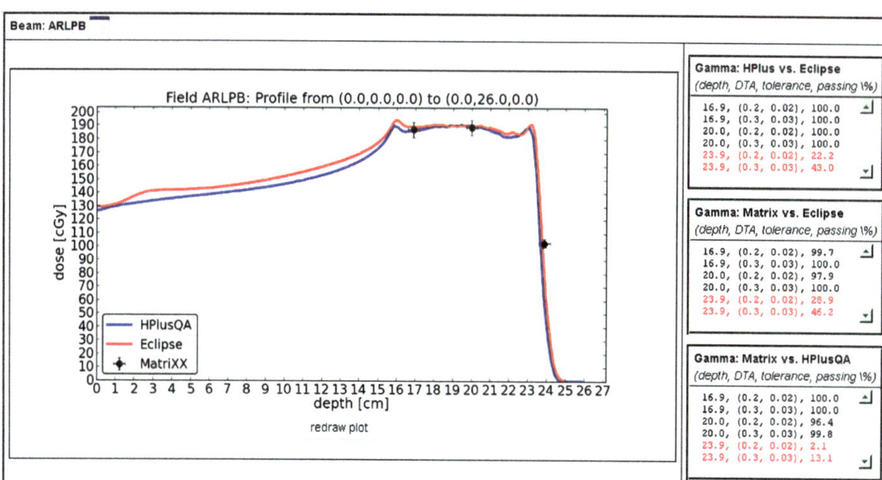

Fig. 6.19 Screenshot of display of results of an analysis of treatment fields labeled ARLPB for a prostate cancer patient from HPlusQA software. The measured dose points are overlaid onto the HPlusQA calculated dose *(blue)* and the Eclipse treatment planning system calculated dose *(red)*. The error bars of the measurements depict a 3%/3 mm variation used for better visualization. On the right, the two-dimensional gamma results are shown. One can see that good agreement is found at the center of spread-out Bragg peak, but there are larger differences at the distal edge because of the sharp dose gradient (3%/3 mm dose/distance agreement may not be applicable in this region). DTA, Distance to agreement.

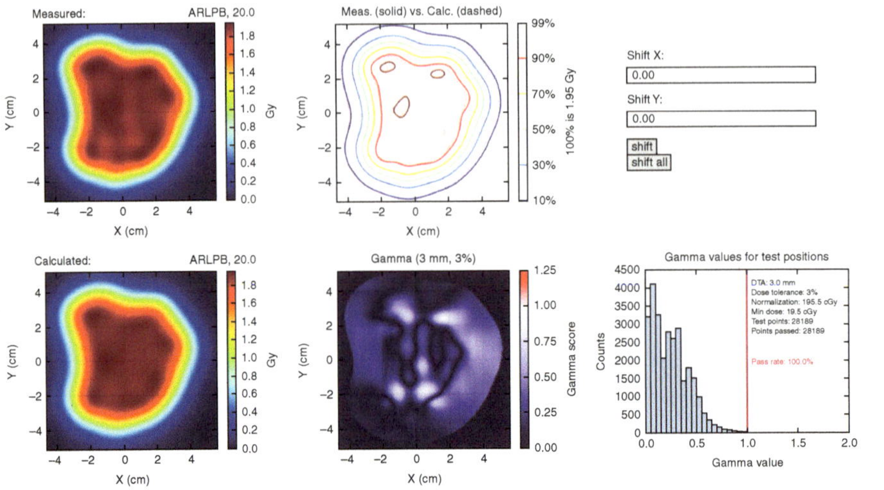

Fig. 6.20 Analysis page of the same patient as in Fig. 6.19 at a depth of 20 cm for a right lateral beam labeled ARLPB. DTA, Distance to agreement.

positions. The QA report is reviewed by a physicist before the patient treatment fields are approved for delivery. If any of the QA metrics are found to be out of their established tolerance limits, additional analysis and measurements and, if necessary, replanning are performed with an aim to have a plan for which the tolerance limits of the QA metrics are met for every field before they are used for treatment.

RESULTS OF PATIENT TREATMENT PLAN–SPECIFIC QUALITY ASSURANCE AT THE UNIVERSITY OF TEXAS MD ANDERSON CANCER CENTER PROTON THERAPY CENTER IN HOUSTON

The results of the PSQA measurements for 249 prostate cancer patients at PTC are published in a paper by Zhu et al.[12] The point dose measurements in the center of the "fishbowl" phantom was found to be within 2% of the TPS calculated values for 248 cases and was within 3% for 1 case only. The gamma pass rates for 3%/3-mm dose/distance agreement criteria for comparing the TPS calculated dose distribution and measured dose distribution both by film and MatriXX were more than 90% for all treatment fields measured at the depths in the flat SOBP regions and proximal to this region. All the measured point doses along the central axis met the 3%/2-mm dose/distance agreement criteria. The results of a large set of PSQA measurements for various sites (309 plans) treated with scanning proton pencil beam at PTC are published in a paper by Mackin et al.[17] The overall gamma passing rate for the 3%/3-mm dose/distal agreement was found to be 96.2% for all cases; the lowest was 95% for treatment plans for targets in the head and neck, and the highest was 100% for treatment plans for the prostate. The gamma pass rate was lower for fields with range shifters (94.8% ± 0.6%) as compared with fields without range shifters (99% ± 0.6%). Gamma pass rates were similar for multifield and single-field optimized plans. Most low gamma pass rates were observed for depths located in the steep dose gradient region and in the region proximal to the SOBP, where the calculated dose distributions were found to be overestimated attributed to the limitations of the analytical dose calculation algorithm used in the TPS. The spot position log analysis has been automatized to alert the physicists to any occurrence of unusual deviation of the delivered spot positions and MUs for every treatment field. No incidence of deviation in the spot MUs have occurred.

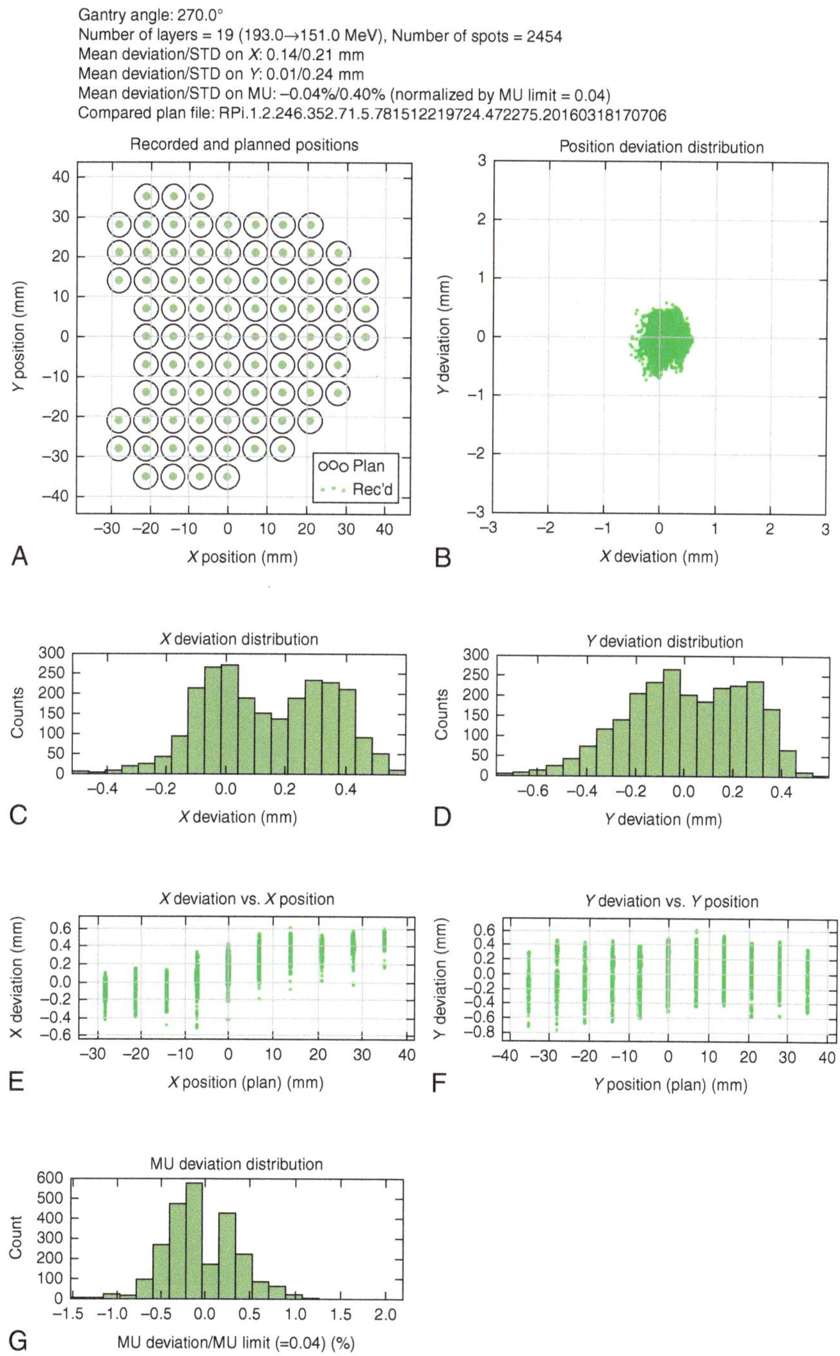

Fig. 6.21 Log file analysis with HPlusQA which compares planned spot position with actually delivered spots, as shown in (A). This tool also provides results of additional statistical analysis for spot position and spot monitor unit *(MU)* deviations from their planned values, as shown in (B) through (F).

TABLE 6.5 ■ **Summary Information About the Deviation of the Delivered Spot Positions and Monitor Units From the Planned Position. The Tolerance for the Mean Deviation for the Spot Position Is 1 mm and for Monitor Units Is 1%.**

Field ID	Gantry Angle (°)	Number of Layers	Number of Spots	Mean Deviation/STD *X* (mm)	Mean Deviation/STD *Y* (mm)	Mean Deviation/STD MU (%)
ARLPB	270	19	2454	0.14/0.21	0.01/0.24	−0.04/0.40
BLLPB	270	21	2456	−0.44/0.22	−0.45/0.27	−0.01/0.44

MU, Monitor Units; *STD*, standard deviation.

Occasional spot position deviations have been noticed because of malfunctioning of specific channels in the spot positioning monitor. This had led to further investigation, including dose measurements and corrective action to ensure proper functioning of the spot position monitor in the scanning proton beam nozzle.

PATIENT TREATMENT PLAN–SPECIFIC QUALITY ASSURANCE AT OTHER INSTITUTIONS

There are only a handful of published results of PSQA for the scanning proton pencil beam in the literature. Papers by Pedroni et al.[18] and Lomax et al.[19] describe the PSQA work performed at the Proton Therapy Center in PSI in Villigen, Switzerland. The doses of the patient treatment fields were verified by measurements of 2D dose distribution using charge-coupled device camera–based scintillator screens and point doses using ionization chamber arrays in water to measure dose profiles at selected depths. Good agreement was seen between the measured and planned point doses, being within 3% tolerance limits. A systemic difference of 1.5 mm in the measured range and planned range was seen in their PSQA checks. Jäkel et al.[20] have reported their methodology and results for PSQA for their scanned ion beam therapy at the German Cancer Research Center in Heidelberg, Germany, using a set of 24 small ionization chambers in a water phantom. Agreement around 3% of the measured dose with the planned dose was reported. Furukawa et al.[21] reported their methodology and results for PSQA for scanning carbon ion beams for treatment fields for 122 patients. Their measurements include 2D dose distribution using PTW Octavius Detector 729 XDR (PTW, Freiburg, Germany) at several depths. A gamma pass rate of 90% for 3%/3-mm dose/distance agreement criteria was met for all of the fields used in this study. They have also developed a multiwire proportional chamber (MWPC) to record 2D fluence images during the beam delivery for QA measurements, which are then used as a reference for constancy checks of delivered fluence recorded in the MWPC during patient treatment sessions. A recent paper by Belosi et al.[22] describes the use of spot delivery log files to reconstruct the delivered dose to patients and quantify any differences between the delivered and planned doses. They have found this tool as very useful as part of plan-specific QA, specifically the check of plan robustness for uncertainties in the delivered spot positions. Such an approach can be easily automatized and be part of any PSQA program for scanning proton pencil beam therapy.

Summary

The machine QA program for scanning proton pencil beam at the PTC has evolved over the past 10 years, and we have a robust QA program to periodically monitor the performance of the delivery system. No major deviations in the results of QA checks have been found over the 10 years except for occasional couch rotational isocentricity going out of tolerance as a result of accidental couch and gantry collisions. The current PSQA program[23] combines measurement with independent dose calculations and makes use of software both for automatized analysis of the results of comparison of measured and calculated dose distributions and for report generation. The automatized log file analysis of deviation of the delivered spot positions from the planned position provides continuous QA checks of the delivered dose to the patient in each fraction. Future enhancements in the PSQA program include Monte Carlo–based independent dose calculation, reduction in the number of measurements for each field to one depth only, and spot log file–based composite dose calculation for the QA session and for the entire treatment course.

References Available Online.

CHAPTER 7

Intensity-Modulated Proton Therapy Patient Treatments

Michael T. Gillin ■ Yoshifumi Hojo ■ Narayan Sahoo ■ X. Ronald Zhu

Introduction

Intensity-modulated proton therapy (IMPT) can begin only after a number of other processes have been completed, including simulation and treatment planning. For both proton and photon treatments, radiation oncology has evolved to the point in which the treatment parameters, defined in the treatment planning process, are included in the radiation oncology electronic medical record (EMR) to be uploaded to the delivery system for each treatment field on each day. At the completion of daily treatment for a specific patient, the delivery system downloads a number of parameters of the treatment delivered on that day. The delivery system may also have its own logs, which contain a history of operations at specific times on a specific day. These treatment delivery logs are the ultimate source of truth because they record the details as to the actions taken by the treatment device. It is necessary on limited occasions to consult the treatment logs to confirm the individual treatment on a specific day.

IMPT is an example of a very complex treatment technique that would be impossible to deliver without the use of an EMR to upload the treatment parameters. In addition to the treatment parameters, patient-specific referenced images are also uploaded to the delivery system so that a comparison can be made to daily patient setup images. It is not unusual that there are devices or systems from multiple vendors involved in the IMPT treatment process. For example, at MD Anderson Cancer Center (MDACC), the treatment delivery system is provided by vendor H (Hitachi), the EMR system by vendor E (Elekta), and the treatment planning system (TPS) by vendor V (Varian). A key to this successful digital communication is the Digital Imaging and Communications in Medicine (DICOM) standard. DICOM was developed by the American College of Radiology and the National Electrical Manufacturers Association to aid the distribution and viewing of medical images. The first version of DICOM was released in 1985. DICOM for radiation therapy came later, in 1995, with DICOM Working Group 7. Information on this industry standard can be found on the DICOM homepage, dicom.nema.org. DICOM is a very successful, mature standard that has evolved over time and continues to evolve. DICOM makes IMPT possible in the multivendor environment.

DICOM defines many basic radiation therapy ion beam attributes, including beam type (static or dynamic), radiation type (photon, proton, ion), scan mode (none, uniform, modulated, modulated spec), and so on. DICOM uses the concept of control points for radiation therapy treatments. Control point 0 has the cumulative meter set weight set to zero and defines all initial parameters (e.g., gantry, table, collimator). Control points are important in IMPT delivery. A new control point is defined for each energy change. Each control point has a specific number of spots and monitor units (MUs).

Treating with individual spots (packets of protons), which change energy and location, is different than treating with large fields, either protons or photons. The concept of dose, energy deposited per unit mass, needs reflection when treating with spots; for example, the unit mass involved and the instantaneous dose rate. One potential unique catastrophic failure would be the corruption of data or failure of devices such that all spots were delivered to the same physical location over and over and over.

Intensity-Modulated Proton Therapy Treatment Delivery

IMPT is a highly conformal radiation treatment in which the intensity of the proton beam is adjusted and shaped to conform to the shape and depth of the tumor. Individual spots of the pencil proton beam can have different energies, different locations, and different intensities (dose). IMPT offers a three-dimensional (3D) approach to sculpt the radiation pattern to match the target.

In 2008, Hitachi provided University of Texas MD Anderson Cancer Center (UT MDACC) Proton Therapy Center in Houston the second clinical spot scanning system in the world. The first clinical spot scanning facility is the Paul Scherrer Institute, a multidisciplinary research institute in Switzerland. Some 94 different proton energies are available with ranges from 4.0 to 30.6 cm. The maximum field size is 30 cm × 30 cm. The maximum MU per spot is 0.04 MU, whereas the minimum MU per spot is 0.005 MU. The full width at half maximum spot size in air at isocenter varies from 12 to 34 mm, depending on the energy. MDACC chose to define the MU in a manner consistent with photon MU definitions, as opposed to the number of protons passing through the dose monitor approach. The definition of the MU was built into the TPS early in the commissioning process.[1]

The MDACC spot scanning nozzle has a very conservative design, as appropriate for an early system. The length of the beam path in the nozzle is greater than 3 m. As the beam enters the nozzle, the beam encounters the profile monitor and then enters a helium chamber. Outside of the helium chamber, there is the Y scanning magnet and then the X scanning magnet. Eventually, the beam passes through two dose monitors and a spot position monitor. Before leaving the nozzle, the beam can pass through an energy filter (ridge filter) and an energy absorber (range shifter), if such devices are in place. Finally, it is possible to insert an aperture for the purpose of reducing the penumbra. The system has worked well for the treatment of patients with discrete spot scanning proton therapy, including the IMPT technique.[2]

Routine patient IMPT delivery requires a treatment plan that contains parameters for each spot (beam energy, location, and the MU/dose per spot), a record and verify/EMR, which uploads the treatment parameters to the delivery system and records the treatment delivered, and the delivery system. Table 7.1 displays treatment field parameters for a multifield optimized treatment plan with three treatment fields for a head and neck patient.

At MDACC, the current TPS system is Eclipse from Varian,[3] the EMR system is Mosaiq from Elekta,[4] and the delivery system is from Hitachi.[5] The software associated with each

TABLE 7.1 ■ **Treatment Field Parameters**

Prescription Isodose Line (%)	CTV60 (cc)	Total Target (cc)	Field	Nominal Range (cm)	Nominal SOBP (cm)	Max E (MeV)	Layers	Total Spots	mu
100.0	32.2	201.4	ALPPB	10.2	10.2	153.2	37	1973	62.94
			BPAPB	20.3	18.6	203.7	47	1910	60.94
			CLAPB	7.5	7.4	143.2	32	3144	109.46

Max E, Maximum energy; *SOBP*, spread-out Bragg peak.

system may change or may remain static. Substantial testing is required when there is a change in software. In the last 10 years, there have been upgrades to Eclipse at approximately 2-year (or longer) intervals and upgrades in Mosaiq at approximately 18- to 24-month intervals. There have been no changes in the Hitachi system delivery system software. This stability in the treatment delivery control system is reassuring, to a point, as upgrades are useful to refine the treatment process. In a large clinic, changes in the radiation oncology practice-wide EMR may be driven by developments outside of protons, which are only supported by newer versions of the EMR software.

Radiation oncology has now evolved to the point at which nearly all patients are treated using the radiation oncology EMR, even emergent patients. Approximately more than 9000 patients have been treated at the UT MDACC proton center, including approximately 3000 spot scanning patients. Zero patients have been treated without the use of the Rad Onc EMR. This enforces a safety discipline on treatment delivery because there are no last-minute rush patients. Before the first fraction is treated, clinical physics must approve the calibration and the chart after reviewing the initial quality assurance (QA) measurements.

The Hitachi treatment delivery system can deliver the beam while in three different modes, namely, treatment mode, physics mode, and service mode. The number of active interlocks changes in the various modes. Service mode is essentially limited to service and almost exclusively used for service purposes. Physics mode is designed for the physicists to perform commissioning, patient-specific and machine QA. The parameters for physics mode tests are stored in folders that are not contained in the EMR. In physics mode, it is easy to run the same file multiple times. In treatment mode, all interlocks are functional, and all field-specific parameters must be uploaded from the EMR each time that the field is run and downloaded from the delivery system after each delivery. Time is required for this information transfer, in addition to the time required to deliver the proton beam. For protons, Mosaiq EMR has a special function for each treatment field, entitled QA. This function is used to upload to Mosaiq the field strength of the last bending magnet so that this parameter can be verified for each treatment. Doses are not recorded in the EMR when Mosaiq QA is used. Patient treatment field delivery using the Mosaiq QA option with the Hitachi system in treatment mode must be performed for each field before patient treatments can be delivered.

Verification of the treatment parameters is performed independently in the Hitachi delivery system and in a joint fashion between the Hitachi system and Mosaiq. The details are important regarding which information is available in which system. For example, the TPS provides the energy of the proton beam required to treat the required depth. The delivery system needs to provide the correct energy from the accelerator and set the correct beam optics parameter to have the desired energy to exit the nozzle. For photons, there is one beam energy per field, for example, 6 MV. For IMPT, there are multiple beam energies per field, for example, 33 different beam energies. The nozzle beam optics must be changed for each beam energy. Thus, the verification of the magnetic field strength for the final gantry bending magnet is an important check to ensure that the delivered spot is appropriate.

Treatment mode of the Hitachi system is not very efficient for physics to deliver the same field multiple times to measure the dose distribution at various depths as part of the pretreatment patient QA process. Thus this part of patient-specific QA work is performed in physics mode. The communication within the Hitachi delivery system between the treatment mode and the physics mode is nonexistent, so the same patient information must be communicated in a different manner, outside of the EMR. The current method of transferring information from the TPS to the treatment device in physics mode is through the use of a memory stick, which is an old-fashioned approach and frowned on by information security.

Both therapists and physicists must interact with the Hitachi system through the human-machine interface. There are three major phases in this interaction, namely, the download phase, the setup phase, and the irradiation phase. Verification in the Hitachi system has two different components, namely, the clinical verification and machine verification. Clinical verification confirms that the verify switch is IMPAC (now called Mosaiq) and that certain basic parameters have been set, including patient, gantry, dose monitor, and 6 degrees of freedom (DOF) couch. The machine verification displays the status of very specific machine parameters that are required to deliver the treatment. Treatments begin with the therapist first interacting with the EMR and downloading patient treatment parameters to the delivery system. The delivery system must internally confirm certain parameters and communicate their correct settings back to the EMR before the next steps can be taken in the delivery system. There is a constant communication check between the EMR and the delivery system.

Treatments do not always proceed as expected in that the treatment delivery system may abort itself during treatment because of electronic noise or encountering some unexpected setting. The ability to recover correctly from an unexpected abort during an IMPT treatment is important. With our system, when an abort occurs and treatments are only partially delivered, the Hitachi system uploads to Mosaiq the number of control points and spots per control point that have been delivered. This is accurate to within one spot. The Mosaiq system has the ability to record the partial treatment and then calculate the remaining control points and spots that remain to be delivered. This partial plan can then be downloaded back to the delivery system and the remaining treatment delivered. MDACC has developed additional software that analyzes the Hitachi logs in the event of an abort. This software provides an independent tool to review the performance of the delivery system and to focus on conditions that may be causing the system to abort during treatments. These conditions include the name of the field being delivered, the gantry angle, and the specifics regarding control points and spot numbers. The exact point where the system aborted (beam energy, spots delivered at this energy) is easily determined. This MDACC-developed software, which sends emails to both proton physics and the Hitachi service and maintenance leaders, is much easier to use and much quicker than reviewing the Hitachi logs. The number of aborts per day varies over the years depending on the conditions of the system. Currently, the system is aborting once or twice per day. Recovery to deliver the remaining dose of a partially treated field could be changeling in treatment mode. The accelerator and EMR vendors are encouraged to optimize the delivery work flow, including recovery of partial treatment. It should be remembered that the inability to deliver the entire spot pattern will result in a portion of the target volume receiving less than the daily prescribed dose. This is different than the situation with scattered protons or photons in which the entire treatment volume may receive less than the desired dose.

In summary, IMPT treatment requires that, before treatment, each treatment field is run to upload specific treatment parameters from the delivery system to the EMR system. Thus QA must always be performed before the first treatment. Generally, but not always, IMPT treatment delivery works well, assuming that the required steps are taken in order. The delivery system does occasionally abort. There are established mechanisms for partial treatment with EMR and treatment delivery system.

Every patient has their own specific IMPT treatment plan. The treatment plan generally has more than one field. Each field has a number of proton energies. Each energy has a number of different spots. Each spot has a specific location and a certain dose (MUs) to be delivered. The net result from each field is a 3D dose pattern, which can be highly modulated. The TPS provides a dose pattern based upon the patient's anatomy. Generally, the first step in patient-specific QA is to convert the dose pattern in the patient to a dose pattern in water phantom. Three-dimensional dosimetry systems are in active development but are not in routine use at MDACC. There are well-established 2D ion chamber array dosimetry systems in routine use, for example, the MatriXX.[6] Multiple 2D measurements can be made to approximate the 3D dose pattern, or

TABLE 7.2 ■ **Gamma Index Passing Rate for Fields Delivered at Treatment Gantry Angles**

Field	Gantry Angle (Degrees)	Snout Position (cm)	SSD (cm)	Depth (cm)	Gamma Index (3%/3 mm)
ALPPB	110	21	268	2.0	95.7%
BPAPB	180	25	265	5.0	99.9%
CLAPB	65	19	268	2.0	90.7%

SSD, Source-to-skin distance.

TABLE 7.3 ■ **HPlusQA Versus Eclipse Gamma Index Passing Percentages**

Field	Depth (cm)	Gamma Index Passing Percentage (3% Dose, 3-mm DTA)
ALPPB	2.0	96.3%
	2.9	97.6%
BPAPB	5.0	98.8%
	9.9	100%
CLAPB	2.0	87.9%
	3.9	98.3%

DTA, Distance to agreement.

measurements can be made at only one depth, which will confirm the spot pattern at that depth. Table 7.2 displays the results of measurements made with the MatriXX versus calculations using a 3%/3-mm dose-distance agreement criteria. Some 90% or more of the pixels passed this criterion.

The entire dose pattern must be delivered for each field. There are no shortcuts, such as limiting the number of MUs delivered. Every 2D measurement may require 2 to 5 minutes per field to deliver. This will limit the number of 2D measurements made for QA and other purposes.[7]

The time required for patient-specific IMPT measurements and the limitations of these measurements serve as an inspiration to consider additional approaches to IMPT QA. One approach, which is in use at MDACC, is to calculate the dose pattern using a second, completely independent system, using the field parameters provided by the TPS.[8] The number of 2D measurements to be made and the number of independent calculations performed per field per patient are ongoing issues. Table 7.3 displays the comparison at different depths of the dose calculated by the MDACC independent dose calculation system, HPlusQA, and the commercial TPS.

The agreement is quite good except for one shallow depth. Monte Carlo calculations are currently being implemented as the secondary independent dose calculation engine to increase the confidence of dose verification.

As part of the routine patient QA program, an analysis is done of the Hitachi treatment logs, which are collected after delivering the treatment fields.[9] The measured spot position location is compared with the spot position from the treatment plan. Table 7.4 presents the analysis of these log files.

TABLE 7.4 ■ **Analysis of Log Files Generated Through Delivering Treatment Fields With Mosaiq in Quality Assurance Mode and Proton Therapy Treatment Control System in Clinical Mode**

Field ID	Gantry Angle (Degrees)	Number Layers	Number Spots	Mean Deviation/STD *X* (mm)	Mean Deviation/STD *Y* (mm)	Mean Deviation/STD MU (%)
ALPPB	110	37	1973	0.26/0.14	0.20/0.35	−0.05/0.54
BPAPB	180	47	1910	0.01/0.17	0.16/0.20	−0.05/0.47
CLAPB	65	32	3144	0.19/0.21	−0.07/0.34	0.03/0.61

STD, Standard deviation.

The spot scanning beam is in use to treat patients from early in the morning (4 a.m.) to late at night (11 p.m.), 5 days per week. The time required to treat one patient depends upon the disease site being treated. Genitourinary (GU) patients can be treated within 15 minutes, whereas head and neck patients require approximately 30 minutes. The three most commonly treated disease sites are head and neck, brain, and GU. There are a small number of patients with other diseases being treated, including gastrointestinal, gynecologic, and lung. Not all patients who are being treated with spot scanning receive IMPT treatments, as some plans are designed using the single-field optimization technique.

Motion Management

Organ motion management in IMPT treatments is an important topic for all treatment sites, but especially for targets in the lung and upper abdomen. Kubiak has recently published a review article on particle therapy of moving targets.[10] This article notes that the main approaches to moving particle irradiation include gating, rescanning/repainting, gated rescanning, and tumor tracking. The author clearly states his opinion that "it is absolutely necessary to minimize the negative influence of target motion on radiotherapy precision by the proper use of motion compensation techniques." The author further opines that standard planning target volume or breath-hold techniques have insufficient usefulness in particle therapy. Another recent article from the Particle Therapy Co-Operative Group (PTCOG) Thoracic and Lymphoma Subcommittee concludes that "Active motion management (e.g., breath hold), beam gating, rescanning, tracking, or adaptive planning may be needed for cases involving significant motion or changes in motion or anatomy over the course of treatment."[11] Motion management with scanned proton beams remains an active area of research and development.

MDACC has used a very cautious approach to the motion management challenge with the scanned proton beam. All patients, for whom motion may be an issue, have four-dimensional computed tomography (4D CT) scans. Patients whose targets demonstrate substantial motion in 4D CT simulation studies are not considered to be good candidates for IMPT. Breathhold with the scanning beam is available for use. However, this approach can result in a very inefficient treatment delivery process and inherently is not a precise approach. MDACC has published its experience on clinical implementation of IMPT for thoracic malignancies with 34 consecutive patients.[12] All patients had a 4D CT scan with motion less than 5 mm. Individualized tumor-motion dose uncertainty analysis was performed for each patient. Plan robustness was optimized using a worst-case scenario method. During treatment, all patients had 4D CT verifications. Substantial work was performed for patients selected for IMPT treatment to address the motion question.

Adaptive planning is important for all proton treatments, including IMPT. The depth of the target can change as a consequence of the early portion of the radiation treatment. Thus the initial plan is adapted to account for changes in the target or in the normal tissue in the beam path. CT simulations, which are repeated, provide the opportunity to develop several adaptive plans during a course of treatment. Of course, every new plan requires a certain level of QA before being delivered to the patient.

In-Room Imaging for Intensity-Modulated Proton Therapy Treatments

The definition of a patient-specific reference point using image guidance is very important for IMPT treatments, as it is for all external beam radiation oncology treatments. In fact, the photon-based treatment systems may have better-integrated imaging systems than the proton systems with the imaging control system as another application of the treatment device. Newer proton systems are often equipped with cone-beam CT (CBCT) systems or with CT-on-rails systems. Older systems, such as the one at MDACC, are generally equipped with orthogonal x-ray systems (x-ray tube and flat-panel detector), which are attached to the gantry. Images are taken with the patient in the treatment position and compared by the therapists against reference images, which are provided by the TPS. Small couch adjustments can be defined, and the couch can be moved to a more correct position. The distances to be moved are uploaded from the patient image analysis system (PIAS) to the couch. A second set of images may or may not be taken. The Hitachi couch is a 6-DOF couch. However, there is a higher level of confidence when the couch motions are restricted to simple translational and rotational motions around the vertical axis. The rotational movements around the other two axes have not being used.

An interesting QA challenge, which can be addressed in part by the in-room imaging system, is couch alignments. Couches can become misaligned, either from routine use or from collisions with the gantries. A properly aligned x-ray system is very useful in confirming couch alignment.

Real-time tumor tracking, developed at Hokkaido University by Shirato et al., has been in clinical use on x-ray treatment devices since 2000. This system is now available on the new Hitachi proton systems. In fact, Hokkaido University Hospital began treatment in May 2016 with real-time image-gated and spot scanning proton beam therapy, using the Hitachi delivery system, and has published their experience with seven lung cancer patients.[13]

Future Intensity-Modulated Proton Therapy Directions at University of Texas MD Anderson Cancer Center Proton Therapy Center in Houston

In the 10 years or more that IMPT has been offered at MDACC, the basic technology is essentially unchanged. The available energies are the same and the spot sizes are the same, while the planning systems have improved. Modest technology changes at MDACC include the routine use of the energy absorber and the use of apertures to provide a sharper edge beam. A constant goal is to understand and to reduce uncertainties. The largest uncertainty is, of course, the uncertainty in human biology. Uncertainty has been reduced as clinical and technical experience has been gained with this unique tool. Motion management remains a challenging task. Limitations of real-time tumor tracking need to be understood. Clearly, patients with tumors in the thorax and in the upper abdomen potentially could benefit greatly from better motion management.

Modern scanning beam delivery systems have better imaging guidance technology, including CBCT and in-room CT on rails and robotic treatment couches, which offer greater flexibility for 3D in-room imaging. Robotic couches result in more flexibility for better treatments on the spot scanning line.

What subset of patients has increased local control and/or decreased toxicity with IMPT? MDACC continues to study this question. One future direction is to increase the number of protocol patients being treated with IMPT. Protocols that compare IMPT with intensity-modulated radiation therapy are of great academic interest and are being developed. Technology protocols are difficult for multiple reasons, for example, technology continues to evolve and may require large numbers of patients to reach a statistically valid answer.

There are interesting differences between treatment with passive scattered protons and spot scanning. With IMPT, treatment plans can be developed in which the beam reaches its range within the target. Thus, the small volume of higher relative biological effectiveness (RBE) can be taken advantage of. The result may be higher local control or lower toxicity. Protocols are being developed that will formally study this well-discussed RBE phenomenon.

One reoccurring solution to technology, for example, IMPT, is more technology. Future plans for IMPT may include additional imaging with positron emission tomography or magnetic resonance (MR). MDACC PTC has an MR unit that is being used for radiation oncology simulation purposes. A patient could be transported to or from the spot scanning beamline to the MR unit within approximately 1 minute. Potentially, this would permit daily MR-based adaptive planning or almost immediate tissue response to radiation. Certainly, imaging holds great potential to improve IMPT treatments. In-room dosimetry systems, for example, prompt gamma emission, potentially could reduce uncertainties in IMPT.

The future clearly will contain new machines. An MRI-guided proton therapy unit was described by Oborn et al. in 2017.[14] There will be other new treatment units. UT MDACC has made major contributions with its IMPT experience. Major contributions will continue to be made, even with 10-year-old equipment. Although the technology is important, the clinical team is more important. Dedicated radiation oncologists, who have a strong support team, are the key reason why IMPT has been successful at the MDACC Proton Therapy Center.

References Available Online.

SECTION III

Disease Sites

CHAPTER 8

Proton Radiotherapy for Breast Cancer

Wendy A. Woodward ■ Falk Poenisch ■ Karen E. Hoffman

Introduction

Numerous planning studies demonstrate superior dosimetry for proton radiotherapy compared with photon-based radiotherapy for breast cancers of all stages, even compared with intensity-modulated radiotherapy.[1] Protons can reduce dose to the heart by a factor of two to three compared with well-designed photon-based three-dimensional conformal plans, and target coverage is improved with protons.[2–9] An ongoing randomized clinical trial is comparing proton therapy to photon therapy to examine the effect on cardiac toxicity (NCT02603341). To date, however, clinical outcome data comparing protons to photons for breast cancer are limited, so translation of this dosimetric advantage remains under investigation, and access and cost may offset the obvious dosimetric gains in some cases. Reports of several hundred patients treated with protons have been published, and these highlight patient satisfaction and good early clinical outcomes in most studies[10–13] but increased skin toxicity and other side effects in others.[11,14–16] A broad range of dose regimens has been used, adding complexity to the analysis of the emerging data (Table 8.1). Here we briefly review the available data on dosimetric, clinical, and value related to proton therapy for breast cancer, highlight cases for whom there is an obvious benefit in the context of the existing data, and touch on planning issues to optimize outcomes. For all plan reviews, plans should be evaluated by physics before review by the radiation oncologist. Physics sign-off should confirm that the plan is robust. When multiple passive fields are used, each beam should be viewed independent of the others for complete coverage. For multiple-field-scanning beam planning, robust optimization, discussed below, should be used before physician review.

Complex Geometry/Locally Advanced Breast Cancer

A commonly spoken misconception about radiotherapy for breast cancer is that it is easy. Some of it is. When it isn't easy, though, breast cancer can present a vast array of unique and complex scenarios that arise from a combination of body habitus, disease factors, and surgical or systemic therapy choices that make tried-and-true breast radiation techniques suboptimal. Regional nodal irradiation (RNI; infraclavicular, supraclavicular, and internal mammary nodal basin coverage) is a primary driver of both lung and cardiac dose. Although these nodal basins can be treated within normal tissue constraints for many patients by using photon electron combinations, meeting the target goals and constraints can be impossible with photon- and electron-based therapy for patients where (1) depth to the internal mammary nodes is large, (2) involved nodal coverage requires significant coverage of internal mammary spaces directly anterior to the heart, or (3) a significant proportion of the overall lung volume lies in the supraclavicular field. Importantly, a meta-analysis of two randomized trials examining the benefits of RNI demonstrated increased overall survival in RNI-treated patients.[17] In complex geometry cases where RNI is warranted, the radiation oncologist often must compromise on the goals, perhaps using intensity-modulated radiation therapy and

TABLE 8.1 ■ **Clinical Breast Proton Data**

Publication	*n*	Median FU (Months)	Gy (RBE)/# Fractions	IBTRFS	Early Skin Toxicity (*n*)	Late Skin Toxicity	Good-Excellent Cosmesis
APBI							
Bush et al.[10]	100	60	40/10 once a day	97% (5 years)	0 MD	7% grade 1 telangiectasia	90%
Chang et al.[14]	30	59	30/5 once a day	100% (5 years)	1 MD		69% (at 3 years)
Galland-Girodet et al.[15]	19	82.5	32/8 twice a day	89% (7 years)	NR	54%–69% late skin toxicities	62% (MD at 7 years); 92% (PRO)
MDACC[a]	113	36	34/10 twice a day	100% (3 years)	0 MD	23% telangiectasia	NR
LABC						***grade 2 esophagitis***	
Cuaron et al.[11]	30	6	50.4/28	NA	8 MD	$n = 8$	1 grade 3 reconstructive complication
MacDonald et al.[12]	12	2	50.4/28 (nodal dose 45)	NA	9 grade 2 skin	$n = 0$	NA
Mutter et al.[13]	12	10	50/25	NA	1 MD, 5 grade 2 skin	$n = 2$	1 small dehiscence
Verma et al.[16]	91	15.5	50.4/28 + 10/5 boost	NA	~7 treatment break	$n = \sim30$	NA
Bradley et al.[19]	18	20	50.4/28 + 10/5–16/8 boost	NA	~4 grade 3 skin tox	$n = 5$	NA

[a]Unpublished.

APBI, Accelerated partial breast irradiation; *FU,* follow-up; *IBTRFS,* ipsilateral breast tumor recurrence-free survival; *LABC;* locally advanced breast cancer; *MD,* moist desquamation; *MDACC,* MD Anderson Cancer Center; *NA,* not applicable; *NR,* not reported; *PRO,* patient-reported outcomes.

accepting a higher heart and lung dose or lowering the dose to the target to achieve safe constraints. Numerous dosimetric studies demonstrate that these challenges can be overcome for patients with complex anatomy by using proton therapy.[1–4,8,9,18–26] Efforts to create objective indications for patients for whom geometric challenges merit proton therapy have been published, including the work by Mailhot Vega et al. demonstrating value for all patients with one or more cardiac risk factors for whom the mean heart dose would otherwise be greater than 5 Gy.[27] This recommendation is based on clear demonstration that protons can reduce left anterior descending coronary artery dose and mean heart dose.[28] The ongoing randomized photon versus proton RadComp trial will determine if improvements in dosimetry from using proton therapy will improve clinical cardiac toxicity from breast radiotherapy among unselected patients receiving RNI (NCT02603341).

Postmastectomy Radiation Planning

Planning begins with obtaining planning computed tomography (CT) images, paying careful attention to setup and immobilization including head position.[20,25,29,30] The physician draws the clinical target volume (CTV), which the physicist edits to create a scanning target volume (STV). The STV excludes 5 mm for the skin rind and includes a distal margin on the CTV calculated based on the range (~3.5%). Reducing the distal margin can avoid overshooting into the lung because the chest wall thickness for those patients is rather small (~5 mm), but it must be balanced with the concern that an adequate dose is delivered to the tissues immediately anterior to the chest wall, and in some cases, the chest wall itself. In most cases, photon/electron treatments of locally advanced postmastectomy targets would fully cover the chest wall in the target, and this should be considered in the patient selection and planning process.

To avoid tangential beam entrance, an en face beam is preferred, and thus often only one beam with one ideal angle is needed. This is achieved by a 30-degree beam from the anteroposterior direction, with ±10-degree variation, depending on the patient's setup. Given the field size limit of 30 cm, in some cases, the full volume cannot be encompassed in one field, and a two-isocenter plan is used with two junctions during the course of treatment. In this case, field-specific targets may be created, and each field would have at least a 4-cm dosimetric overlap to have a smooth transition at the junction of both beams.

Robust optimization should be performed to ensure that coverage is not overly affected by variation in setup and anatomy. If a single-field plan is used, robust optimization may have little benefit.

SILICONE IMPLANTS

Implants are a major driver of complex geometry in patients with locally advanced breast cancer. We have demonstrated that implants and reconstruction can compromise optimal electron/photon plans.[31–33] This could be overcome with the dosimetric advantages of protons. Because the silicone material is very uniform and the range prediction is very good, the planning is very similar to that for the mastectomy case discussed earlier, taking a correction for the stopping power of silicone into account.

To determine this correction, we tested three different silicone types (smooth, rough surface, and profiles) from two different vendors (Mentor and Allergan). The first step was to determine the water-equivalent range of the different types of tissue expanders (TEs). The silicone material stopping power does not lie on the CT calibration curve (Hounsfield unit [HU]-to-stopping power conversion curve) for human tissue because of its rather high Z number (14) compared with human tissue, which has an average Z-number of 7. Thus its HU value in CT is overestimated, and the HU value must be overridden to avoid underranging the proton beam and thus missing the distal target.

To obtain the HU value, we scanned all implants by using a Siemens Definition Edge CT scanner and its clinical CT protocol used for patient treatment planning CT scans. The devices were positioned along the CT's *z*-axis in such a way that they do not overlap and thus do not cause any attenuation artifacts. The material properties and the measured HU numbers are shown in Table 8.2. The overestimated relative stopping powers based on HU values are shown in the last column.

The experimental setup is shown in Fig. 8.1. The result of the measured dose and its different depth in water is shown in Table 8.3. The ratio between the water difference and the thickness of the spacer results in the relative water-equivalent stopping power. The weighted

TABLE 8.2 ■ **Parameters and Properties of Silicone Implants**

	Surface	Shape	Volume (cc)	Measured Hounsfield (HU)	Estimated. Relative Stopping Power
	Rough	Teardrop	445	92 ± 3	1.0828
Mentor	Smooth	Round, high profile	650	90 ± 4	1.0811
Allergan Naturelle	Smooth	Full round	445	93 ± 3	1.0836

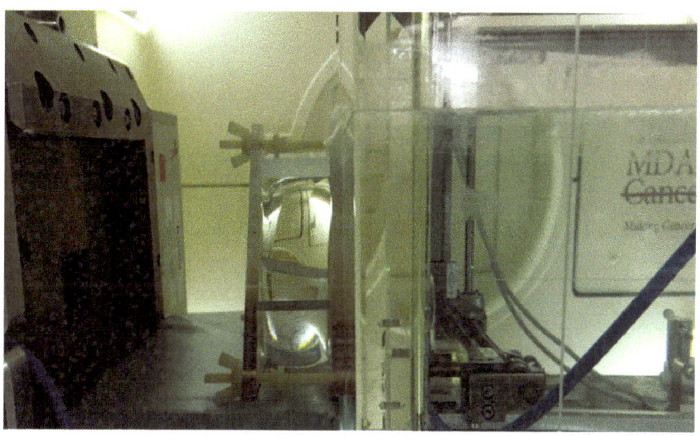

Fig. 8.1 Experimental setup to determine water equivalent thickness using a 5 × 5 cm^2 field aperture block, a snout position of 20 cm, and a source-to-skin distance setup of 270 cm. The silicon was squeezed slightly inside a homemade vice that had and defined acrylic spacer, thus providing two parallel acrylic surfaces. A 160-MeV beam of range of 13 cm and 10-cm spread-out Bragg peak were used, and the percentage depth dose curve was measured.

TABLE 8.3 ■ **Relative Stopping Power Measurement**

Measured Range (cm)	Range Difference in Water (cm)	Spacer Thickness (cm)	Relative Stopping Power
6.962	3.987	4.318	0.9233
6.307	4.642	4.967	0.9345
6.908	4.041	4.318	0.9358

average of the water-equivalent value for silicon is about 0.933 ± 0.010. This corresponds to the HU value in our HU-to-stopping power conversion table of −89. This is the correct override factor to be used by the dosimetrist to override any silicone implants. The variation between those three samples is around 1%. Thus, our range prediction in Eclipse and its agreement with the actual dose to the patient is very accurate, and the distal margin can be very small (1–2 mm).

TISSUE EXPANDERS

TEs represent the greatest challenge to treatment planning because of the presence of metal inside the surrounding irradiation area. In proton therapy planning, passing a proton beam through an area of metal is undesirable. The design of TEs is fairly consistent across vendors. They consist of an injection dome, a needle damper, a needle guard, and a magnet. Therefore knowing the model and make of a TE does not affect the planning strategy. Drawings provided by some manufacturers can help to understand the thickness of the different components because those cannot be measured by the CT because of large CT artifacts. An x-ray image taken for setup before treatment provides a better understanding of the dimension without distortion from artifacts (Fig. 8.2). A CT image of a TE is shown in Fig. 8.2C. The magnet appears as a circular object instead of a narrow rectangle (see Fig. 8.2B). In Eclipse version 13.7, we override to a CT value over 2500 HU because the HU-stopping power table is not linear above that HU threshold. Because the overridden area is bigger than the actual dimension of this object, we need to avoid the proton beamlet passing through this contour. Beamlets can, however, stop in front of this structure. In addition, one can see the outer thin-walled stainless structure, where the HU value is below 2500 attributed to a partial volume effect. Therefore, this structure is not overridden. The soft tissue artifacts, however, are overridden to HU = 0.

Two treatment planning system optimization algorithms are used to determine the spot position as well as weights of the spots: (1) the proton convolution superposition (PCS), and (2) the newer nonlinear universal proton optimizer (NUPO) that supports robust optimization, which has been available since Eclipse version 13.7. The NUPO algorithm avoids sharp gradients and can produce a robust plan with regard to setup and range uncertainty. However, whether those uncertainties are met must always be verified by calculating plan uncertainty doses. A NUPO plan can be as poorly robust as a traditional PCS plan, and a PCS plan could be more robust than

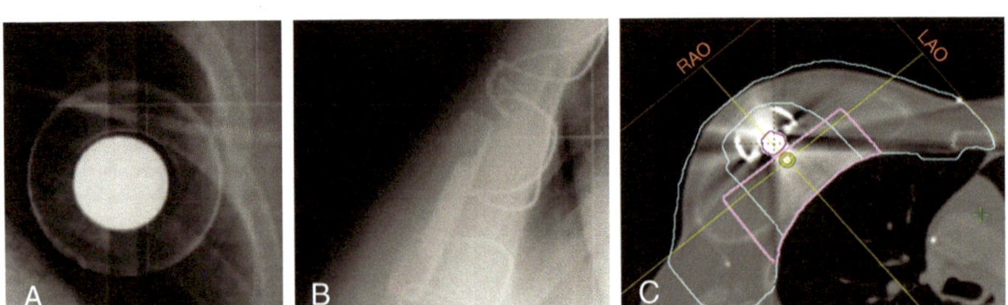

Fig. 8.2 X-ray image of tissue expander: (A) Anteroposterior direction, and (B) lateral. The outer light-gray ring is 36 mm diameter and consists of a 0.25-mm-thick wall; the center white circle is caused by the neodymium magnet, which is about 13 mm in diameter. (C) Transaxial computed tomography slice through the central portion of the tissue expander: the magenta contoured object is the neodymium magnet with a very high Z of 60, thus producing very large artifacts.

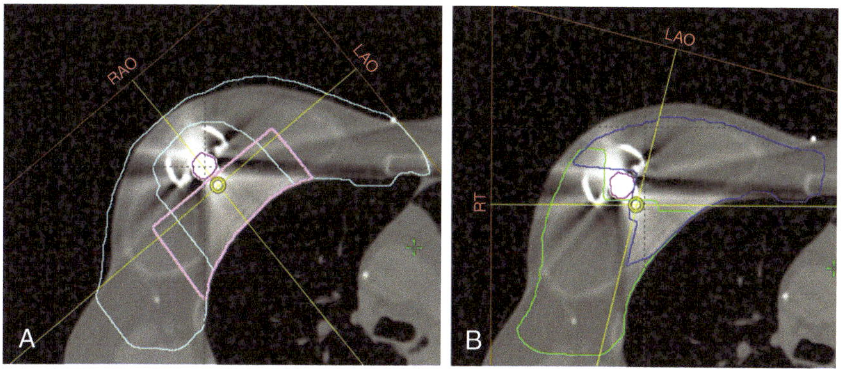

Fig. 8.3 (A) Field arrangement for 1+1 patch field: the primary field is the right anterior oblique *(RAO)* beam (treating the *cyan-colored* target), and the left anterior oblique *(LAO)* beam (treating the *purple* target) fills in the patch from the missing dose behind the tissue expander. (B) Field arrangement for the two oblique fields. The right lateral beam (treating the *green* target) and the LAO beam (treating the *blue* target) treat about the same total volume. There are small overlap areas anteriorly and posteriorly to the port ensuring full target coverage. *RT*, right.

a NUPO plan; it depends on anatomy, beam angle selection, field target selection, and planning objective. Furthermore, the NUPO plans do have fewer dose gradients and therefore do not produce good results when a gradient caused by a heterogeneous object (e.g., metal) is present. On the other hand, the NUPO method is the preferred technique, and one should create a plan first with this method and check whether it is robust. If the results are not good, the PCS algorithm can be used.

Because of the presence of metal, at least two beams with enough hinge angle to cover the target behind the port are used. This requires the use of a multifield optimization technique, where both individual fields have heterogeneous dose but, combined, provide a uniform dose. Examples:

1+1 patch field technique: This approach consists of two fields (Fig. 8.3A) in which the en face beam treats almost the entire breast, excluding a 5-cm-diameter cylindrical area behind the TE. This rather small cylindrical volume is treated by the left anterior oblique (LAO) beam. The LAO beam has a slightly steeper angle than the port. The marked targets are the area where spots can be placed from the individual beam. In this figure, there is an area around the port that is not covered by either target. This results in cold spots there. This is not an issue clinically because this is artificial, nonbiologic material.

Two-field oblique technique: The two-field oblique technique uses two beams that have a hinge angle of more than 100 degrees (Fig. 8.3B). This is the preferred technique because it is more robust as a result of the transition area being in homogenous material. Fig. 8.3B shows two overlapping fields (anterior and posterior to the port) that create a smooth transition and thus a smaller dose gradient in this overlap area. The advantage is that the tissue behind the port (around the chest wall) is treated with at least one beam that did not penetrate any metal object.

Dosimetric Results

The 1+1 patch plan shows the most homogenous dose distribution and the best dose-volume histogram in the nominal plan (Fig. 8.4). However, plans must be compared in regard to their robustness. Eclipse allows calculation of plan uncertainty doses that can include either setup or range uncertainty or a combination of both. Although the range uncertainty is the most sensitive

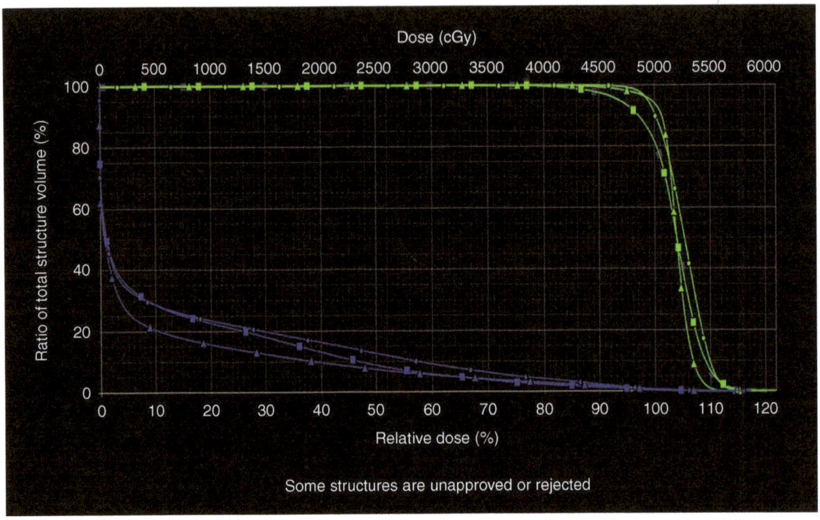

Fig. 8.4 Dose-volume histogram comparing three plans: 1+1patch_PCS *(triangle)*, 2Obl_PCS *(circle)*, and 2Obl_NUPO *(square)*.

one when doing patching fields, we also analyzed the setup uncertainty (Fig. 8.5). The 1+1 patch plan produces a very large hotspot of over 140% inside the ribs and in the lung. The 2Obl_NUPO plan, however, does not show such an effect. The 2Obl_PCS is not as robust as the NUPO plan, but the coverage is better. Another planning aspect is the lung dose, which is generally quite high for the ipsilateral lung because the target abuts it. For planning, it would help to create a separation between lung and target.

Accelerated Partial Breast Irradiation

Numerous efforts have been directed toward increasing the convenience of postlumpectomy radiotherapy for breast cancer. One approach is to offer accelerated partial breast irradiation (APBI) to appropriate candidates. National consensus guidelines define candidates for APBI based on oncologic variables. Technical feasibility is a second critical element for choosing APBI candidates. The APBI approach seeks to target the tumor bed plus margin for the postlumpectomy site with short, high-dose regimens, typically 1 week or shorter. The rationale is that cosmesis will not be compromised if the high-dose regimen is localized to a small component of the total breast. Thus the first critical technical factor is the ability to clearly identify the tumor bed. The second is the ability to adequately cover the tumor bed while sparing a significant portion of the nontarget breast tissue. Protons facilitate targeting of eccentric or irregular tumor bed volumes, an advantage over catheter-based approaches, without significant dose to nontarget tissue, an advantage over photon-based APBI.[3,7,8,20,26] In some patients with small cup sizes, this is sometimes the only external beam approach that meets standard dose constraints, thus affording the patient a partial breast treatment option.

APBI has been offered on protocol to patients at several institutions over the past decade, and 5-year clinical outcomes have now been reported.[10,14,15] Doses, outcomes, and toxicity are noted in Table 8.1. Galland-Girodet et al. report that single fields are associated with greater skin toxicity. Both Chang et al. and Galland-Girodet et al. conclude that multiple fields are recommended to

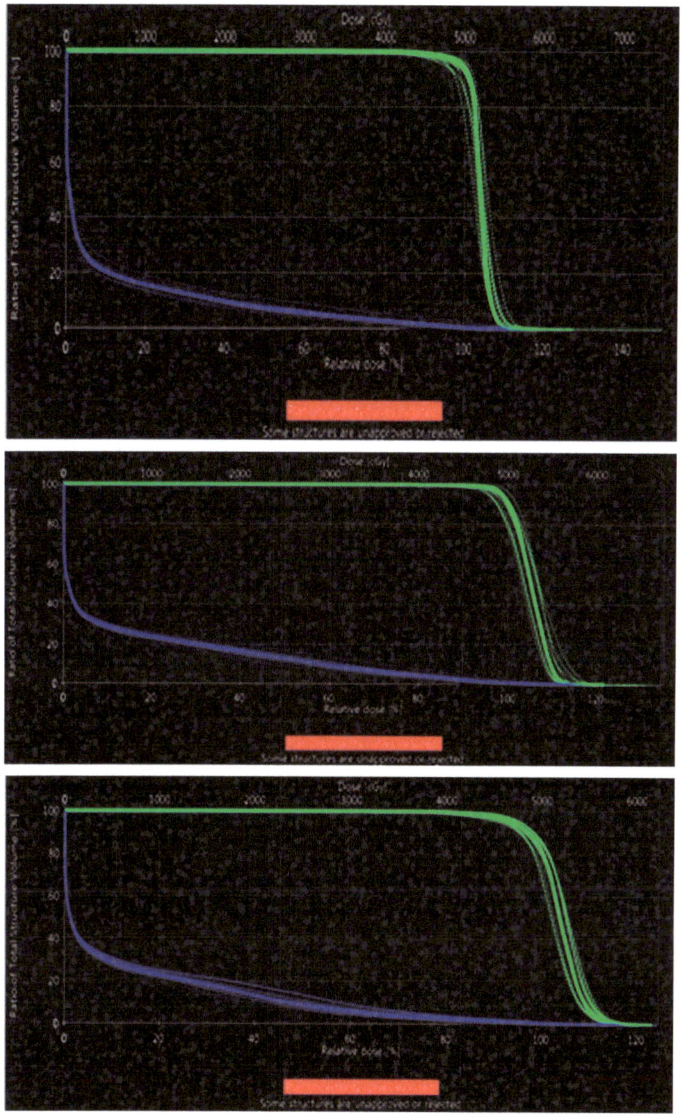

Fig. 8.5 Plan uncertainty dose-volume histogram using 3-mm setup uncertainty or 3.5% range uncertainty. The dotted lines are the uncertainty plan; the solid line, the nominal plan. *Top:* 1+1Patch_PCS, *Middle:* 2Obl_PCS, *Bottom*: 2Obl_NUPO.

reduce late skin toxicity, predominantly telangiectasia and hyperpigmentation. Recht et al. identified dose-volume constraints that predict increased rates of pneumonitis if coplanar beams are used.[34] As a whole, the literature points to the benefit of multiple, en face, noncoplanar beams to reduce side effects, and all 1-week regimens report notable skin toxicity. In the face of excellent patient satisfaction, this may not deter the use of APBI but should be discussed with patients. Notably, most published studies used passive-scattered proton therapy, and future studies are likely to use scanning beam technology, which may change the toxicity profile.

Simulation and target delineation: Setup and immobilization are critical for all proton therapy cases. Several immobilization techniques have been described.[20,24,25,35] An optimal APBI setup would immobilize the breast into the most spherical shape possible to facilitate ideal planning using multiple en face beams. Tangential proton beams are not considered robust, as small differences in setup can have a significant effect on coverage.[8] For this reason, using a supine setup, if the arm can be positioned down to mound up the breast, is preferred. An extra-large vac-loc cradle facilitates stability of the adducted elbow. For laterally positioned breast lumpectomy scars, the arm must be raised. In this case, consideration can be given to a slight lateral decubitus positioning to mound the breast as much as possible. At all times, personalized positioning based on anatomy and target knowledge is needed. Given that the target for APBI is anterior to all bony structures and is often mobile, bony anatomy is not a useful surrogate for set up. As depicted in Fig. 8.6, placement of radio-opaque markers, including a wire on the scar and small metal balls (BBs) on the breast mound, ensure that the soft tissues of the breast are appropriately localized before treatment. In general, published CTVs are similar to those for photon-based APBI described in RTOG 0413 (NCT00103181). CTV expansions are limited by the chest wall and 5 mm rind of skin and range from 1 to 1.5 cm.

Planning: Using radio-opaque markers, a 5-mm radial planning target value (PTV) margin is adequate for most APBI patients.[25] Range-specific distal PTV margins are calculated. Three beam plans are preferred, and noncoplanar beams are selected to optimize en face dosimetry, taking collision issues and skin sparing into account. Ideally, the beams will not overlap completely on the skin. If passive planning is used, compensators are designed to place the thinnest area in the center of the aperture and to create isolines that are symmetric with total compensator thickness less than 4 cm.

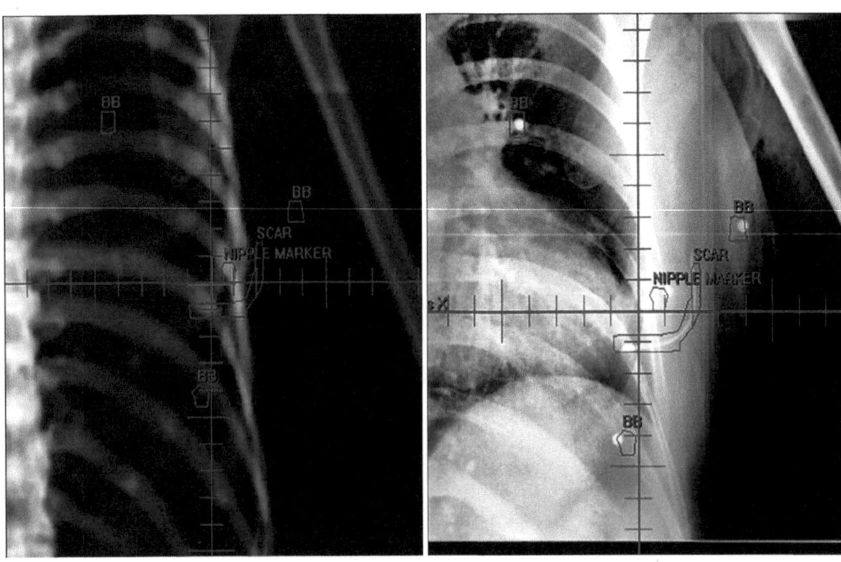

Fig. 8.6 Radio-opaque wires and BBs are placed on the skin at the simulation. The scar is wired precisely. BBs are placed on the nipple and three nonlinear points on the breast mound, preferring patient skin features such as freckles or moles when present and appropriate. These marks are photographed and, when needed, noted on the skin with a marker for future reference. The same marks are placed at the time of treatment to obtain optimal positioning but removed before turning the beam on.

Value

A major challenge to the routine use of protons is the question of value. Is the benefit for what it costs comparable to other options? In the case of complex geometry where protons create a safe treatment that is not feasible with another modality using national guidelines for both coverage and normal tissue constraints, the answer is yes. Most of the time, however, the issue is not black and white; a safer solution may be afforded by protons, but whether that improvement is clinically meaningful has not been proven. Efforts to define predictors for and measurements of value have been published.[27,36–40] For APBI, the case is more straightforward. Several studies of charges demonstrate that APBI with protons is similar in cost to accepted standard-of-care approaches, including catheter-based APBI and hypofractionated whole breast irradiation.[7,39] Beyond APBI, Swedish oncologists estimate the percentage of Swedish breast cancer patients for whom benefit of protons adds value is around 10%, or 300 annually.[41] Lundkvist et al. report a cost per quality-adjusted life year (QALY) gained of 67,000 euro for the base case analysis of an average breast cancer patient. The cost per QALY gained would, however, be considerably lower if a population with a high risk of developing cardiac disease was treated.[36] In sum, most studies suggest value based on dose reductions if patients are properly selected for excess cardiac and pulmonary risks by using criteria such as those suggested by Mailhot Vega.[27]

Future Studies

Publication of additional clinical experiences will confirm or refute technical strategies to minimize telangiectasia in APBI and add confidence regarding optimal regimens. The RadComp trial will provide definitive evidence for or against the case for cardiac-sparing benefits with protons. Other important areas for study include the potential benefit in avoiding nontarget nodal basins both to reduce lymphedema risk and to leave these important immune system mediators undisturbed.

References Available Online.

CHAPTER 9

Adult Central Nervous System Tumors

David R. Grosshans

Introduction

For both primary and metastatic brain tumors, radiation therapy (RT) remains one of the standard treatment modalities. Although RT techniques using photons have greatly improved in recent decades, substantial concerns remain among both physicians and patients regarding the potential for long-term side effects after RT to the brain.

Adverse effects after RT to the brain are numerous. In consenting when patients give consent for therapy, potential damage to specific structures such as the optic chiasm, optic nerves, or spinal cord is often cited, which could result in vision impairment, paralysis, and so on. Thankfully, such side effects are relatively infrequent. However, subtler long-term side effects may be problematic for both patients and their families. This includes the potential for long-term cognitive deficiencies. Although deficits in memory formation are the most commonly studied in the field of radiation oncology, deficits in attention or other executive functions may be equally as debilitating. Remarkably little is known regarding the biological basis for the side effects. However, progress is being made in the pharmacologic prevention of side effects and with use of advanced photon techniques, such as hippocampal-sparing intensity-modulated RT (IMRT).[1–3] Proton therapy may offer much greater normal tissue sparing and thereby further decrease the incidence of the side effects.

Particle therapy, including proton therapy, is hoped to expand the therapeutic index of radiation for primary brain tumors. Unlike photons, as the proton beam passes through tissue, protons continuously slow down, and the rate at which they deposit dose increases along their path. The point at which all energy is depleted is termed the Bragg peak. Past the Bragg peak, virtually no extra dose is delivered, and hence, normal tissues distal to the target should receive virtually no radiation exposure. Based on these principles, assuming target volumes are adequately covered, RT with protons should offer equivalent disease control but with superior normal tissue sparing and hence a reduction in long-term adverse effects.

Presently within the United States alone, nearly 30 proton centers are in operation, with many more in the planning or development stage. Although proton therapy has been used in the treatment of a variety of primary brain tumors, no published randomized studies exist to document its clinical superiority in comparison with advanced photon techniques. In the setting of increased scrutiny from insurance providers, this may limit patients' access to proton therapy. In this review, we highlight the technologies used to deliver proton therapy as well as preliminary clinical studies of primary brain tumors, including gliomas, meningioma, and others. Finally, areas for additional study, including the use of advanced treatment planning techniques, are offered.

Gliomas: Low and High Grade

LOW-GRADE GLIOMAS

Gliomas have a broad spectrum of disease types with associated differences in outcomes.[4] Our understanding of the molecular profiles of these tumors continues to evolve rapidly and is now informing us which patients may achieve long-term survival. Mutational profiling is now the standard of care for lower-grade gliomas, including the World Health Organization (WHO) grades II and III. Broadly speaking, patients may be grouped as those having or not having mutations in isocitrate dehydrogenase (IDH). Although a descriptor of grade II or III may be assigned by pathologists, evidence suggests little difference in outcomes based on grade, but the presence of an IDH mutation indicates favorable prognosis.[5,6] Conversely for patients with grade II or III tumors where no IDH mutation is identified, these tumors may be classified as a "molecular glioblastoma (GBM)," and patients may experience rapid disease progression similar to that seen with grade IV GBM.

RT has an integral role in the treatment of low-grade gliomas, and although mutational status is now influencing therapeutic decisions, historically, treatment decisions have been based on tumor grade. For WHO grade II gliomas, combined-modality therapy has contributed to improved survival rates, and early RT is associated with improved progression-free survival.[7,8] However, the timing of RT that is, whether it is delivered as adjuvant or salvage therapy, remains controversial. The existing controversy centers on the negative effects of radiation on cognitive function and quality of life, which are of special importance in patients with a long life expectancy. For patients with WHO grade III tumors, adjuvant RT is considered standard, although, as noted, mutational profiling allows the prediction of favorable outcomes for subsets of patients. In particular, grade III gliomas with an IDH mutation have favorable outcomes, and numerous patients will achieve long-term survival similar to that seen for patients with WHO grade II tumors.[5,6,9] As such, these patients are at substantial risk for cognitive decline after RT.

Cognitive decline after cranial irradiation is especially problematic for brain tumor survivors, as it is associated with reduced quality of life.[10,11] Historically, the overwhelming majority of radiation treatments have been delivered using photon-based techniques. Douw et al. retrospectively evaluated patients with low-grade gliomas treated with or without RT and found RT use to be associated with impaired attentional functioning and executive function.[12] Gondi et al. prospectively evaluated the effects of radiation on cognitive function in adult patients with low-grade brain tumors treated with advanced photon radiation techniques, including IMRT.[13] The trial included both baseline and postradiotherapy assessments including formal neurocognitive tests. Exposure of the bilateral hippocampi to doses as low as 7.3 Gy was associated with long-term memory impairment.

Such evidence has led practitioners to believe that proton therapy may be ideally suited for the treatment of these tumors. In addition to compelling dosimetric studies, initial clinical studies of proton therapy have suggested efficacy.[14] Investigators from Massachusetts General Hospital (MGH) first used mixed photon/proton treatments for dose-escalation studies including patients with WHO grades II and III gliomas.[15] Investigators from the University of Heidelberg, which uses scanning beam proton delivery technology, have also reported on 19 patients treated for low-grade gliomas. Similar to photon-based treatments, their initial results suggest high rates of tumor control and acceptable toxicity rates.[16] The group at The University of Texas MD Anderson Cancer Center has also reported on outcomes after IMRT or proton therapy for these tumors.[17] Although the latter was a retrospective study, disease control outcomes were similar. However, patients with oligodendroglioma treated with protons developed pseudoprogression sooner than those treated with photons.[17] Formal cognitive testing outcomes were unfortunately not available. In a recent study, Shih et al. reported results of a prospective trial that enrolled patients with grade II gliomas.[18] In addition to reporting excellent disease control rates, they assessed cognitive function and quality of life after proton therapy. Twenty patients, all with supra-tentorial tumors, were enrolled. With a median follow-up time of 5.1 years, measures of cognitive function were stable to improved relative to baseline, with no patients experiencing cognitive failure. Sherman et al. reported that compared with normative practice effects, these patients exhibited less improvement in the domains of processing speed, executive function, and verbal memory.[19] However, because this was an uncontrolled, noncomparative trial, it is unclear if this relative stability reflects the absence of an expected practice effect in this treated population.

To provide the best evidence supporting the benefits of proton therapy in comparison with the best photon therapy (IMRT), randomized trials are needed. Historically, with a few exceptions, in the field of photon therapy, randomized trials have not been done to compare radiation techniques such as three-dimensional conformal versus IMRT. However, given that proton therapy is a fundamentally different form of radiation, it is not unreasonable that such trials be conducted. Currently, an ongoing randomized phase II trial is being conducted through the NRG Oncology Group, BN005 (clinicaltrials.gov identifier: NCT03180502). The schema for this trial is presented in Fig. 9.1. Eligible patients include those with an IDH mutant grade II

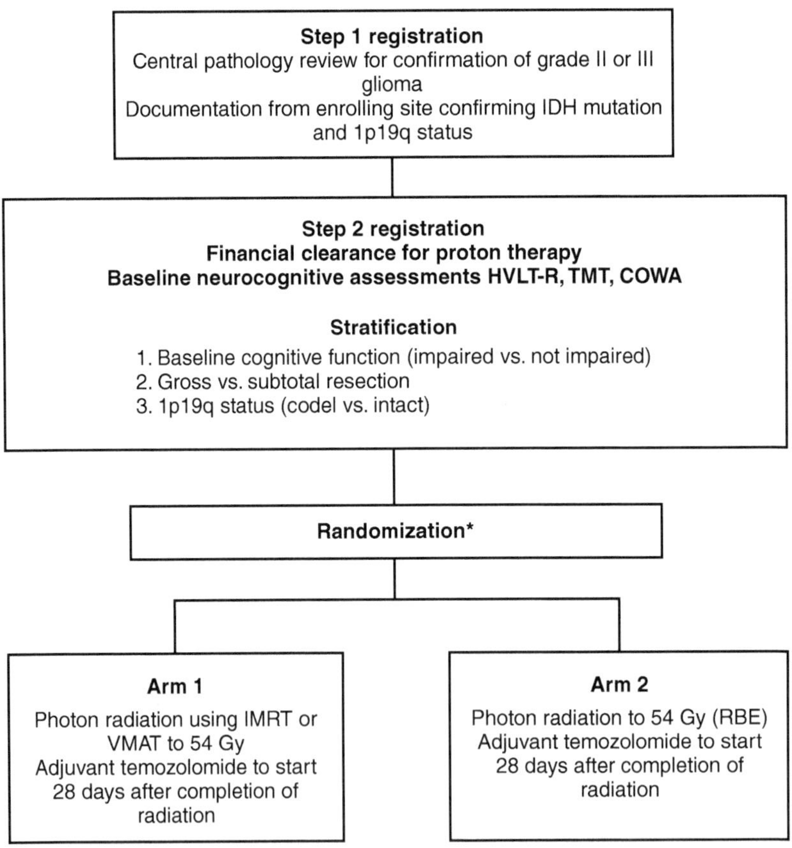

*Randomization is 2:1 in favor of protons
Impaired cognitive function requires a Clinical Trials Battery composite score <–0.5.

Fig. 9.1 Schema for NRG BN005, a phase II randomized trial of proton versus photon therapy (intensity-modulated radiation therapy; *IMRT*) for cognitive preservation in patients with IDH mutant, low- to intermediate-grade gliomas. *RBE*, Relative biological effectiveness.

or III glioma and are randomized to receive protons versus photons. The central hypothesis is that the normal tissue-sparing offered by proton therapy will lead to superior preservation of cognitive function and reduced symptom burden relative to patients treated with photon-based therapy.

HIGH-GRADE GLIOMAS

Glioblastoma multiforme (GBM) is the most common primary malignant brain tumor in adults. In contrast to grade II or III glioma, or grade IV glioma with mutations in IDH, GBM has a very poor prognosis. With the current standard postsurgical temozolomide-based chemoradiotherapy, overall median progression-free survival time is approximately 7 months, with overall survival time of 15 months.[20] Despite poor outcomes, even here, trials using proton therapy have been conducted.

Current recommendations for radiation include dosages up to 60 Gy given in daily fractions of 2 Gy to the enhancing area of the tumor with 1- to 2-cm margins. When this standard radiotherapy regimen is used, 80% to 90% of tumors recur within 2 cm of the original lesion. In an effort to improve tumor control, several groups have used proton therapy to escalate doses up to 90 Gy (relative biological effectiveness [RBE]) (Gy[RBE]). MGH treated 23 patients with GBM by using a combination of photons and protons to a total dose of 90 Gy(RBE) to the gross tumor volume, 64.8 Gy to the 2-cm margin encompassing the gross tumor volume, and 50.4 Gy(RBE) to areas of surrounding edema plus 2-cm margins using accelerated fractionation.[21] When patients were stratified by Radiation Therapy Oncology Group (RTOG) prognostic classes, this plan consistently increased median survival time. Dose escalation up to 90 Gy(RBE) yielded median survival times of 23, 17, and 14 months for RTOG classes III, IV, and V, respectively. This compares with the 17.9, 11.1, and 8.9 months median survival time for the respective classes seen in previous RTOG trials using standard doses of RT with chemotherapy.[22] Of the 23 patients, only one patient had tumor recurrence within the dose-escalated region. Despite the good control and increased median survival time, all 7 patients from whom tissue was obtained developed radiation necrosis, and most patients experienced neurological deterioration.

A more recent study from Tsukuba also escalated the dose to 96.6 Gy(RBE) over 56 fractions in 21 patients, most with RTOG class IV GBM, and obtained a median survival time of 21.6 months.[23] When stratified by the size of the enhancing tumor, acute side effects were found to be tolerable for patients with smaller tumor volumes. However, this study could not comment on late effects of the radiation because of the difficulty in distinguishing between tumor recurrence and necrosis on imaging. These studies demonstrate that dose escalation up to 96 Gy(RBE) with proton therapy provides effective local control and promising increases in median survival time.

NRG BN001 also incorporates proton therapy (clinicaltrials.gov identifier: NCT02179086) as part of a national trial. Although no direct randomization is done between protons and photons, BN001 uses either advanced photon or proton therapy to dose-escalate in patients with GBM. Secondary objectives of the trial will include indirect comparisons of the two radiation types in an attempt to determine if dose escalation may be more safely achieved with proton therapy. Notably, a randomized trial of protons versus photons has also been performed and indeed completed in patients with GBM. This was a single-institution trial performed at MD Anderson Cancer Center (clinicaltrials.gov identifier: NCT01854554). Patients with GBM were randomized to protons or photons and underwent serial cognitive testing, with preservation of cognitive function being the primary outcome. The results of this trial have not yet been reported. However, when assessing cognitive dysfunction, the presence of tumor in the brain parenchyma has dramatic negative impacts on cognitive function.[24] Indeed, evidence indicates that higher-grade or IDH nonmutant tumors are more likely to be associated with greater cognitive deficits at baseline.[25]

Meningioma

Meningiomas are the most common benign central nervous system tumors in adults and portend a generally favorable prognosis, as 90% are classified as WHO class I. Surgery is the mainstay of therapy, but radiation is used as adjuvant therapy in cases of partial resections and high-grade or recurrent lesions. RT can also be used as a definitive treatment for lesions in locations where resection is not possible. Long-term control rates with current RT techniques are greater than 90%.[26] Given the expected long-term survival, improving functional status and limiting toxicities are the objectives of treatment.

Given the proximity of skull base meningiomas to critical structures, particle therapy provides an opportunity to reduce toxicities. Wenkel et al. studied 46 patients with benign skull base meningiomas treated with a combination of photon and proton, and reported recurrence-free rates of 100% at 5 years and 88% at 10 years.[27] Four patients in this series experienced ophthalmic toxicity. In retrospect, doses to the optic nerves of these patients were found to exceed the threshold of 54 Gy when doses were recalculated after a recalibration of the particle accelerator. Patients who did not receive >54 Gy to the optic nerve did not experience any ophthalmic toxicity. Neol et al. studied functional outcomes of 51 patients with skull base meningiomas treated with a combination of photons and proton therapy.[28] Four-year local control and overall survival rates were 98% and 100%, respectively. Two patients (3.9%) suffered from grade III side effects. In addition, 68.8% of the eye-related symptoms improved after RT, and 67% of other miscellaneous symptoms improved, which compares favorably with photon studies reporting functional outcomes.[29–32]

Weber et al. from the Paul Scherrer Institute, which uses a pencil beam scanning–based proton treatment, studied 39 cases treated with only protons as part of RT.[33] At least 10 patients in this series had WHO grade II/III meningiomas, and the average tumor volumes were larger than most other series. Five-year local control and overall survival rates were 84.8% and 81.8% for all histology types and 100% for benign histology. The 5-year grade III/IV toxicity-free survival rate was 84.5%. Patients who experienced late-grade toxicity were those with large tumor volumes and optic tract meningiomas. Initial outcomes seem to support the use of particle therapy for meningiomas, especially for lesions in close proximity to critical structures. However, the study by Wenkel et al. demonstrates the need for careful planning to avoid adverse effects.

Unlike WHO grade I tumors, grade II or III meningiomas, although rare, may be more prone to local recurrence. This has prompted consideration of dose escalation for such tumors.[34] Investigators at MGH have begun enrollment on a prospective study of dose escalation using proton therapy for these aggressive malignancies (clinicaltrials.gov identifier: NCT02693990). As part of this phase I/II trial, intensity-modulated proton therapy (IMPT) for sequential dose escalation for patients with atypical or WHO grade III (malignant) meningiomas.

Pituitary Tumors and Vestibular Schwannomas

Pituitary adenomas are benign tumors found in the sella turcica. RT is typically used after medical and surgical therapies have failed; RT offers the potential for cure, even if the lesion is unresectable. Moreover, medical therapy may require lifelong treatment, or tumors may become refractory to medical management.

Two primary dose schedules are commonly used in RT for pituitary adenomas. Stereotactic radiosurgery (SRS) delivers a high-dose single-radiation treatment (typically 15–20 Gy), whereas fractionated schedules deliver 45 to 54 Gy over 5 to 6 weeks. It has been suggested that SRS normalizes hormone levels of functional adenomas faster than conventional fractionated RT.[35] However, the use of SRS may be limited in tumors located in close proximity to critical structures, such as the optic chiasm, because of the high doses prescribed.

Some institutions have started performing SRS with protons. Similar to fractionated proton therapy, proton SRS (PSRS) exhibits low entry dose and no exit dose, resulting in decreased risk of toxicity. MGH has studied PSRS in the treatment of adrenocorticotropic hormone– and growth hormone (GH)–secreting tumors. A total of 22 patients with residual GH-secreting tumors after transsphenoidal resection were treated using PSRS with a median dose of 20 Gy (RBE).[36] A complete response (CR), defined as sustained (≥3 months) normalization of insulin-like growth factor 1 levels, was seen in 59% of patients after a median of 42 months after radiotherapy. In another study, 38 patients with Cushing disease or Nelson syndrome were treated with PSRS for persistence of symptoms and cortisol levels after transsphenoidal resection.[37] At a median follow-up time of 62 months, CR was achieved in 100% (5 of 5) cases Nelson syndrome (5 out of 5) and in 52% (17 of 33) cases of Cushing disease. The median time to CR was 18 months after PSRS. In both studies, the portion of patients achieving CR and time to CR were comparable with previous SRS studies.[38–46] Also, no evidence of visual disturbances, seizures, or clinical signs of brain injury were noted. However, both studies experienced slightly higher rates of hypopituitarism after PSRS when compared with other SRS studies. Still, PSRS is a promising RT technique.

Like most pituitary tumors, vestibular schwannomas are benign intracranial tumors. These lesions are believed to arise from the myelin-forming cells of the vestibulocochlear nerve. Observation is a reasonable option for many patients, as many vestibular schwannomas are found only incidentally on imaging, and only 43% to 46% of tumors show any growth, with an average rate of 1.2 to 1.9 mm/year.[47] For tumors requiring treatment, surgery and RT can both be used as first-line treatments. Surgery offers excellent control rates and tends to be used to treat larger tumors with mass effects. Definitive RT is also a therapeutic option that offers excellent tumor control rates of greater than 90%. Although vestibular schwannomas treated with RT may have a reported lower incidence of adverse effects, including hearing loss or facial nerve palsies, compared with microsurgery, direct comparisons are difficult to make because tumors treated with microsurgery tend to be larger.[48]

Harsh et al. used a PSRS protocol prescribing 12 Gy(RBE) to the tumor and limiting the brainstem dose to 12 Gy(RBE) and found control rates of 94%, trigeminal and facial nerve preservation of 95.3%, and hearing preservation of 33.3%.[49] Low rates of hearing preservation were thought to be attributed to the patients being older (mean age = 67 years) and resections being done before RT, which may increase susceptibility to cranial nerve damage. Bush et al. used a fractionated protocol prescribing 54 to 60 Gy(RBE) in 30 to 33 fractions.[50] At a mean follow-up time of 34 months, the control rate was 100%, no trigeminal and facial nerve toxicities were observed, and 31% maintained useful hearing. Using the α-β model to compare doses in fractionated stereotactic RT and SRS studies, the protocol prescribed roughly 40% more radiation at standard fractionation. Prescribing an equivalent dose may have resulted in better-preserved hearing. Vernimenn et al. suggest that hypofractionated proton therapy may also be an option for large, inoperable tumors.[51] The average tumor volume in this series was 5.3 cm^3, which is among the highest studied. The protocol prescribed 26 Gy(RBE) over 3 fractions and reported a 5-year local control rate of 98%. At a mean follow-up time of 72 months, hearing preservation rate was 42%; trigeminal and facial nerve preservation rates were 93% and 90.5%, respectively. Baummert et al. compared dose distributions of photon and particle therapy and found that conformality was equal, but proton therapy reduced the integral dose. Because greater dose sparing is realized in larger lesions, particle therapy may be particularly useful for larger lesions.

Medulloblastoma and Other Malignancies

Although more common in pediatric patients, diseases such as medulloblastoma, ependymoma, and craniopharyngioma can also occur in adult patients. For pediatric patients, it is generally assumed that protons will be superior and lead to less long-term adverse effects, as children are likely more sensitive to radiation-induced normal tissue toxicity than adults. For each of the previously listed tumor types, survival outcomes are expected to be good to excellent for adult patients presenting with these tumors. As such, proton therapy is increasingly used for adult patients with these tumors.

For patients treated on the craniospinal axis, such as those with medulloblastoma, data are available to support the notion that proton therapy may have quantifiable benefits. Retrospectively comparing patients treated with photon or protons, Brown at al noted a decreased incidence in nausea and esophagitis with protons.[52] Importantly, patients treated with protons also had better maintained hematologic profiles.[52] With pediatric patients, practitioners typically treat the entire vertebral body to prevent late-growth asymmetries. However, with adults, this is not necessary; rather, in addition to anterior structures such as the heart and thyroid, most of the bone marrow can be spared, likely helping to maintain white blood cell counts.[53] This could be because these patients are likely to receive adjuvant chemotherapy and therefore may better be able to tolerate this treatment.

Diseases such as craniopharyngioma and ependymoma arising in adult patients are rare, and there are few reports of these treated with proton therapy. However, in pediatric patients, these tumors may be successfully treated with protons, and again, the low-dose sparing is expected to translate into a reduction in adverse effects.[54,55]

Radiation Techniques and Treatment Planning

Although the clinical studies reviewed earlier provide initial evidence in support of proton therapy for the treatment of primary brain tumors, most of these patients have been treated with what some may call antiquated proton technology. Similar to advances made in photon therapy in recent decades, proton therapy is a rapidly evolving technology.[56] Since 2010, the number of active centers treating patients, and publishing outcomes, has been small. Moreover, virtually all these centers used passive-scattered proton therapy (PSPT). With PSPT, physical elements are introduced into a broad proton beam to shape the distal and lateral edges. Nearly all new centers now offer only scanning beam proton therapy. With scanning proton therapy, small pristine proton beams are scanned magnetically to conform to the lateral edges of the target volume and energy changes control the depth of penetration. Scanning beam proton therapy allows maximally conformal, not only low-dose, but high-dose radiation (Fig. 9.2). Indeed, in comparing PSPT with IMRT, IMRT plans often may have better high-dose conformity. Scanning beam

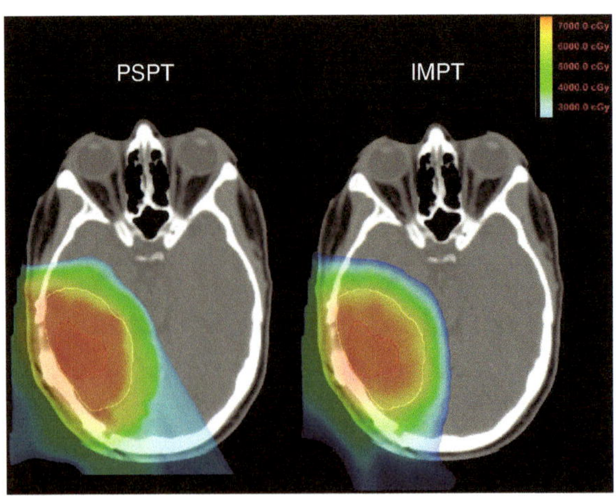

Fig. 9.2 Passive-scattered proton therapy *(PSPT)* and intensity-modulated proton therapy *(IMPT)* plans for a patient with glioblastoma with dose escalation. Note improved high-dose conformality with IMPT.

proton therapy also allows the delivery of true IMPT. With true IMPT, the optimizer has the flexibility to manipulate all beamlets within each proton field simultaneously to deliver a maximally conformal treatment plan. This review of the literature should account for the fact that most patients were treated with what may be considered first-generation proton therapy delivery techniques in which the normal tissue sparing in high-dose regions is not maximized.

Biological Consequences

New laboratory evidence is emerging that, biologically, protons are very different from photons.[57] However, in current clinical practice, protons and photons are considered to be very similar. The simplistic assumption is that the RBE of protons compared with photons is a constant of 1.1. In other words, it is assumed that protons are roughly 10% more effective in killing cancer cells than photons. In reality, as laboratory experiments have demonstrated, the biological effects of protons are very complex and can differ as a function of many factors. New evidence indicates that the capacity for proton beams to cause biological damage is substantially higher near the distal, high–linear energy transfer (LET) region.[58,59] As described earlier, in the current clinical practice of proton therapy, techniques such as PSPT are routinely used. For centers using a scanning beam, single-field optimized plans are frequently used, in which each beam covers the entire target volume. With such techniques, the distal high-LET regions of beams are nearly always in normal tissues distal to the target volume. In support of the status quo, it is commonly cited that no clinical data are available to suggest that the proton RBE is other than 1.1. However, in pediatric brain tumor patients, evidence is emerging that high-LET regions may be associated with increased rates of subclinical radiation damage.[60,61] In years to come, as investigators extract dose and LET information by using Monte Carlo or analytic techniques, understanding the impact of variable RBE in both pediatric and adult patients is anticipated to improve. Notably, true multi-field-optimized IMPT may allow high-LET regions to be selectively confined within the tumor volume, further sparing normal tissues from the damaging effects of radiation. However, to accomplish this, improved biologic effect models, as well as novel optimization techniques, are needed.

Conclusions and Future Directions

When this chapter was written, for adult brain tumor patients, only one randomized trial had been completed, and two others were ongoing. Although many practitioners question the need for randomized studies, proton therapy is relatively expensive, and increasingly, insurers are demanding evidence to support its use. As a community, it will likely be important to RT practitioners to support such endeavors if the field is to be advanced. As the cost to construct proton therapy facilities decreases, the hope is that more centers will have access to this technology. The expectation is that disease control rates will be similar to photon-based therapy and the hope is that toxicities will be less. Still, evidence is needed to support this notion and support the continued expansion of proton therapy centers.

In addition to considering new randomized studies, much can be learned about proton therapy from cohort or single-arm translational studies. The compact dose distributions offered by proton therapy may be effective in reducing radiation-induced lymphopenia, a treatment-related side effect not commonly appreciated.[62] Lymphopenia is increasingly being associated with poor outcomes. By sparing normal tissues that may harbor sensitive lymphocyte populations, proton therapy may reduce the incidence of treatment-related lymphopenia and even improve survival outcomes. Lymphocyte sparing may be of special importance as we begin to incorporate immunotherapy with radiation. Also within the research spectrum, opportunities remain for novel proton treatment planning and delivery techniques. This includes RBE- or LET-based optimization. Preferentially placing highly biologically damaging portions of the beam within the tumor volumes may improve tumor control or even increase immunogenicity while simultaneously lowering normal tissue exposure. Finally, overall tumor response may differ based on the genetic profile of the cancerous cells. If true, it could be possible to select patients, based on tumor genetic makeup, who might be expected to have a greater response to proton radiation than photon. All such studies should be carefully conducted in prospective trials.

Acknowledgments

Portions of this chapter have been adapted from Dinh JQ, Mahajan A, Pamler MB, Grosshans DR, *Particle therapy for central nervous system tumors in pediatric and adult patients*, Translational Cancer Research 2012;1(3):137-149 and Grosshans DR, Mohan R, Gondi V, Shih HA, Mahajan A, Brown PD, *The role of image-guided intensity modulated proton therapy in glioma*, Neuro-Oncology 2017;129(suppl 2):ii30-ii37.

References Available Online.

CHAPTER 10

Gastrointestinal

Emma B. Holliday ■ Prajnan Das

Introduction

Proton beam radiation (PBR) has the potential to improve the therapeutic ratio in the treatment of several gastrointestinal malignancies by decreasing the dose to nontarget critical structures. In general, radiotherapy to the abdomen and pelvis is challenging because of the inherent sensitivity of gastrointestinal organs to radiation toxicity.

GASTRIC

The Role of Radiation Therapy

Postoperative radiotherapy for gastric cancer was once the established standard of care on the basis of the Intergroup 0116 study showing the survival benefit of adjuvant fluorouracil-based chemoradiation (CRT) compared with surgery alone.[1] When CRT is administered, the prescribed dose is 45 to 50.4 Gray (Gy) in 1.8-Gy fractions, with higher doses sometimes considered for positive margins or gross residual disease. However, patients treated at most centers in Western countries are more likely to receive perioperative chemotherapy, which has also been shown to improve survival over surgery alone.[2] In Eastern countries, the practice is to routinely perform more extensive surgery, including D2 lymph node dissection, and chemotherapy is the preferred adjuvant treatment.[3] Patients with node-positive disease and intestinal-type histology did seem to benefit from adjuvant CRT when compared with adjuvant chemotherapy,[4] and this subset of patients is the subject of an ongoing trial.

Completion rates for adjuvant CRT and chemotherapy are historically poor, with 15% and 10% of patients not able to complete adjuvant CRT and chemotherapy, respectively, as a result of toxicity.[1,3] For this reason, a neoadjuvant therapy approach is currently favored at the University of Texas MD Anderson Cancer Center. In a cooperative group phase II trial, the pathologic complete response (pCR) rate and margin-negative resection (R0) rates were 26% and 77%, respectively, and 98% of patients were able to complete all therapy per protocol.[5]

The Rationale for Proton Therapy

Other efforts to decrease acute toxicity and improve the tolerability of CRT for gastric cancer have centered on the use of more conformal radiation techniques to minimize the normal tissue irradiated. Current US guidelines state that intensity-modulated radiation therapy (IMRT) may be used to reduce dose to organs at risk.[6] Studies have shown IMRT to be feasible and well tolerated in both the neoadjuvant and adjuvant settings.[7,8] However, IMRT leads to a larger volume of normal tissue receiving low radiation doses, which raises the concern for increased secondary malignancy rates.[9] PBR has the potential to improve nontarget tissue sparing and further improve the tolerability and therapeutic ratio for gastric cancer. Furthermore, PBR has the potential to reduce the secondary malignancy rates that have been reported in higher numbers after adjuvant CRT when compared with surgery alone on long-term follow-up.[10]

Dosimetric Studies

In the postoperative setting, PBR has been shown to reduce the volume of several normal organs receiving low to moderate doses.[11] One treatment planning study showed the median volume of small bowel receiving 15 Gy (V15) was 133 cc with IMRT and 82 cc with 2- to 3-field double-scattered-uniform scanning technique proton therapy. Mean liver and kidney doses were also lower with PBR compared with IMRT. Perhaps more importantly, a significantly lower mean heart dose was achieved with PBR compared with IMRT (7.4 Gy relative biologic effectiveness [RBE], assuming an RBE of 1.1 for protons compared with photons, vs. 9.5 Gy).[12] With data from long-term breast cancer survivors suggesting that the rates of major coronary events increase linearly with mean heart dose at a rate of 7.4% per Gy with no apparent threshold,[13] this suggests a meaningful reduction in late toxicity may be afforded by PBR in this population. Dionisi et al. also showed the robustness of PBR in the postoperative treatment of gastric cancer by reporting that target coverage on repeat verification computed tomography scans was within ±2% of the initial simulation scan.[12] This is important because one of the challenges of using PBR in the treatment of gastric cancer is the variability of gastric volume, contents, and the presence of gas. Appropriate volumes to account for uncertainties in day-to-day target volumes, as well as dietary management, such as following a low-residue diet and fasting for a defined period before treatment, are essential for the accurate and effective treatment of gastric cancer.[14]

Clinical Studies

The potential for both feasibility and clinically meaningful toxicity in the preoperative or inoperable settings can be extrapolated from work done in esophageal and gastroesophageal junction cancers. pCR rates and near-pCR rates were high with few severe toxicities in a prospective study performed at MD Anderson evaluating proton-based preoperative CRT to a dose of 50.4 Gy equivalents (GyE) for esophageal cancer.[15] A retrospective study of definitive proton-based CRT to 60 GyE performed at the University of Tsukuba likewise showed good control rates and very low rates of serious acute toxicities. Two case reports in the 1990s demonstrate the feasibility of using definitive PBR for inoperable advanced gastric cancer[16,17] and showed clinical CRs after 61 GyE in 35 fractions and 83 to 86 GyE, respectively. The potential dosimetric and clinical benefits of PBR for gastric cancer certainly merit further study. The specific location, size, and extent of tumor will likely influence the magnitude of benefit (Fig. 10.1).

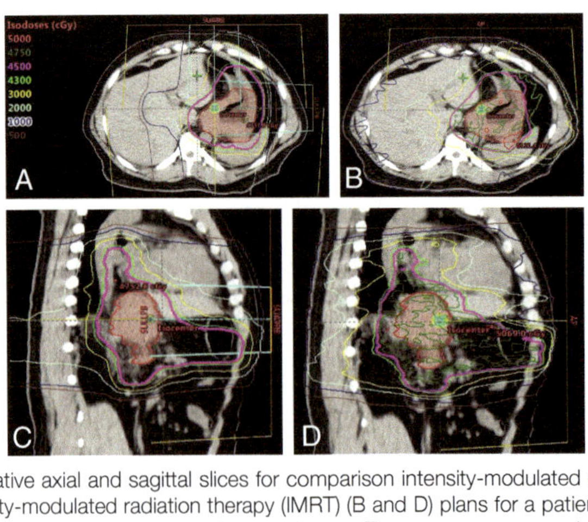

Fig. 10.1 Representative axial and sagittal slices for comparison intensity-modulated proton therapy (IMPT) (A and C) and intensity-modulated radiation therapy (IMRT) (B and D) plans for a patient with an 8-cm T3N1 gastric adenocarcinoma with extension into the esophagus. Target coverage was similar between the two plans, but the mean heart dose was 17.5 GyE in the IMPT plan compared with 22.2 Gy in the IMRT plan, and the mean liver dose was 9.4 GyE in the IMPT plan compared with 19.8 Gy in the IMRT plan.

PANCREAS

The Role of Radiation Therapy

Pancreatic adenocarcinoma is a particularly aggressive disease with surgical resection as the only current curative option, but median overall survival (OS) time after surgery alone is only 20 months.[18] Systemic therapy has been shown to improve disease-free survival,[19–21] but the use of radiotherapy in general for pancreatic malignancies is somewhat controversial.[20,22–24] A currently open randomized trial is evaluating whether concurrent fluoropyrimidine-based CRT improves survival for patients who have received 5 months of adjuvant chemotherapy after surgical resection of pancreatic adenocarcinoma.[25] Because completion rates of adjuvant therapy are low,[19] interest is growing in a neoadjuvant approach.[26,27] This neoadjuvant treatment approach is currently favored at MD Anderson. Neoadjuvant CRT can help convert borderline-resectable cancer to potentially operative disease,[28] improve the margin-negative (R0) resection rates,[29,30] and potentially reduce costs associated with care.[31] Stereotactic body radiotherapy (SBRT) has emerged as an alternative to standard fractionated radiotherapy. A currently accruing trial by the Alliance for Clinical Trials in Oncology (A021501) is comparing neoadjuvant therapy consisting of either chemotherapy alone or chemotherapy followed by either SBRT (33–40 Gy in 5 fractions) or hypofractionated image-guided radiation (25 Gy in 5 fractions).[32] Finally, despite the lack of an OS benefit demonstrated in the randomized trial evaluating consolidative CRT given after 4 months of induction chemotherapy, CRT did result in improved local control (LC) with no increased rates of grade 3 to 4 toxicity except for nausea.[22] Studies have shown that local progression is the leading cause of death for patients with locally advanced pancreatic cancer after 15 months.[33] As systemic therapy improves distant control, local treatment modalities, such as CRT, may have the chance to prove their value.

The Rationale for Proton Therapy

The pancreas is located in an anatomically challenging part of the body surrounded by radiosensitive organs, such as the stomach, duodenum, jejunum, kidneys, and liver. Radiation to the pancreas can cause acute side effects, such as fatigue, nausea, vomiting, diarrhea, and abdominal cramping. Radiation is only one part of a multidisciplinary approach, so it is important to minimize the side effects of this component to improve the completion rates for all therapy. PBR may be able to improve the therapeutic ratio by both allowing dose escalation while minimizing toxicities from unintended dose to adjacent normal organs.

Dosimetric Studies

One early dosimetric study showed the potential benefit of PBR for the treatment of inoperable pancreatic cancer necessitating large fields. Zurlo et al. showed that for four patients for whom IMRT plans conferred a 5% higher risk of toxicity to the kidneys, liver, or bowel, proton plans were able to deliver the same target coverage without the excessive risk of morbidity.[34] Other treatment planning studies have also shown the benefit of PBR for reducing low to moderate doses to normal tissue.[35] One small study showed the feasibility of PBR to safely dose escalate to 59.4 GyE while reducing mean dose to the spinal cord, left kidney, right kidney, and liver by 78%, 73%, 42%, and 55%, respectively.[36] Another treatment planning study performed at MD Anderson showed that PBR could allow safe dose escalation to 72 GyE with reduction in the V15 of the stomach and small bowel (48% vs. 5% and 61% vs. 9%, respectively).[37] In the postoperative setting, treatment planning studies have also shown the ability to reduce dose to the small bowel, stomach, and kidneys with PBR.[38,39] However, there are some concerns regarding the robustness of PBR plans for the treatment of pancreatic cancer. One study showed that proton plans were highly susceptible to interfractional anatomic change, with coverage of the clinical target volume reduced by 8% as a result of the daily variability.[40] A worst-case optimization strategy, which has been studied in carbon ion therapy for pancreatic cancer, may be useful to mitigate risks posed by

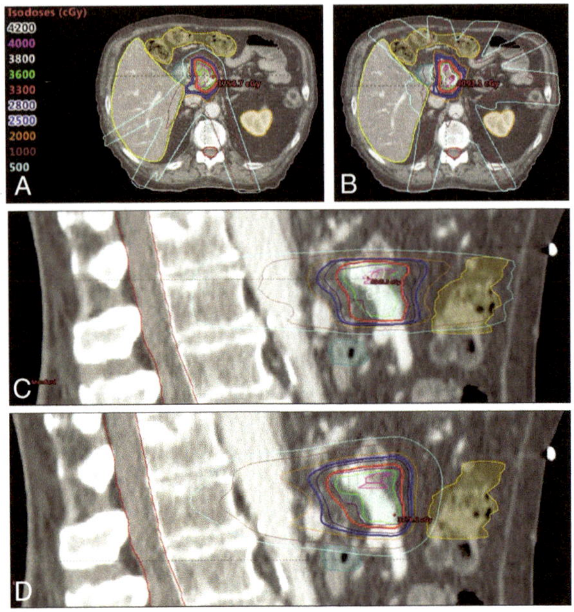

Fig. 10.2 Representative axial and sagittal slices for comparison intensity-modulated proton therapy (IMPT) (A and C) and intensity-modulated radiation therapy (B and D) plans for a patient with borderline resectable pancreatic adenocarcinoma treated with stereotactic radiation therapy to a total dose of 33 Gy (or Gy [relative biological effectiveness]) in 5 fractions. The maximum dose to the duodenum was similar, but the volume of bowel receiving lower doses (5, 10, and 15 Gy) was significantly lower with IMPT.

interfractional anatomic changes.[41] Fig. 10.2 shows IMRT and IMPT comparison plans for a patient receiving neoadjuvant SBRT for borderline-resectable pancreatic cancer.

Clinical Studies

Results from a phase I study at Massachusetts General Hospital showed no dose-limiting toxicities at any of the four dose levels of PBR tested in patients with localized, resectable adenocarcinoma of the head of the pancreas. Radiation regimens ranged from 3 Gy(RBE) × 10 fractions (dose level 1) to 5 Gy(RBE) × 5 fractions over 1 week (dose level 4), and 5 Gy(RBE) × 5 fractions was established as the maximum tolerated dose (MTD). Concurrent capecitabine was given, and surgical resection was performed 4 to 6 weeks after completion of radiotherapy. Of the 15 patients enrolled, 4 had G3 toxicities (pain, stent obstruction, and infection), and 11 went on to undergo surgical resection. There were no unexpected postoperative complications.[42] The same group performed a subsequent phase II study on which 35 additional patients were enrolled and treated with the established MTD of 5 Gy(RBE) × 5 fractions. The treatment was well tolerated with an acute G3 toxicity rate of 4.1%. The median progression-free survival time was 10 months, and the median OS time was 17 months. Locoregional failure occurred in 16.2% of patients, and distant failure was the predominant pattern of failure at 72.9%.[43] These LC and OS results are slightly better than those reported in photon-based SBRT series (median survival time of 14.5 months and 1-year LC rate of 61%),[44] but this may be related to patient selection, and randomized clinical studies are still needed to compare the two modalities.

PRIMARY LIVER

The Role of Radiation Therapy

Transplant and surgical resection are considered to be the only curative options for patients with hepatocellular carcinoma (HCC),[45] but a minority of patients are anatomically and medically eligible for a curative surgical approach at diagnosis.[46] The National Comprehensive Cancer Network guidelines list ablation, arterially directed therapies, and external beam radiation therapy (EBRT) as locoregional therapy options for those patients for whom resection is not feasible or a bridge to transplant is desired.[47] EBRT is recommended with the category of 2B (based on lower-level evidence, with consensus that the intervention is appropriate). However, current patterns of practice data suggest that radiation is an underused modality for these patients. Data from the Surveillance, Epidemiology, and End Results (SEER) program suggest that only 9% of Medicare patients diagnosed with HCC between 1998 and 2007 were even seen by a radiation oncologist.[48] Radiation is also not a first-line treatment in the treatment of intrahepatic cholangiocarcinoma (IHC). The mainstay of curative treatment is surgical resection, with no conclusive data to guide adjuvant therapy recommendations.[49] Chemotherapy consisting of cisplatin and gemcitabine remains the mainstay for metastatic or unresectable disease, but a currently active trial is evaluating the role of radiation therapy for patients in this setting.[50]

The Rationale for Proton Therapy

One barrier to the use of radiotherapy in the treatment of HCC and IHC is concern about radiation-induced liver disease (RILD) and other toxicities to nearby organs, such as the bowel, bile duct, and kidneys.[51] However, more recent data from the current treatment era suggest radiation can be delivered safely by using more conformal techniques and may provide valuable LC benefits that may translate into improved OS survival for patients with unresectable HCC and IHC.[52,53] The physical properties of PBR allow a more favorable therapeutic ratio by reducing exit dose through healthy, functional liver tissue. Thus PBR can offer a better therapeutic ratio, particularly for IHC HCC patients who might otherwise have unacceptable hepatic toxicity from photon-based radiation.

Dosimetric Studies

The use of PBR for tumors in the liver has been studied more extensively than for cancers in any other gastrointestinal site. Early treatment planning studies confirmed that PBR had the ability to significantly reduce the dose to the normal liver as well as to other organs at risk compared with both three-dimensional (3D)-conformal techniques and IMRT. Dose escalation on the order of 20% to 30% was also possible with PBR while achieving lower doses to nontarget tissues.[54]

Clinical Studies

Most of the early data on the use of PBR for HCC has come from Japan, where HCC is endemic. Results from hypofractionated regimens (16–25 fractions) to ablative doses for large tumors are similar to those after surgical resection, with 5-year LC and OS rates of 90% and 50%, respectively. The group at Tsukuba University has published extensively on the use of PBR to safely treat larger tumors to larger doses per fraction.[55] The same group published on a more recent cohort of 318 patients with HCC treated between 2001 and 2007, and the 5-year OS rate was 44.6%. Treatment regimens were more standardized in this cohort, with patients with peripheral tumors away from the gastrointestinal mucosa and porta hepatis receiving 66 Gy(RBE) in 10 fractions, tumors within 2 cm of the porta hepatis receiving 72.6 Gy(RBE) in 22 fractions, and tumors within 2 cm of the gastrointestinal mucosa receiving 77 Gy(RBE) in 35 fractions. These regimens were very well tolerated, with no reported cases of RILD and few serious toxicities.[56] Other case series from Asian centers show similar outcomes,[57,58] which have been shown to vary based on patient and tumor characteristics, including liver function, disease burden, and portal vein tumor thrombus (PVTT). Encouraging response rates and acceptable toxicity profiles were seen as well when PBR was used for advanced HCC with PVTT.[59] A more recent report showed feasible and promising results from a risk-adapted simultaneous integrated boost technique using PBR for patients with HCC and PVTT. Median OS time was 34.4 months in this cohort of 41 patients treated with 50 to 66 Gy(RBE) in 10 fractions depending on gross tumor volume and distance from gastrointestinal mucosa.[60]

Several prospective studies have also been conducted and published in this setting. Mizomoto and colleagues reported on 266 patients treated in three prospective protocols developed at the Proton Medical Research Center in Tsukuba, including 66 GyE in 10 fractions for tumors more than 2 cm away from the portal region, 72.6 GyE in 22 fractions for tumors within 2 cm of the hilum, and further reduction to 77 GyE in 35 fractions for tumors adjacent to the gastrointestinal tract. Most of the tumors were less than 5 cm. The average 3-year LC and OS rates were 87% and 61%, respectively, with no significant differences in LC among the three different fractionation schemes used. Toxicity rates were low, suggesting that appropriate selection of dose and fractionation based on tumor location can improve the therapeutic ratio.[61] Long-term outcomes for patients treated at Tsukuba were recently reported and showed favorable long-term control with no grade 3 or higher toxicities. This update also showed 5-year LC and OS rates of 90% and 34%, respectively, for patients with PVTT, suggesting that PBR may be a viable treatment strategy for this subset of patients with historically poor outcomes.[62]

In the United States, a phase II trial from Loma Linda evaluated PBR for 76 patients with inoperable HCC and cirrhosis. Some 18 patients in this cohort eventually underwent liver transplant, and 33% of those explants showed a pCR after 63 Gy(RBE) delivered over a 3-week period.[63] MD Anderson participated in a multi-institutional trial headed by Massachusetts General Hospital, which included patients with unresectable HCC or IHC. PBR was used to deliver up to 67.5 Gy(RBE) in 15 fractions to tumors from 2 to 12 cm (median 5 cm). Most of the included patients had cirrhosis, and 79.5% were Child-Pugh B. Despite the unfavorable characteristics of this cohort, LC rates at 2 years were 94.8% for HCC patients and 94.1% for IHC patients; OS rates at 2 years were 63.2% and 46.5%, respectively.[64]

Two randomized clinical trials involving PBR for HCC are currently underway. At Loma Linda, patients with HCC who met either the Milan or the San Francisco transplant criteria were randomized to receive PBR or transarterial chemoembolization (TACE). In the PBR arm, the dose was 70.2 Gy(RBE) in 15 fractions over 3 weeks. In an interim analysis reported recently, the 2-year OS rate was 59% for the cohort, with no difference between the groups. Approximately one-third of the patients in each arm went on to transplant and the pCR rate after PBR was 25% compared with 10% after TACE, although the difference was not statistically significant. A trend toward was noted improved LC rates in the PBR arm (88% vs. 45% at 2 years; $P = .06$). There were fewer hospitalization days also after PBR when compared with TACE, which the authors suggest may indicate reduced toxicity.[65] The NRG Oncology cooperative group recently opened a phase III trial randomizing patients with HCC to receive definitive treatment with either photons or protons.[66] With a primary outcome of improved OS, hopefully this trial will generate the necessary data to cement the benefit of PBR for this population of patients.

METASTATIC LIVER

The Role of Radiation Therapy

The definitive management of liver metastases is common practice for treating patients with colorectal primaries, as long-term survival, and even cure, are possible. With surgical resection of liver metastases coupled with the development of more effective chemotherapy regimens, the median survival time for these patients has increased to 20 months, with 20% to 25% of patients still alive 10 years later.[67] However, not all patients are surgical candidates, either because of the location of the disease, medical comorbidities, or the hepatoxicity of prior chemotherapy or other liver-directed therapies. Thus interest has been growing in the use of radiotherapy for the treatment of these patients. SBRT is of particular interest, given the relative radioresistance of colorectal metastases to standard dose/fractionation regimens.[68,69]

The Rationale for Proton Therapy

Most SBRT studies have primarily included patients with small metastatic tumors less than 3 to 6 cm in maximum dimension. The limiting factor for treating larger volumes remains the risk of RILD and other toxicity of nontarget tissues. As is the case with primary liver tumors as described above, PBR has the potential to allow to dose escalation while sparing nontarget liver and other at-risk organs.

Dosimetric Studies

Dosimetric benefits of PBR for the treatment of hepatic metastases are largely extrapolated from treatment planning and clinical studies of primary liver tumors. However, given the potential for long-term survival after successful treatment of isolated hepatic metastases, there is additional concern for radiation-induced secondary malignancies that result from unnecessary dose to nontarget tissues. A group from the University of Stockholm performed a treatment planning study that showed using IMPT for liver SBRT significantly decreased the calculated risk of secondary malignancy by decreasing dose to skin, lungs, esophagus, and healthy functional liver.[70]

Clinical Studies

A single-arm phase II trial was recently completed in which 89 patients with liver metastases from a variety of primary tumors were treated with PBR-based SBRT to 30 to 50 Gy(RBE) in 5 fractions depending on the effective volume irradiated. No G3–5 toxicities were reported, and the median survival time was 18.1 months. LC rates at 1 and 3 years were 71.9% and 61.2%, respectively. SBRT was found to be successful in this population, even when tumors were larger than 6 cm.[71] At MD Anderson, we have also used PBR to perform a "radiation hepatectomy" for patients with bilobar colorectal liver metastases who were initially deemed candidates for a two-stage hepatectomy but who were not able to undergo the second stage of treatment. For this unique group of patients, ablative doses of PBR (biologically effective dose >89.6 Gy[RBE]) were delivered to the entire right hemiliver. All five patients treated with this regimen experienced a partial or complete radiographic response and had in-field LC at latest follow-up. Two patients remain alive without evidence of disease, and two experienced distant progression outside the liver.[72]

A currently accruing phase I–II trial at Loma Linda is evaluating toxicity and LC rates after proton-based SBRT for liver metastases. The radiation regimen consists of 3 fractions to total doses of 36, 48, or 60 Gy(RBE) in an escalating fashion.[73] The hope is that the dosimetric advantages of PBR in the liver can help to safely escalate dose while maintaining a safe toxicity profile.

RECTAL

The Role of Radiation Therapy

For patients with T3, T4, or node-positive rectal adenocarcinoma, the current standard of care in the United States is to administer neoadjuvant CRT to a total dose of 45 to 50.4 Gy in 25 to 28 fractions before total mesorectal surgical excision followed by adjuvant chemotherapy.[74] An alternative strategy is to administer 25 Gy in 5 fractions followed by surgery.[75] Radiation is also sometimes used for recurrent disease, either before reresection or definitively to palliate symptoms of the local recurrence. Hyperfractionation is commonly used for reirradiation, with the regimen commonly used at MD Anderson consisting of 39 Gy in 1.5-Gy fractions delivered twice daily with a 6-hour interfraction interval.[76]

The Rationale for Proton Therapy

Similar to what has been demonstrated for other pelvic malignancies, PBR has the potential to reduce dose to organs at risk while maintaining adequate dose coverage to the intended target.

Dosimetric Studies

Several benefits, including bone marrow, bowel, and bladder sparing, have been demonstrated when using PBR for whole-pelvis irradiation for gynecologic and prostate malignancies.[77,78] Similarly, Colaco et al. from the University of Florida demonstrated that PBR was able to reduce the volume of bone marrow receiving 5, 10, 15, and 20 Gy(RBE). Also, the volume of small bowel receiving 30 and 40 Gy(RBE) and the volume of bladder receiving 40 Gy(RBE) could also be reduced with PBR when compared with traditional 3D conformal RT plans delivering 45 Gy to the pelvis followed by a boost of 5.4 Gy to the tumor plus margin.[79] Other treatment planning studies have found similar benefits.[80] Some dosimetric analyses have suggested that the decreased volume of small bowel irradiation may make treatment escalation possible, either with increased radiation dose or with an intensified chemotherapy regimen, which may improve pCR rates and increase LC.[81,82]

Clinical Studies

For recurrent rectal cancer, some studies have shown the potential benefits of PBR. At the University of Pennsylvania, seven patients with recurrent rectal cancer after prior CRT and surgery were treated with PBR to a mean dose of 61.2 Gy with concurrent fluorouracil. Only one patient experienced a CR, and the toxicity rates were significant, with three cases of G3 diarrhea, one case of G3 abdominal pain, two cases of small bowel obstruction, and one rectovaginal fistula.[83] Data were also presented in abstract outlining the treatment of six patients with pelvic recurrences after prior radiation with a more modest dose of 39 to 45 Gy using PRB with a single posteroanterior beam or opposing lateral fields. No G3+ toxicities were reported with a median follow-up time of only 1 year, and no in-field failures were reported.[84] One trial is currently active and recruiting patients at the Samsung Medical Center that is prospectively evaluating the efficacy and toxicity of salvage CRT with PBR for patients with previously irradiated recurrent rectal cancer. The primary outcome measure is 3-year LC rate, with secondary objectives that include adverse events, response rate, survival, and quality of life.[85]

ANAL

The Role of Radiation Therapy

The current standard of care for squamous cell carcinoma of the anal canal was established by Radiation Therapy Oncology Group (RTOG) 9811 and includes definitive CRT with fluorouracil and mitomycin-C (MMC).[86] However, studies have shown equivalent results from fluorouracil with cisplatin as concurrent treatment,[87] so that regimen is also used at some centers, including MD Anderson.[88] IMRT emerged as the new standard of care in the treatment of anal cancer when RTOG 0529, a phase II study, prospectively showed that IMRT could significantly reduce G2+ hematologic and G3+ dermatologic toxicity.[89]

The Rationale for Proton Therapy

The landmark studies establishing CRT as the standard of care used 3D treatment techniques. As such, large volumes of bowel, bladder, external genitalia, and skin received significant doses. On the MMC arm of RTOG 9811, G3–4 hematologic and nonhematologic acute toxicity rates were 61% and 74%, respectively.[86] Although IMRT was shown to reduce toxicity, patients receiving IMRT with concurrent fluorouracil and MMC on RTOG 0529 still experienced 77% G2+ gastrointestinal, 73% G2+ hematologic, and 23% G3+ dermatologic toxicity rates. Emerging data also suggest that bone marrow dose may actually be higher with IMRT.[90] The importance of bone marrow dose in predicting the risk of hematologic toxicity for patients receiving CRT for anal cancer has been established. Specifically, the volume of pelvic bone marrow receiving 5, 10, 15, and 20 Gy were all significantly associated with decreased white blood cell and absolute neutrophil count nadirs.[91] PBR has the potential to preferentially spare bone marrow from unnecessary dose and potentially increase the tolerability of treatment. Additionally, PBR has the potential to decrease dose to the external genitalia, bowel, and bladder, which may further improve acute and long-term quality of life for patients receiving CRT for anal cancer. Hematologic, gastrointestinal, and dermatologic toxicity are common reasons patients need breaks during treatment. Because prolonging the overall treatment duration with breaks can worsen oncologic outcome,[92] PBR thus has the potential to improve the efficacy of treatment.

Dosimetric Studies

Two small treatment planning studies published in 2015 evaluated the potential benefits of pencil beam scanning proton beam therapy (SPBT) for anal cancer.[93,94] The first, performed at the Mayo Clinic, compared plans for eight patients with squamous cell carcinoma of the anal canal. The gross tumor volume plus margin received 54–60 Gy, and the elective nodal volumes received 45–50.4 Gy. They found no difference between target coverage between IMRT and SPBT. The SPBT plans were also robust to uncertainties, as evidenced by acceptable coverage even with the worse-case dose values. However, the mean doses to the bone marrow, bladder, small bowel, and genitalia were all significantly lower with SPBT than with IMRT. Specifically with regard to the bone marrow, SPBT reduced the pelvic bone marrow V10 by 54% ($P = .008$), V20 by 56% ($P = .008$) and V30 by 44% ($P = .008$).[94] Another treatment planning study performed at the University of Pennsylvania also compared IMRT and pencil beam SPBT plans for patients with anal cancer. They similarly found no difference in target coverage, but they showed significant reductions in doses of up to 35 Gy to the small bowel ($P = .008$), up to 29 Gy to the genitalia ($P = .008$), and up to 30 Gy to the bone marrow ($P = .008$).[93] Fig. 10.3 shows the bone marrow and anterior viscera sparing achievable with IMPT compared with IMRT.

Clinical Studies

Few clinical results have been published on the use of PBT for anal cancer. The group from the University of Pennsylvania treated eight patients with PBT on a registry study from 2013 to 2014. They published dosimetric results of their treatment planning study,[93] but they have not yet published any clinical results regarding efficacy or toxicity. They did publish results of their robustness assessment because concerns have been raised regarding day-to-day variations leading to uncertainties in target coverage and dose to normal structures. In this registry study, they performed verification scans every 1 to 2 weeks during treatment. The dose received by 98% of the clinical target volume was evaluated on each verification scan, and they found deviations ranging between 0.1% and 0.43%.[93] Other clinical data include case reports, including one describing a man with an anal cancer presenting after prior brachytherapy for prostate cancer. Protons were used to spare the urethra and minimize further toxicity from reirradiation.[95] A second case study described PBT used as a 24.2-Gy boost to the primary after 45 Gy of photon-based RT was delivered to the primary plus elective nodal volumes with concurrent chemotherapy. The patient had a complete clinical response and no evidence of disease 5 years later.[96]

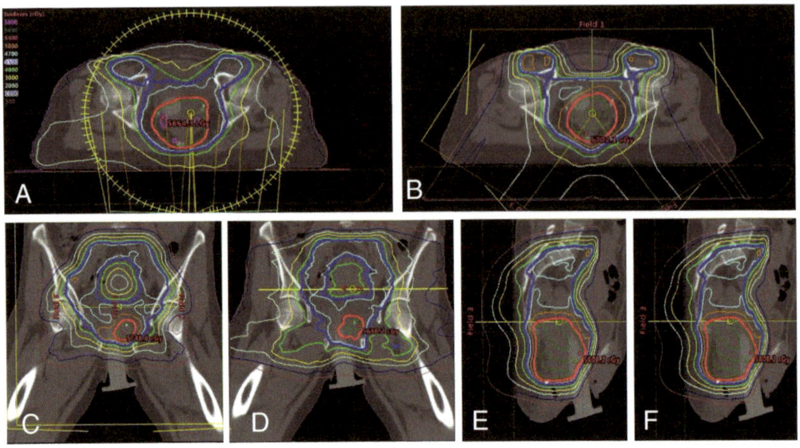

Fig. 10.3 Representative axial and sagittal slices for comparison intensity-modulated proton therapy (IMPT) (A, C, and E) and intensity-modulated radiation therapy (IMRT) (B, D, and F) plans for a patient with T2N0 squamous cell carcinoma of the anal canal. The mean dose to the pelvic bone marrow was 29.4 Gy with IMRT versus 23.8 Gy (relative biological effectiveness [RBE]) with IMPT. The volume of pelvic bone marrow receiving 10 Gy or Gy(RBE) was over 90% with IMRT versus 66% with IMPT.

Two studies are currently evaluating the potential role of PBT to reduce toxicity in the treatment of anal cancer. The University of Cincinnati is recruiting patients to a pilot study with the primary end point of G3+ hematologic, gastrointestinal, genitourinary, and dermatologic toxicity. Doses of PBT are based on disease stage and range from 50.4 to 54 Gy to the primary in 28 to 30 fractions, with 42 to 54 Gy to the elective nodal volumes in 28 to 30 fractions. The concurrent chemotherapy consists of fluorouracil and MMC.[97] Another joint pilot study at the University of Pennsylvania and Massachusetts General Hospital is ongoing but not actively recruiting participants. Similarly, the end point is G3+ toxicity, and the concurrent chemotherapy consists of fluorouracil and MMC.[98]

Conclusion

In conclusion, proton therapy may help to improve the therapeutic ratio in the treatment of many gastrointestinal malignancies by allowing safe dose escalation and by limiting dose to sensitive organs at risk. This is an exciting area of much ongoing study, and the hope is that future data will better define the value of proton therapy in this setting.

References Available Online.

CHAPTER 11

Proton Therapy for Gynecologic Malignancies

Lillie L. Lin

Introduction

Each year more than 90,000 women are diagnosed with a gynecologic (ovarian, vulvar, vaginal, cervical, uterine, fallopian tube, or primary peritoneal) cancer in the United States.[1] Radiotherapy is often used with curative intent with or without concurrent chemotherapy for locally advanced vulvar, vaginal, or cervical cancer. Women with high-risk features after surgery for cervical, uterine, or vulvar cancer may also receive adjuvant radiotherapy.[2–7] The standard of care for women with locally advanced cervical cancer is external beam radiotherapy (EBRT) and intracavitary brachytherapy in conjunction with concurrent chemotherapy to increase local control and overall survival.[8] For women with high-risk stage III/IV endometrial cancer, adjuvant pelvic or extended-field radiotherapy may be recommended, usually combined with systemic chemotherapy delivered either in a sandwich or sequential manner with or without concurrent radiosensitizing chemotherapy.[6]

The target volume in women requiring pelvic radiotherapy includes the pelvic lymph nodes (obturator, external and internal iliac, and common iliac) as well as the presacral nodes in women with cervical cancer or those with endometrial cancer and cervical involvement. The primary target in women after hysterectomy includes the operative bed, which consists of the upper vagina and paravaginal tissues. For women with cervical cancer, the primary target would include the gross tumor volume, uterus, entire cervix, and parametrial tissues. The target would extend and cover the entire mesorectum with parametrial involvement.[9] For women with involved or suspicious paraaortic lymph nodes, the field would extend to cover these nodes up to the level of the renal hilum.

EBRT was initially delivered with two or four fields to the pelvis or to the pelvis/paraaortic region, oftentimes with concurrent chemotherapy, for gynecologic cancers. Such a treatment combination can result in acute hematologic, gastrointestinal, and genitourinary toxic side effects as well as late morbidity. Recent randomized studies of intensity-modulated radiotherapy (IMRT) compared with three-dimensional conformal radiation therapy (3DCRT) for both uterine and cervical cancer after hysterectomy have demonstrated that IMRT can reduce the incidence of acute bowel toxicities.[10] Importantly, acute hematologic toxicity in the setting of concurrent chemotherapy can result in dose reductions or delays in chemotherapy, which may result in compromised outcomes. Hematologic and gastrointestinal toxicities often limit the ability to deliver combined-modality therapy, as was observed when Duenas-Gonzalez et al. attempted to add weekly gemcitabine to weekly cisplatin concurrent with radiotherapy for locally advanced cervical cancer.[11] Proton therapy for gynecologic malignancies has the potential to widen the therapeutic window and allow the testing of treatment intensification with novel therapies; it may also allow for potentially more conformal dose delivery and the possibility of dose escalation.

After Hysterectomy

The radiotherapy technique for gynecologic malignancies has evolved in the last several decades. Initially, patients were treated with opposed fields or four-field conventional photon therapy, with fields defined by bony landmarks. With computed tomography (CT) imaging, the organs at risk (OARs) can be defined to reduce dose to nearby normal tissues. However, this still results in high doses of bowel irradiated. The recently completed NRG Oncology/Radiation Therapy Oncology Group TIME-C study (RTOG 1203) sought to test whether IMRT could reduce normal tissue toxicities in patients receiving posthysterectomy radiotherapy for either cervical or uterine cancer compared with 3DCRT.[10] The primary end point was patient-reported bowel toxicity measured with the bowel domain on the EPIC (Expanded Prostate Cancer Index Composite) instrument. Results demonstrated that the EPIC bowel domain scores at 5 weeks of therapy for women receiving IMRT were higher (meaning less toxicity) than for women receiving 3DCRT. Given that smaller volumes of bowel receive radiation with protons, particularly in the low-dose region, it seems reasonable to test the hypothesis that proton therapy may further reduce bowel toxicity.

Lin et al. published the first clinical report on the use of pencil beam scanning (PBS) proton therapy for women who have undergone hysterectomy for either cervical or uterine cancer.[12] In their series, 11 patients received PBS proton therapy using uniform scanning. They were treated using opposed lateral, two lateral and posterior, or two posterior oblique fields. Improved sparing in the low-dose region was noted for organs such as the small bowel, pelvic bone marrow, and bladder. Weekly or biweekly CT simulation scans were also obtained to confirm robustness relative to setup uncertainties.

Xu et al. reported on seven patients with endometrial cancer who were treated with PBS to an extended field to include the pelvis and paraaortic region.[13] They demonstrated that dosimetrically, PBS resulted in lower volumes of exposed pelvic bone marrow, small bowel, and bladder. No significant (grade 3 or higher) toxicities were observed in this population. All patients were treated with two posterior oblique fields. These early studies demonstrate the feasibility of treating patients with proton therapy. Other prospective studies are ongoing.[14] Fig. 11.1 shows a patient who received PBS proton therapy after radical hysterectomy for a FIGO (Fédération Internationale de Gynécologie et d'Obstétrique) stage IIB cervical carcinoma. She also had a pelvic kidney that necessitated proton therapy to minimize the dose to that kidney.

INTACT CERVICAL CANCER

The use of brachytherapy is the standard of care in women with locally advanced cervical cancer receiving definitive chemoradiotherapy. Omission of brachytherapy has been associated with decreased survival. However, some rare situations may preclude the use of brachytherapy, such as a patient with bicornuate uterus (although interstitial brachytherapy may be an option), disease that obstructs the cervical os, or a patient who cannot tolerate sedation for the procedure. Arimoto et al. published the results of a series of 15 patients with gynecologic malignancies treated with high-energy proton beam radiotherapy in lieu of brachytherapy at Tsukuba University in the mid-1980s.[15] Results at 2 years demonstrated local control rates and overall survival rates of 92.3% and 93.3%, respectively. All tumors were controlled if the dose was greater than 78 Gy. Two patients experienced transient radiation proctitis at 7 and 9 months after radiation. Clivio et al. also evaluated the use of intensity-modulated proton therapy (IMPT) in lieu of brachytherapy for locally advanced cervical cancer in a conceptual feasibility study. IMPT was planned with 5 fractions of 6 Gy to the cervix, including the macroscopic tumor as defined on magnetic resonance imaging (MRI) with a 5-mm margin. The doses to OARs, including the rectal wall, sigmoid wall, and bladder wall, were acceptable and within the dose constraints recommended by the GEC-ESTRO (Groupe Européen de Curiethérapie the European SocieTy for Radiotherapy and Oncology).[16,17] Given the toxicities associated with combined-modality therapy, it is reasonable to investigate radiotherapy techniques that would potentially reduce dose to OARs. Fig. 11.2 shows a represen-

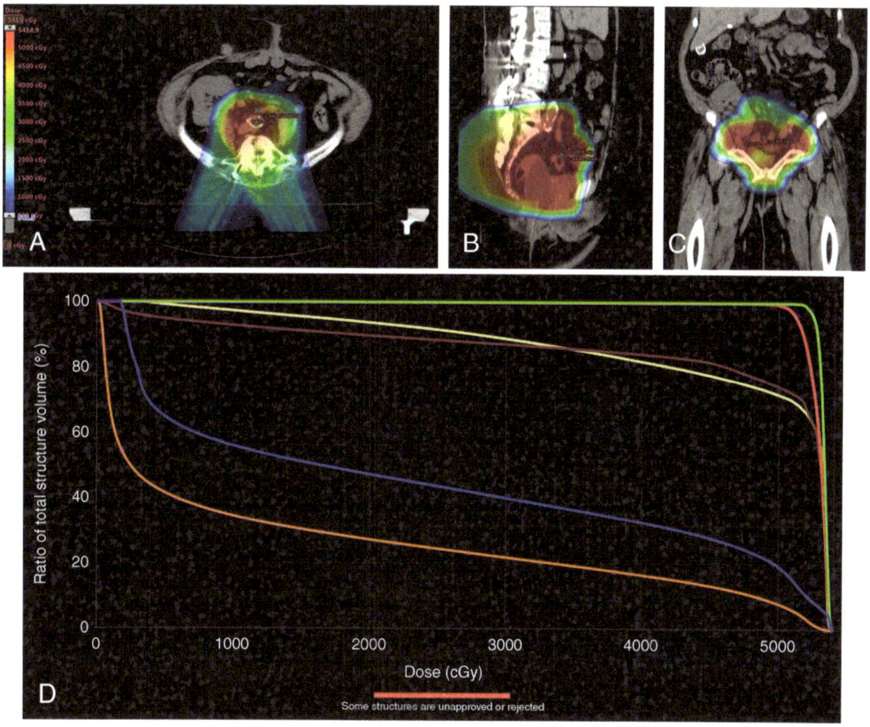

Fig. 11.1 Axial (A), sagittal (B), and coronal (C) color-wash views of a proton therapy treatment plan for a patient with FIGO (Fédération Internationale de Gynécologie et d'Obstétrique) stage IIB cervical carcinoma who underwent radical hysterectomy and required postoperative radiotherapy. She had a history of renal failure s/p kidney transplantation. Given the location of her pelvic kidney, proton therapy was used to reduce the dose to that kidney. (D) Dose volume histogram of her kidney *(orange)*, small bowel *(blue)*, bladder *(yellow)*, rectum *(brown)*, planning target volume *(red)*, and clinical target volume *(green)* are shown.

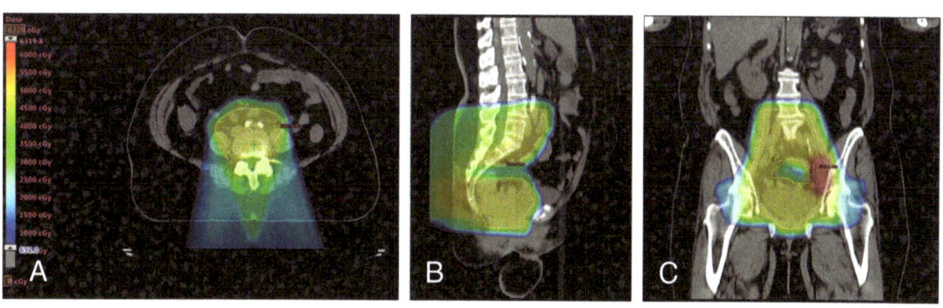

Fig. 11.2 Axial (A), sagittal (B), and coronal (C) color-wash views of a proton therapy treatment plan of a patient with FIGO (Fédération Internationale de Gynécologie et d'Obstétrique) stage IIIB cervical cancer with positive pelvic nodes. She was treated with pencil beam scanning proton therapy followed by brachytherapy and a nodal boost.

tative example of a patient who was treated with PBS proton therapy for a FIGO stage IIIB cervical carcinoma. Posterior oblique beams were chosen with no exit radiation dose to the anterior abdominal organs. A multinational phase III study of concurrent cisplatin[11] and gemcitabine with radiotherapy followed by consolidative cisplatin and gemcitabine for two cycles resulted in significantly higher toxicities and hospitalizations than the weekly cisplatin and radiotherapy, the standard of care. If we are to identify incremental improvements in combined-modality therapies for locally advanced cervical cancer, methods to reduce radiotherapy toxicities will be necessary.

Reirradiation

For patients who develop recurrent disease or a second primary after prior full-dose radiation to the pelvis, options may include surgical resection versus primary radiotherapy versus systemic therapy. Surgical resection may be possible depending on the clinical situation and has been used for other malignancies, including lung, esophageal, rectal, and breast cancer.[18,19] A patient with a central recurrence of cervical cancer treated with primary concurrent chemoradiotherapy may be a candidate for an exenterative procedure. However, a patient with a sidewall recurrence would not be a suitable candidate for surgery, but may be a candidate for reirradiation, depending on the extent of local disease as well as the status of disease elsewhere. Chemotherapy alone for gross disease is rarely curative on its own. The decision to deliver radiotherapy in an area of prior radiotherapy should consider multiple factors, including (1) length of time since prior treatment, (2) performance status, (3) options for alternative therapies, and (4) burden of disease. During the decision-making process, the potential for morbidity and increased late complications that this process could entail. Depending on the timing of the in-field recurrence, the disease could be considered a recurrence versus a new primary, and the ability to render curative therapy may also depend on the time course of the disease recurrence. Eifel et al. found that the hazard ratio for relapse peaked at the first year of follow-up and then fell off. They observed better survival rates among women who relapsed 3 years after initial therapy.[20] Li et al., in a case report, described the treatment of a patient with a history of FIGO stage IIB cervical squamous cell carcinoma treated in the 1980s with conventional radiotherapy and low-dose-rate brachytherapy alone who subsequently developed a new vaginal squamous cell carcinoma in 2011.[21] She was treated with limited opposed lateral passive scattering fields to treat just the primary fluorodeoxyglucose (FDG)-avid disease on positron emission tomography (PET)/CT imaging. She also received brachytherapy and now, more than 6 years after therapy is without evidence of disease; she did experience grade 3 radiation proctitis.

Simulation, Target Delineation, and Treatment Planning

A noncontrast CT simulation scan should be performed for dose calculation purposes, as contrast can shift the Hounsfield units (HUs) and compromise proton range calculations.[22] If helpful, a contrast CT scan can be obtained subsequently and fused to the initial treatment planning scan for delineation of nodal volumes. Oral contrast may be given as well on subsequent imaging to aid in the definition of the large and small bowels.

Options for immobilization include a knee and foot lock indexed device that limits hip rotation and encourages flexion at the knees and hips when the patient is to be treated in the supine position. Arm positioning should be such that it does not interfere with beam paths and is reproducible on a daily basis. Use of a ring on the superior chest for a patient to hold is one option, as is use of a wing board with arms overhead. Although a prone position can result in a greater displacement of bowel, it may not be tolerable for patients. Such positioning also may not be reproducible on a daily basis without optimal immobilization. Devices such as alpha cradles or vacuum lock bags are not routinely used for proton therapy setups, as they may increase the proton range uncertainty and thereby compromise the precision of the beam.

To minimize rectal and bowel gas, the recommendation to the patient is to consume a low-fiber or low-residue diet before simulation and during therapy if possible. Prophylactic use of antigas tablets such as simethicone can also help promote regular emptying and reduced gas. For simulation and subsequent treatments, an endorectal balloon can also be used (filled with 50–100 mL of water).

Given the significant inter- and intrafraction variability in bladder filling,[23] simulation with both a full and empty bladder is appropriate, with daily treatment given with a full bladder. This can be achieved by asking the patient to void fully and then drink 16 to 24 ounces (470–700 mL) of water approximately 45 minutes before their simulation and scheduled treatment time.

Target Delineation

In patients requiring posthysterectomy pelvic radiotherapy, fiducials may be placed at the vaginal apex before simulation to better identify the vaginal apex for target delineation. Any artifacts caused by the fiducials or any high-Z materials, such as surgical clips, should be overridden for treatment planning purposes.

Depending on the clinical situation, MRI and PET/CT imaging may be useful for identification of gross disease, extent of invasion, and local recurrence. If these techniques are to be used for treatment planning for proton therapy, the scans should be performed while the patient is in the treatment position, ideally at the time of CT simulation with the identification immobilization device and fused with the noncontrast CT scan.

Clinical target volume and OAR contouring for a patient receiving proton therapy in the posthysterectomy setting is identical to that for a patient receiving IMRT. We recommend using the RTOG guidelines with the inclusion of the obturator nodal region, which should stop inferiorly when the obturator vessels enter the obturator canal.[24] The nodal clinical target volume (CTV) should include the pelvic lymph nodes (external, internal, and common iliac), obturator, and presacral nodes when treating cervical cancer and endometrial cancer when there is cervical or parametrial involvement. Several groups have demonstrated significant vaginal motion depending on bladder/rectal filling. We therefore recommend using both full and empty bladder scans to delineate a vaginal internal target volume (ITV). Significant differences in rectal filling are possible as well, and we have treated patients with an endorectal balloon in place, both at the time of simulation and daily during treatment, filled with the same volume.[12] Taku et al. have also demonstrated that with a daily endorectal balloon, the range of vaginal motion is smaller.[25] Most patients tolerate this reasonably well. The other option is to simulate with and without an endorectal balloon and then treat daily without one, as is preferred at some institutions. A third option is to forego a balloon, but if the rectum is empty at the time of simulation, the anterior border of the ITV should be extended into the bladder by 2 cm, and if the rectum is full, the posterior border of the ITV should be extended into the rectum and within 1.5 cm of the posterior rectal wall. The proximal vaginal cuff should be included in the vaginal ITV.

The OARs to be contoured include small and large bowels, rectum, pelvic bone marrow (including bone marrow in the lower pelvis, ilium, and lumbosacral spine), kidneys, femoral heads, and bladder. The small and large bowels should be contoured within the field and 2 cm above the field.[26]

Treatment of the paraaortics may be necessary for some women with either cervical or endometrial cancer, depending on the clinical situation. Treatment may be included as part of an extended-field treatment, or the clinical situation may be such that only the paraaortic region needs treatment. Typically, the fields are from the posterior direction and exit anteriorly into the bowel. This may not be a concern for patients who are receiving 45 to 50 Gy to treat subclinical disease. However, for patients with gross lymph nodes, the dose may be higher, upwards of 66 Gy. In those situations, the bowel relative to the CTV should be reviewed carefully on diagnostic imaging. If the small bowel, including the duodenum, is approximating the CTV, the neighboring bowel will receive the prescription dose, as the beam uncertainties at the end of the range are higher. In these situations, we may elect to treat with IMRT. We try to maintain the V55 of the duodenum to less than 15 cm^3.

A margin of 7 to 8 mm should be added to the nodal CTV to generate a planning target volume. This margin would account for variations in patient positioning and daily setup. The margin on the vaginal or primary ITV may be institution-specific, as it depends on how the ITV is contoured, but can range from 7 to 15 mm.

As discussed elsewhere throughout this book, proton beam ranges have uncertainties. To limit the effects of this uncertainty, robust optimization can be used, or a PBS-specific optimization structure can be created for planning purposes when a single-field optimization planning technique is used. Typically, this structure is created by adding to the CTV a margin of 3.5% of the beam range in the beam direction.

Treatment Planning

Several-specific treatment-planning issues can affect proton range uncertainty and robustness that must be considered. Imaging artifacts must be minimized, as they can influence proton range calculations. For instance, high-HU markers placed on the skin surface to help mark the isocenter can influence range calculations, particularly because they will not be on the skin during daily treatment. Any surface markers therefore must be contoured and overridden with the HU for air (−1000). Other artifacts in tissue caused by other high-density materials (i.e., calcifications, surgical clips, vaginal fiducials) should be contoured and overridden with the average HU of the tissue that is immediately adjacent.

Bowel gas within the treatment field should be contoured and overridden with the average HU of neighboring tissue. Bowel gas will increase the proton range if it persists during treatment; however, the rationale for contouring the gas is that it will provide robust target overage in the event that the gas is replaced with tissue. In clinical scenarios involving significant bowel gas, using the HU override technique is suboptimal, and beam angles should be chosen to avoid the areas of high gas.

Weight changes can occur during course of therapy and particularly in patients requiring pelvic or abdominal treatment; this can change their anterior or lateral wall contours. For patients receiving pelvic radiotherapy for gynecologic malignancies, the preference for beam selection is posterior or posterior oblique, and therefore, this is less of a concern, but nonetheless it must be monitored. Berger et al. demonstrated that weight changes in patients receiving fractionated radiotherapy for cervical cancer did not result in significant changes to targets and OARs when a four-field (two laterals and two posterior obliques) IMPT plan was used, demonstrating the feasibility of IMPT.

As for beam angle selection, anterior fields are typically avoided to minimize the anatomical uncertainties in the beam path. Although lateral fields may be appropriate for pelvic treatments, they are not feasible for most paraaortic fields. Also, large patients with shifting abdominal tissue are not ideal candidates for lateral beams because the amount of soft tissue in the beam path could change on a daily basis. When lateral fields are matched to a superior posterior field, a smeared match line can be used to avoid match line changes. The match between these fields can be created by dose painting shallow gradients from each field at the match line using multiple optimization volumes.[27]

Treatment Delivery

If available, daily cone-beam or CT-on-rails imaging is appropriate. Weekly or biweekly CT imaging to evaluate potential changes in anatomy may also be sufficient if cone-beam CT imaging is unavailable. Daily kilovoltage imaging would be appropriate as well, with matching to bony anatomy or fiducials as clinically appropriate. Kilovoltage imaging may be sufficient to identify an endorectal balloon if used.

Conclusions

Proton therapy may benefit women with gynecologic malignancies by widening the therapeutic window. Future studies are needed to clarify the group of women who would benefit from proton therapy and to measure the benefits relative to other radiotherapy techniques.

References Available Online.

CHAPTER 12

Proton Therapy for Prostate Cancer

Seungtaek L. Choi ■ Quynh-Nhu Nguyen

Introduction

The use of proton therapy for the treatment of cancer was first proposed by Robert Wilson in 1946.[1] A beam of protons gives most of its dose at a fixed depth in the tissue known as the Bragg peak, with very little dose deposited beyond that depth. As a result of this physical characteristic, protons are better able to deliver high doses of radiation therapy with less scatter dose to nearby critical structures. Because of this perceived advantage, the use of proton beam radiation therapy has increased significantly in the past decade. Currently, 68 proton centers are in operation around the world, with 27 of them located in the United States.[2]

Several studies have demonstrated the importance of dose escalation in the treatment of prostate cancer, with a higher radiation dose to the prostate leading to improved biochemical relapse-free survival and freedom from clinical failure rates.[3–5] However, higher doses mean a higher risk of side effects. Because patients with prostate cancer can often expect to live for long periods after diagnosis and treatment, it is crucial that any treatment minimize the risk of side effects and negative effects on quality of life (QoL) for patients undergoing that treatment. As mentioned, the physical characteristics of proton beam therapy allow dose escalation to the tumor with less scatter and exit dose to the surrounding normal tissues, which, for prostate cancer, include the rectum and bladder.

This chapter summarizes the physics of proton therapy and recent technical advances in the delivery of proton beams, reviews clinical results, and describes the treatment protocol used at our institution for the treatment of prostate cancer.

Physics of Proton Beam Radiation Therapy

The proton is a positively charged particle; therefore, it has a more limited range in matter than x-rays. A beam made up of protons deposits most of its energy at a fixed depth known as the Bragg peak, with very little dose deposited beyond that depth (Fig. 12.1). In contrast, an x-ray beam deposits its maximum dose just inside the patient's body and then continues to travel through the body, depositing dose until it exits the body. The depth of the Bragg peak is based on the energy of the proton beam, with greater depths of deposition having higher doses. Normally, the Bragg peak is too narrow to treat an entire tumor. Therefore the width of the Bragg peak is spread out to cover the entire target volume with margin. This is known as the spread-out Bragg peak.

For patients with prostate cancer treated with protons, the most common beam arrangement is two beams coming in from the right lateral and left lateral directions. In contrast, x-rays with intensity-modulated radiation therapy (IMRT) use multiple angles or arcs to concentrate the radiation dose to the prostate, which results in low-dose scatter to the rest of the pelvis, including the bladder and rectum, with IMRT. Using proton therapy significantly reduces this scatter dose (Fig. 12.2).

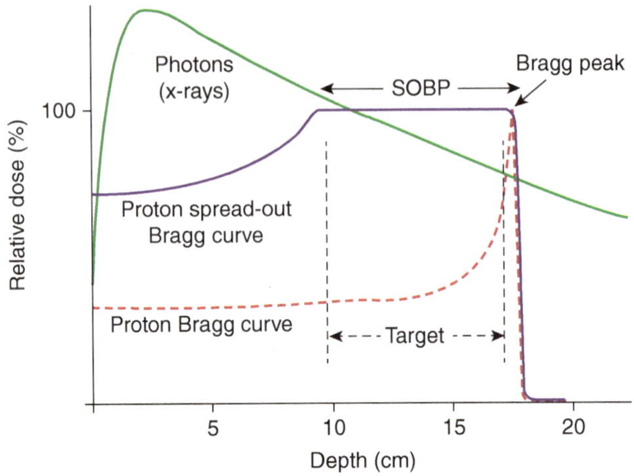

Fig. 12.1 Dose deposition characteristics of protons versus x-rays. *SOBP,* Spread out Bragg peak. (From Mohan R, Mahajan A, Minsky, BD. New strategies in radiation therapy: exploiting the full potential of protons. *Clin Cancer Res*. 2013;19(23);6338-6343. ©2013 AACR.)

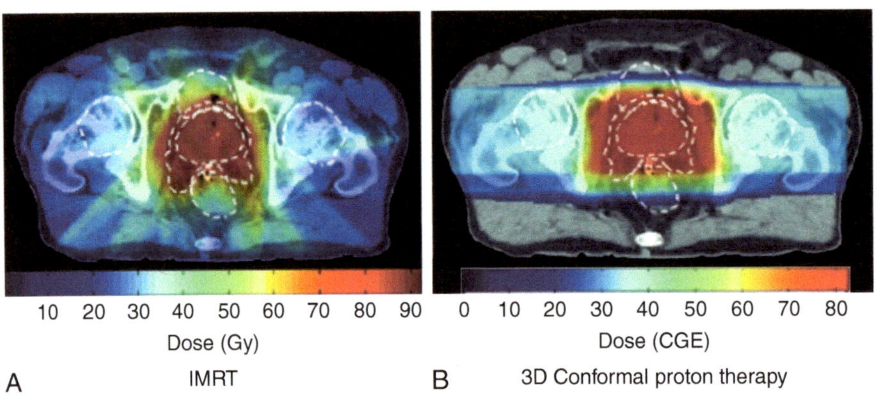

Fig. 12.2 Prostate treatment with protons versus intensity-modulated radiation therapy *(IMRT)*. *3D*, Three-dimensional; *CGE*, cobalt Gy equivalent. (From Trofimov A, Nguyen PL, Coen JJ, et al. Radiotherapy treatment of early-stage prostate cancer with IMRT and protons: a treatment planning comparison. *Int J Radiat Oncol Biol Phys*. 2007;69(2):444-453.)

Modes of Proton Delivery

Currently, there are two types of proton therapy delivery: passively scattered proton therapy and pencil beam proton therapy. Passively scattered proton therapy consists of a monoenergetic beam of protons, which is then passed through a scattering system to create a larger beam of protons. At MD Anderson, the passively scattered beam used to treat patients comes in three sizes: small (10 × 10 cm), medium (18 × 18 cm), and large (25 × 25 cm). As mentioned before, the Bragg peak is usually spread out by using a range modulator wheel to cover the entire tumor with the margin in the direction of the beam. This beam is then further shaped by using two additional custom devices: a brass aperture and an acrylic tissue compensator. The aperture determines the shape of the radiation field (akin to multileaf collimators for x-rays), and the compensator shapes the distal edge of the proton beam dose to the shape of the target volume (Fig. 12.3). These devices are created for each patient by milling machines located on-site at the Proton Therapy Center.

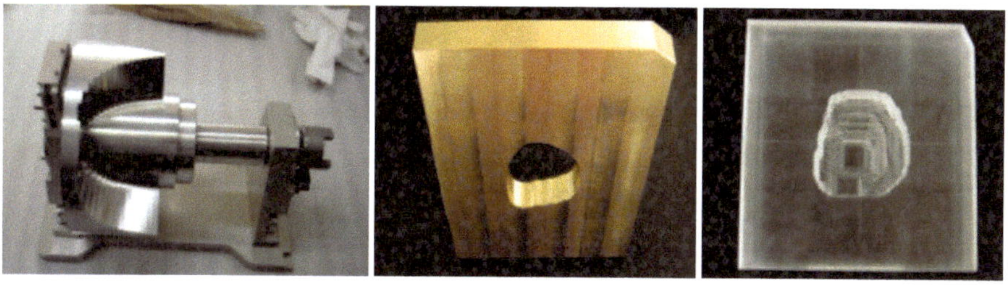

Fig. 12.3 Hardware used for passively scattered protons (from left, range moderator wheel, aperture, tissue compensator).

Pencil beam proton therapy (also known as active scanning proton therapy or spot scanning proton therapy) uses a narrow proton beam ("pencil beam") to deliver dose by sequentially layering multiple pristine Bragg peaks (or "spots") over the target volume. An electromagnetic field is used in the pencil beam to scan the protons in both directions perpendicular to the beam direction (i.e., *x*- and *y*-axes) without the need for a scattering device or an aperture.[7–9] The depth of dose deposition (i.e., *z*-axis) is controlled by changing the energy of the protons in the pencil beam and delivering multiple layers of dose. Because this layering of dose allows better conformity of the proximal edge of the target volume compared with passively scattered proton therapy, normal tissue sparing is improved.

Pencil beam proton therapy has several other advantages over passively scattered proton beam therapy. Pencil beams therapy allows improved conformality of the proton dose, with improved tumor coverage and normal tissue sparing, especially around curved structures. The pencil beam does not require the use of brass apertures and acrylic compensators, which saves the time and effort normally needed to manufacture such hardware. It also makes it easier and faster for radiation therapists to treat the patient because they no longer need to mount the hardware on the treatment machine. Each beam angle with the passively scattered proton therapy needs its own set of aperture and compensator, therefore the number of beam angles that can be used per patient is limited. Pencil beams have less of a limit on how many beam angles can be used for treatment. Furthermore, the hardware in the pathway of the passively scattered proton therapy (which includes the range modulator wheel, aperture, and tissue compensator) leads to increased neutron production. As a consequence, pencil beam proton therapy also has the advantage of lower neutron doses, which should decrease the risk of secondary cancers and decrease the potential effect on implanted medical devices. Finally, pencil beams are required for intensity-modulated proton therapy (IMPT) with multifield optimization. IMPT allows further improvements in dose conformality and simultaneous integrated boosts to the gross tumor. However, pencil beam proton therapy requires more advanced planning and rigorous quality assurance to make sure that the dose delivered matches the treatment plan.

Fig. 12.4 illustrates a comparison of a pencil beam plan and a passively scattered plan for the treatment of a patient with prostate cancer.[6] As can be seen, the radiation dose lateral and posterior to the prostate is much more conformal with the pencil beam. Most proton therapy centers now have pencil beams available for treatment. In fact, the newest proton therapy centers are being built with only pencil beam capability (and will no longer be able to treat with passively scattered proton beams).

Clinical Outcomes

Numerous studies have shown the benefit of dose escalation in the treatment of prostate cancer. Kuban et al. randomized 301 patients with stage T1b to T3 prostate cancer to either 70 or 78 Gy delivered with x-ray therapy. At a median follow-up time of 8.7 years, the patients who received

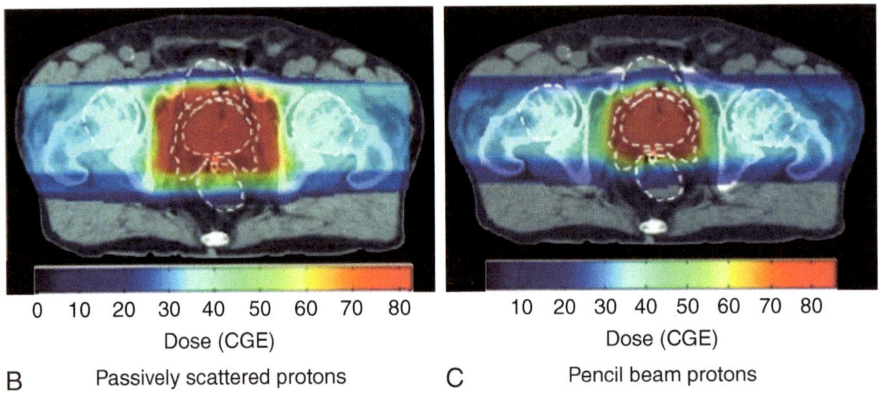

Fig. 12.4 Prostate treatment using passively scattered protons versus pencil beam protons *CGE*, Cobalt Gy equivalent. (From Trofimov A, Nguyen PL, Coen JJ, et al. Radiotherapy treatment of early-stage prostate cancer with IMRT and protons: a treatment planning comparison. *Int J Radiat Oncol Biol Phys.* 2007;69(2):444-453.)

78 Gy had better rates of freedom from biochemical or clinical failure (78%) than the 59% for patients who received 70 Gy ($P = .004$).[4] The clinical failure-free survival rate in the 78-Gy arm was better than that in the 70-Gy arm (93% vs. 85%; $P = .014$), but no overall survival benefit was noted. Unfortunately, the 78-Gy dose was also associated with higher toxicity, with the rate of Radiation Therapy Oncology Group (RTOG) grade 2 or higher gastrointestinal (GI) toxicity being 26% versus 13% ($P = .013$). No significant difference was found between groups in RTOG grade 2 or higher genitourinary (GU) toxicity (13% vs. 8%).

The Dutch Multicenter Trial randomized 669 patients with localized prostate cancer to either 68 or 78 Gy delivered with x-ray therapy. After a median follow-up time of 70 months, the 7-year freedom from failure rate was better in the 78-Gy arm than in the 68-Gy arm (54% vs. 47%; $P = .04$).[10] Once again, late grade 2 or higher GI toxicity was higher in the 78-Gy arm than in the 68-Gy arm (35% vs. 25%; $P = .04$), but no significant difference was noted in late grade 2 or higher GU toxicity (40% vs. 41%; $P = .6$).

The Proton Radiation Oncology Group (PROG) 95-09 study randomized a total of 393 patients with stage T1b–T2b with prostate-specific antigen (PSA) levels less than 15 ng/mL treated at either Loma Linda University Medical Center (LLUMC) or Massachusetts General Hospital (MGH). All patients received three-dimensional conformal x-ray therapy to the prostate and seminal vesicles to a dose of 50.4 Gy, followed by a proton boost of either 28.8 cobalt Gy equivalent (CGE) or 19.8 CGE. Therefore the patients were randomized to either 79.2 CGE or 70.2 CGE. At LLUMC, patients were treated while supine with opposed lateral 250-MeV proton beams. At MGH, patients were treated in the lithotomy position with a single transperineal 160-MeV proton beam. At a median follow-up time of 8.9 years, patients who received 79.2 CGE were significantly less likely to have local failure, with a hazard ratio of 0.57. The 10-year biochemical failure rates according to the American Society of Therapeutic Radiation Oncology definition were 16.7% and 32.4% for the 79.2 CGE and 70.2 CGE arms, respectively ($P \leq .0001$).[5] Patient-reported outcomes using the Prostate Cancer Symptom Indices and Distress Scales were published separately. At a median of 9.4 years, no difference in urinary obstruction/irritation ($P = .36$), urinary incontinence ($P = .99$), bowel problems ($P = .70$), or sexual dysfunction ($P = .65$) were noted between dose groups.[11] Unfortunately, PROG 95-09 was not a randomized comparison of protons and x-rays; all of the patients received a combination of photons and x-rays. However, no increased GI toxicity was seen with dose escalation in this study when proton therapy was used for boost dosing.

Several single-institution reports have been published on outcomes after proton therapy for prostate cancer. Slater et al. published the LLUMC experience of 1255 patients treated between October 1991 and December 1997. Patients with 15% or greater risk of having pelvic lymph node metastasis according to the Partin tables were treated with a conformal "boost" with protons to a dose of 30 CGE in 15 fractions given to the prostate and seminal vesicles, followed by a conformal treatment with x-rays to a dose of 45 Gy to the prostate, seminal vesicles and the first- and second-echelon lymphatics. Patients who did not have this risk were treated with proton therapy only to a total dose of 74 CGE in 2-CGE fractions. These patients were treated with a rectal balloon placed daily, usually with one field per day. With a median follow-up time of 62 months, the overall biochemical disease-free survival rate was 73%[12] and depended on both the initial PSA and the PSA nadir reached after the treatment. In patients with an initial PSA of level 4.0 ng/mL or less, the biochemical disease-free survival rate was 90%, and in patients with posttreatment PSA of 0.5 ng/mL or less, 87%. The actuarial 5-year and 10-year rates of freedom from grade 3 and 4 GI toxicity were both 99%. The actuarial 5-year and 10-year rates for freedom from grade 3 and 4 GU toxicity were also both 99%.

Bryant et al. published the outcomes of 1327 patients treated with protons at the University of Florida Jacksonville between 2006 and 2010. With a median follow-up time of 5.5 years, the 5-year freedom from biochemical progression rates were 99%, 94%, and 74% in low-risk, intermediate-risk, and high-risk patients, respectively.[13] The actuarial 5-year rates of late grade 3 or higher on the Common Terminology Criteria for Adverse Events, version 4.0 (CTCAE 4.0) for GI and GU toxicity were 0.6% and 2.9%, respectively. No significant changes were noted in median and mean Expanded Prostate Cancer Index (EPIC) summary scores for the bowel, urinary irritative/obstructive, and urinary incontinence domains. Only sexual function summary scores declined from baseline to 5 years in patients who did not receive hormone ablation therapy.

Pugh et al. reported patient-reported outcomes of 291 patients after proton therapy at MD Anderson Cancer Center who had a minimum follow-up of 2 years. All patients were treated with opposed lateral beams to a total dose of 76 CGE in 2-CGE fractions. Interestingly, 226 patients were treated with passively scattered proton therapy, and 65 patients were treated with pencil beam proton therapy. Cumulative rates of grade of 2 or higher GU and GI toxicity at 24 months were 13.4% and 9.6%, respectively.[14] One patient had grade 3 GI toxicity, but none had grade of 4 (or higher) toxicity. No patients had grade 3 (or higher) GU toxicity. Patients receiving passively scattered proton therapy had a slightly higher rate of argon plasma coagulation compared with pencil beam proton therapy, but that apparent difference was not statistically significant (4.4% vs. 1.5%; $P = .21$).

Several retrospective comparisons of protons and IMRT[15] have been made. A Surveillance, Epidemiology, and End Results (SEER)-Medicare analysis by Sheets et al. showed a lower rate of GI morbidity (relative risk [RR]: 0.66) with IMRT than with protons in a propensity score–matched comparison. However, this analysis was severely limited, as any GI procedure performed after the treatment was coded as a morbidity. Hoppe et al. compared patients undergoing either proton therapy or IMRT by using prospectively collected QoL data from the EPIC; 1243 proton patients were treated with 76 to 82 CGE and 204 IMRT patients were treated with 75.6 to 79.4 Gy. No difference was seen between the two groups for the bowel, urinary incontinence, urinary irritative/obstructive, and sexual domains.[16] However, more patients in the IMRT group reported moderate/big problems with rectal urgency ($P = .02$) and frequent bowel movements ($P = .05$) compared with patients in the proton therapy group. Fang et al.

compared 181 proton therapy patients and 213 IMRT patients treated between 2010 and 2012 in terms of maximum acute and late GI/GU CTCAE-graded toxicities. On multivariate analysis, no statistically significant differences were found in the rates of acute/late grade 2 GU (or higher) and GI toxicities between the two groups.[17] Yu et al. analyzed a Medicare database of 27,647 men and found that patients who received proton therapy had significant less GU toxicity at 6 months compared with IMRT (5.9% vs. 9.5%; P = .03); however, the difference disappeared by 12 months (18.8% vs. 17.5%; P = .66).[18] No difference was found in GI or other toxicity at 6 or 12 months.

Proton therapy may also reduce the risk of secondary cancer when compared with IMRT. Several analyses have predicted that IMRT would increase the risk of secondary cancer, whereas proton therapy would decrease the risk.[18–21] A retrospective matched cohort analysis of 558 proton patients and 558 x-ray patients in the SEER registry published by Chung et al.[22] showed that proton therapy was associated with a significant reduction of secondary cancer risk (RR: 0.52; P = .009) relative to x-ray therapy. However, the limitations of this retrospective study led the authors to state that these results should be considered as hypothesis-generating.

These results show that proton therapy is an effective and safe method for the treatment of prostate cancer. However, because no randomized trial has directly compared proton therapy with IMRT, it is difficult to know if protons are superior to IMRT in terms of efficacy or risk of side effects. One randomized trial is currently ongoing, the Proton Therapy versus IMRT for Low or Intermediate Risk Prostate Cancer (PARTIQoL). However, we will need to wait several years until the results of that trial are available.

Proton Treatment at MD Anderson Cancer Center

PATIENT SELECTION

Although the results of the PARTIQoL trial are not yet available, there are probably several specific instances where proton therapy may be especially beneficial. For instance, we recommend proton therapy for younger patients (although the definition of "younger" can vary significantly among clinicians) and for patients with larger prostates, especially a large medial lobe. Trying to cover a large medial lobe with IMRT usually leads to irradiating a much larger area of the bladder than with proton therapy. However, we routinely recommend that men with a very large medial lobe consider having that lobe surgically removed via a transurethral resection of the prostate or greenlight laser enucleation before radiation therapy. If a patient were to undergo such a procedure, we recommend waiting for 2 to 3 months before starting radiation therapy to allow adequate healing to minimize the risk of urinary incontinence after the radiation therapy.

As is true for IMRT, we do not recommend proton therapy for patients with certain collagen vascular diseases (such as lupus and scleroderma) or inflammatory bowel disease (i.e., Crohn disease and ulcerative colitis). We also do not treat patients with metal in the pelvis (most often artificial hips) in the pathway of the proton beam, for two reasons. The first reason is that the metal can significantly block the proton beam, which could decrease the dose delivered to the prostate. The second reason is that artifacts from the metal make treatment planning less accurate because of increased uncertainty in tissue density calculation from the planning computed tomography (CT) scan. We also discourage patients who are pacemaker dependent from undergoing proton therapy because of the neutron dose from the protons and their potential effects on the pacemaker. When we do treat patients with pacemakers (or any other implanted electronics), we treat them with the pencil beam to try to minimize the neutron dose as much as possible.

Fiducial Placement

Once a patient is deemed to be a candidate for proton therapy as the definitive treatment for prostate cancer, fiducial placement and treatment simulation are planned.

At MD Anderson, the fiducials are inserted transrectally under ultrasound guidance by either the radiation oncology or urology teams. However, at other institutions, fiducials may be placed by interventional radiologists. Fiducial placement may be more[23] important for proton therapy than for IMRT because of the risk of shadowing of the proton dose from the fiducials. Tables 12.1 and 12.2 show the actual amounts of dose attenuation from various types of fiducials. Of the three types of fiducials listed, gold fiducials have the highest proton attenuation, and so we use the carbon/ZrO_2 fiducial at (Fig. 12.5) at MD Anderson. We usually place two fiducials in the prostate (as opposed to three for IMRT) to minimize the risk of dose shadowing in tumor areas. We also try to place the fiducials in areas where little or no cancer is present.

Once the fiducials have been placed, ideally 7 days should elapse before the simulation is done to allow the fiducials to settle. However, because many of our patients are from out of town, we often perform the simulation on the same day as the fiducial placement. In the event of concern about migration of the fiducials, we perform a verification CT during the treatment.

We have just begun to use SpaceOAR hydrogel spacers between the prostate and rectum for patients undergoing proton therapy. Currently, this procedure is done in the operating room. Also, fiducials are placed transperineally at the same time as the SpaceOAR insertion.

TABLE 12.1 ■ **Maximum Dose Perturbations from Small and Large Gold Fiducials in Two Orientations and at Various Implantation Depths**

Marker	Orientation	Zc (cm)	ΔD_{max} (%)	Zs (cm)
Small gold	Perpendicular	19.5	−15	>0.93
Small gold	Perpendicular	23.5	−17	0.58
Small gold	Perpendicular	26.5	−24	Fluctuates
Small gold	Perpendicular	27.5	−46	0.46
Small gold	Parallel	19.5	−37	0.35
Small gold	Parallel	23.5	−41	0.35
Small gold	Parallel	26.5	−67	0.00
Small gold	Parallel	27.5	−86	0.00
Large gold	Perpendicular	19.5	−21	>0.93
Large gold	Perpendicular	23.5	−25	0.93
Large gold	Perpendicular	26.5	−42	1.04
Large gold	Perpendicular	27.5	−69	0.46
Large gold	Parallel	19.5	−43	0.69
Large gold	Parallel	23.5	−48	0.46
Large gold	Parallel	26.5	−83	0.00
Large gold	Parallel	27.5	−91	0.00

Summary of the maximum dose perturbation (ΔD_{max}) resulting from the small and large gold fiducials in two orientations and at various implantation depths (*zc*). The distance of the maximum shadow from the downstream edge of the marker (*zs*) is also given. In addition, "fluctuates" indicates that the measured dose fluctuated for a certain region downstream of the fiducial and did not exhibit a distinctive trough to determine the definitive *zs* for the given fiducial (see Fig. 12.5). The uncertainty of the maximum dose perturbation is on the order of 5%.

From Cheung J, Kudchadker RJ, Zhu XR, et al. Dose perturbations and image artifacts caused by carbon-coated ceramic and stainless steel fiducials used in proton therapy for prostate cancer. *Phys Med Biol.* 2010;55(23):7135-7147.

TABLE 12.2 ■ **Maximum Dose Perturbations from Carbon-Coated Zirconium Dioxide Fiducials in Two Orientations and at Various Implantation Depths**

Marker	Orientation	*Zc* (cm)	ΔD_{max} (%)	*Zs* (cm)
C/ZrO_2	Perpendicular	19.5	—	—
C/ZrO_2	Perpendicular	23.5	−8	0.35
C/ZrO_2	Perpendicular	26.5	−7	Fluctuates
C/ZrO_2	Perpendicular	27.5	−18	0.58
C/ZrO_2	Parallel	19.5	−10	0.58
C/ZrO_2	Parallel	23.5	−15	0.35
C/ZrO_2	Parallel	26.5	−21	0.12
C/ZrO_2	Parallel	27.5	−38	0.23
PEEK/stainless steel	Perpendicular	19.5	—	—
PEEK/stainless steel	Perpendicular	23.5	—	—
PEEK/stainless steel	Perpendicular	26.5	−2	Fluctuates
PEEK/stainless steel	Parallel	19.5	−7	0.58
PEEK/stainless steel	Parallel	23.5	−8	0.58
PEEK/stainless steel	Parallel	26.5	−12	0.35

Summary of the maximum dose perturbation (ΔD_{max}) resulting from the carbon-coated zirconium dioxide (C/ZrO_2) and polyethe rether ketone (PEEK)-encapsulated stainless steel fiducials in two orientations and at various implantation depths (*zc*). The distance of the maximum shadow from the downstream edge of the marker (*zs*) is also given. Note that where no value is given means that there was no observable dose perturbation in the radiochromic film for that given depth. In addition, "fluctuates" indicates that the measured dose fluctuated for a certain region downstream of the fiducial and did not exhibit a distinctive trough to determine the definitive *zs* for the given fiducial (see Fig. 12.5). The uncertainty of the maximum dose perturbation is of the order of 5%.

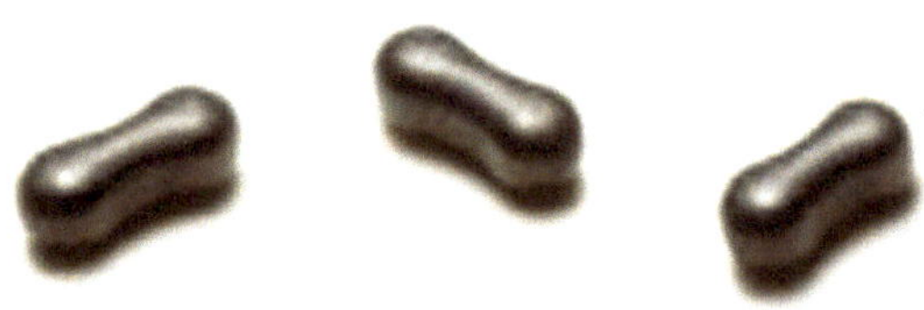

Fig. 12.5 Carbon-coated zirconium dioxide fiducials.

No fiducials are placed for patients receiving adjuvant or salvage treatment after radical prostatectomy.

Simulation

For treatment simulation, the patient is placed in a supine position and the endorectal balloon is placed in the rectum. We then inflate the balloon with 60 to 80 mL of warm water based on the size of the balloon that is used (either "short" or "long"). Once the balloon is placed, we immobilize the patient's legs in a foot-knee indexed cradle. After ensuring that the patient is straight and not rotated, a noncontrast planning CT scan of the pelvis is obtained. Some concerns have been raised about the effect of patient rotation on daily proton treatments. Sejpal et al. and Meyer et al. showed that patient rotational setup errors up to 5 degrees on either side do not significantly change the dose to the target volume or critical structures when passively scattered proton therapy or pencil beam proton therapy are used.[24–25]

The rectal balloon is used to immobilize the prostate in the pelvis. Having a consistent tissue path that the protons must traverse to reach the prostate is important because a change in this path length can affect the dose deposition of the proton beam. The rectal balloon can also push the posterior aspect of the rectum, as well as the sigmoid colon and small bowel, away from the prostate, which likely decreases the risk of toxicity to these structures. However, at the same time, the anterior wall of the rectum is often placed next to the prostate more consistently by the rectal balloon, which may negate some of the benefit of pushing the rest of the rectum away. We do not use a rectal balloon for patients being treated with the SpaceOAR hydrogel.

For postoperative patients, rectal balloon use is determined on an individual basis, because there is no prostate to immobilize. In some patients, the balloon can help to push the sigmoid and bowel away, whereas in others, it can lead to more rectum getting irradiated because the balloon deforms the prostate fossa more posteriorly and laterally around the rectum.

We have a dedicated magnetic resonance imaging (MRI) simulator at the Proton Therapy Center. Currently, we are using this MRI simulator for patients having SpaceOARs inserted to confirm the hydrogel placement and to delineate the hydrogel for treatment planning (the hydrogel is difficulty to distinguish from the prostate and rectum on CT cans). These patients undergo treatment simulation with both CT and MRI. We are also studying the possibility of generating a synthetic CT scan from the MRI, which would eliminate the need for CT simulation.

Contouring

At MD Anderson, the clinical target volume for the definitive treatment of prostate cancer is based on the National Cancer Center Network risk classification for prostate cancer as follows: prostate only for low risk, prostate-proximal seminal vesicles (SV) for intermediate risk, and prostate and entire SV for high risk. Proximal is defined as the proximal 1.5 cm of the SV. Pelvic lymph nodes are generally not treated, even in high-risk prostate cancer, at MD Anderson.

Dosing

The standard dose is 78 CGE, given in 2-CGE daily fractions. We do consider using a slower fractionation scheme (i.e., 77.4 or 79.2 CGE in 1.8-CGE daily fractions) for patients with previous treatments to the prostate (i.e., cryotherapy, high-intensity focused ultrasound) to minimize the risk of urethral toxicity.

We are also evaluating a hypofractionation protocol in which 55.5 CGE is given in 3.7-CGE fractions given 3 times per week (for a total of 15 fractions).

Image Guidance

Daily image-guided radiation therapy is achieved by using daily kV imaging with fiducials (Fig. 12.6). For postoperative patients, we use daily kV imaging of the pelvic bony anatomy.

Conclusions

Proton therapy is an effective and safe treatment modality for the treatment of prostate cancer. Pencil beam proton therapy and the advent of IMPT have allowed further improvements in treatment

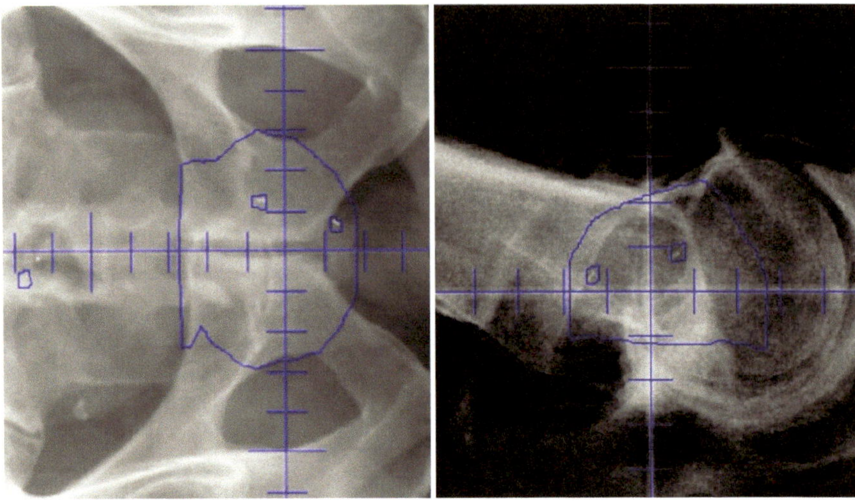

Fig. 12.6 Daily kV imaging of carbon fiducials for proton therapy.

planning and dose delivery. However, a randomized trial is still needed to directly compare protons and x-rays to establish the potential benefit of proton therapy in the treatment of prostate cancer.

In the future, we at MD Anderson aim to incorporate more MRI into the treatment planning process by using an MRI simulator, which, when combined with IMPT, will allow us to target dominant lesions. We will also likely move more toward hypofractionated proton therapy and perhaps even stereotactic body proton therapy to the prostate.

References Available Online.

CHAPTER 13

Head and Neck

Steven J. Frank ■ G. Brandon Gunn

Introduction

Radiation therapy, whether used as definitive treatment or as an adjuvant to surgery, is an essential component of treatment for many patients with head and neck cancer (HNC). Both photon (x-ray) therapy and proton therapy are standard forms of radiation therapy, and both have evolved over time with the advent of technological advances. Proton therapy has evolved from two-dimensional (2D) and three-dimensional (3D) passive scatter to the current state of the art, which is active (spot) scanning intensity-modulated proton therapy (IMPT). With ongoing improvements in terms of the sophistication of both planning and delivery, IMPT is considered likely to advance further in terms of dose distributions in the near future.

One of the main benefits of photon (x-ray) intensity-modulated radiation therapy (IMRT) relative to traditional 2D or 3D radiation therapy techniques for HNC is the ability to conform the therapeutic dose distributions around targets. This ability allows the parotid glands (as one example) to be spared relative to the dose given to the tumor, which translates to reduced xerostomia and improved quality of life compared with the traditional 2D or 3D approaches. However, despite the demonstrated clinical advantages and rapid and widespread adoption of IMRT, the all-too-common problematic acute toxic effects (e.g., mucositis, pain, odynophagia, dysphagia, fatigue, nausea/vomiting, and dysgeusia/ageusia) and late treatment-related toxic effects (e.g., xerostomia, fatigue, dysphagia, and osteonecrosis), with their associated symptoms and negative effects on important functions (e.g., swallowing, cognition, vision, voice, speech, and general activity) and overall quality of life, still remain significant problems for many patients being treated for HNC.

Moreover, clinicians are increasingly recognizing the dosimetric trade-offs and negative clinical consequences of applying the multiple oblique beams (e.g., 7–9 static fields or even 360-degree volumetric arcs) required to generate contemporary parotid-sparing IMRT plans. IMRT techniques inherently increase the irradiated volumes, and their beams traverse numerous nontarget normal tissues that are outside the treatment portals and essentially unirradiated in the pre-IMRT era.[1] Numerous studies have shown that the dose delivered to nontarget structures by IMRT has negative clinical consequences ("beam-path toxicity"), especially for structures that are posterior or anterior to the targets.[2] For example, even intermediate- or low-dose radiation to the brainstem to levels generally considered to be safe correlate with increased nausea and vomiting[3] and fatigue.[2,4] Also, radiation doses to the (nontarget) anterior mandible correlate with anterior oral cavity mucositis and with dysgeusia, ageusia, minor salivary gland function, and long-term perceptions of oral moisture and oral comfort.[2] Other investigators have also highlighted the potential negative effects of technique-driven photon (x-ray) IMRT on unnecessary dose to the skin,[5] larynx,[6] and esophagus and the associated toxic effects.[6,7]

Numerous dosimetric comparison studies have demonstrated that proton therapy—active (spot) scanning IMPT in particular—can achieve better dose distributions than photon (x-ray) IMRT for numerous HN tumor subsites.[8–11] In general, IMPT has been shown to achieve conformality of high-dose regions around targets that is comparable with that from IMRT but with the advantage of further reducing or even eliminating the unnecessary low-to-intermediate-range integral dose to numerous adjacent critical organs and normal tissues. The unique inherent physical properties of protons, with their lower entrance dose and zero exit dose, plus the advantage of a sharper lateral penumbra (particularly with aperture use), translate into fewer beams being required for proton therapy than for IMRT and reduction in beam competition effects relative to that for IMRT plan optimization. Thus, clinicians have sought to exploit the highly conformal and more compact dose distributions from proton therapy for treating HNCs, with the goals of further improving patient outcomes through the safer delivery of therapeutic doses to targets while minimizing or even eliminating the beam path toxicity associated with IMRT.

Passive scatter proton therapy was the first iteration of proton therapy to be used for HNC; over the past several years, more treatment centers are coming online with more advanced active (spot) scanning and IMPT capabilities, and the implementation of proton therapy for HNC has expanded. At the University of Texas MD Anderson Cancer Center, our clinical proton therapy program was initiated after the development of center-specific proton therapy planning strategies,[12,13] completion of dosimetric comparison studies,[9,11] and advancements in plan-specific quality assurance measurement methods.[14] The first HNC patient was treated at our center with passive scatter protons in 2007 and active (spot) scanning IMPT in 2010.[15] As the number of proton therapy centers continues to expand and as clinical follow-up data continue to mature, the number of clinical studies and trials, with corresponding publication of clinical outcomes, is anticipated to increase sharply. Further, the American Society for Radiation Oncology has updated its model policy with recommendations for medical insurance coverage for proton therapy,[16] and the National Comprehensive Cancer Network (NCCN) Clinical Practice Guidelines in Oncology for HNC now recognize proton therapy as a standard option for advanced conformal radiation therapy that can be considered for multiple indications.[17]

The remainder of this chapter is organized by an anatomic HN tumor subsite, concluding with a brief section on the use of proton therapy for reirradiation of recurrent or second primary HNC. Each site-specific section reviews the (1) dosimetric advantages of proton therapy (particularly IMPT) over IMRT in terms of critical organ protection and normal tissue sparing, with illustrative case examples; (2) clinical outcomes reported to date, both in terms of disease control and toxicity reduction; (3) published comparisons of results after proton therapy with those after photon-based approaches; (4) ongoing prospective studies of proton therapy for HNC; and (5) opportunities for further improvement and future directions for the field.

Base-of-Skull Tumors: Chordoma and Chondrosarcoma

Skull-base tumors were the first tumors of the HN region to be routinely treated with proton therapy, with the initial clinical rationale of their challenging location, their proximity to critical structures, and poor outcomes after conventional treatments owing to resistance to the doses that could be safely delivered with photon-based approaches while respecting normal tissue tolerances. Proton therapy is currently widely accepted as the preferred modality for radiation treatment of skull-base chordoma and chondrosarcoma after numerous retrospective series demonstrated substantially superior outcomes relative to historical results (Table 13.1). Given the location of such tumors and their proximity to critical central nervous system structures (namely brainstem, brain, and optic pathways), the use of advanced patient setup/immobilization techniques and robust planning strategies is essential to minimize and account for biophysical uncertainties (e.g., proton range). Future directions to further improve outcomes for these and other classically radioresistant tumors include optimizing the linear energy transfer distribution of proton therapy plans[18] and identifying ways to exploit the enhanced relative biological effectiveness (RBE) of protons at the end of their range.[19]

TABLE 13.1 ■ **Studies Evaluating Proton Therapy for Chordoma and Chondrosarcoma**

References	Patients (*n*)	Type	Site	Treatment	Outcome	Toxicity	Conclusion
Rombi et al.	26	Retro	Skull base and axial skeleton chordoma (19) or chondrosarcoma (7)	Surgery/biopsy, PBR using spot-scanning technique, mean dose 74 CGE for chordoma and 66 CGE for chondrosarcoma at 1.8–2 CGE per fraction	5-y LC: 81% (chordoma), 80% (chondrosarcoma); 5-y OS: 89% and 75%	No high-grade acute or late toxicity	Spot-scanning results in excellent LC with acceptable rates of late toxicity
McDonald et al.	16	Retro	Skull-base and spinal chordoma treated with surgery (15/16) and EBRT	Retreated with PBR to 71.2–79.2 CGE	2-y LC: 85%; 2-y CSS: 88%; 2-y OS: 80%	3 patients with bitemporal lobe necrosis, 1 patient with CSF leak and meningitis, and 1 with ischemic brainstem stroke	Reirradiation is a feasible option for patients with recurrent chordoma of the skull base or spine
Ares et al.	64	Retro	Skull-base chordoma (42) and chondrosarcomas (22)	Surgery/biopsy followed by spot-scanning PBR; mean 68.4 CGE 1.8–2 CGE per fraction 4 days/week	5-y LC: 81% (chordoma), 94% (chondrosarcoma); 5-y DFS: 81% and 100%; 5-y OS: 62% and 91%	94% 5-y freedom from high-grade toxicity; 2 patients experienced grade 3–4 optic neuropathy, 2 patients experienced grade 3 symptomatic temporal lobe damage	Spot-scanning is safe with efficacy and toxicity rates similar to passive scatter
Rutz et al.	10	Retro	Skull-base and spinal chordoma (6) and chondrosarcoma (4)	Surgery followed by spot-scanning PBR; median 66–74 CGE with/without chemotherapy	100% 3-y LC, DFS, and OS	Only grade 1 acute toxicity reported. Late toxicity in 3/10 patients: pituitary, alopecia, and radiographic brain changes and auditory changes	IMPT has similar safety and efficacy as passive scatter but may allow dose intensification

Continued on following page

TABLE 13.1 ■ **Studies Evaluating Proton Therapy for Chordoma and Chondrosarcoma** (Continued)

References	Patients (*n*)	Type	Site	Treatment	Outcome	Toxicity	Conclusion
Noël et al.	100	Retro	Skull-base or cervical spine chordoma	Surgery/biopsy, combined proton-photon RT; median dose 67 CGE	2-y LC: 86%; 4-y LC: 54%; 2-y OS: 94%; 5-y OS: 81%	42 with late complications: 11 with vision loss, 11 with neuropsych complications, 21 with decreased hearing, 16 with pituitary dysfunction	Homogeneity of dose in the target volume is an important predictor of control
Munzenrider et al.	519	Retro	Skull base chordoma and chondrosarcoma	Surgery/biopsy followed by 66–83 CGE proton-photon RT	5-y LRFS: 73% (chordoma), 98% (chondrosarcoma); 5-y OS: 80% and 91%	3 patients died of brainstem injury, 8 patients had temporal lobe injury; other toxicities reported were hearing loss, cranial neuropathy, endocrinopathy	Postoperative treatment with PBR is the best management strategy for patients with base-of-skull chordoma and chondrosarcoma

CGE, Cobalt Gray equivalent; *CSF,* cerebrospinal fluid; *CSS,* chordoma-specific survival; *DFS,* disease-free survival; *EBRT,* external beam radiation therapy; *IMPT,* intensity-modulated proton therapy; *LC,* local control; *LRFS,* local relapse-free survival; *n,* number; *OS,* overall survival; *PBR,* proton beam radiation; *Retro,* retrospective; *RT,* radiation therapy; *y,* year.

Modified from Holliday EB, Frank SJ. Proton radiation therapy for head and neck cancer: a review of the clinical experience to date. *Int J Radiat Oncol Biol Phys.* 2014;89(2):292–302. With permission.

Sinonasal Tumors

Building on the clinical rationale for the aforementioned skull-base tumors, many centers have implemented proton therapy as a preferred radiotherapy approach for a variety of sinonasal malignancies of various histologic types, and clinical outcomes have been encouraging (Table 13.2). The largest of these single-institution studies evaluated 102 patients with tumors of various histologic subtypes, treated with or without surgery followed by postoperative or definitive combination photon-proton therapy from 1991 through 2002. With a median follow-up interval of more than 5 years for surviving patients, the local control rates after treatment that incorporated proton therapy were excellent: 95% for those who underwent complete surgical resection, 82% for partial, and 87% for those with nonresected or intact tumors. The most common pattern of recurrence was distant, occurring in about 30% of patients at 5 years. The extent of surgical resection was, unsurprisingly, associated with distant metastasis and long-term outcomes.[20] In another study, Truong et al. reported an excellent local control rate of 86% at 2 years after high-dose (median, 76 Gy [RBE]) proton therapy for sphenoid sinus tumors, a particularly challenging tumor location.[21]

Notable findings in the studies summarized in Table 13.2 are the high rates of both local control and survival for patients with unresected mucosal melanoma after proton therapy. In general, toxicity rates for these types of tumors at this site tend to be high, reaching 20% for higher-grade toxicity; yet these rates were still comparable with those from existing photon data and were likely biased by selecting the most challenging cases to be treated with proton therapy. A meta-analysis by Patel et al. summarized a largely retrospective body of evidence and provided the strongest comparative effectiveness data for particle- and photon-based treatments for sinonasal disease. These results revealed a survival advantage for particle or proton therapy; at a median follow-up interval of about 40 months, overall survival rates were higher for those who received particle- versus photon-based treatment at 5 years (relative risk [RR]: 1.51; $P = .0038$) and were also higher at the longest follow-up interval (RR: 1.27; $P = .037$). Local-regional control rates were no different at 5 years (RR: 1.06; $P = .79$) but were higher for the particle therapy group at the longest follow-up interval (RR: 1.18; $P = .031$). The studies included in this meta-analysis were somewhat limited by the usual biases inherent in retrospective single-institution series. However, given the power and consistently favorable outcomes reported across the series, particle or proton therapy should be considered a valid option for sinonasal malignancies,[22] and this recommendation has been incorporated into the 2017 and 2018 NCCN guidelines for HN cancer.[17] A case study involving postoperative proton therapy for a paranasal sinus (maxillary) tumor is shown in Fig. 13.1; a case study of IMPT for a nasal cavity/anterior skull-base tumor that involved using an aperture to spare the anterior eyes and corneas is shown in Fig. 13.2.

Pharyngeal and Oral Tumors

Because most patients presenting with pharyngeal cancers (particularly human papillomavirus–associated oropharyngeal cancer [OPC]) are relatively young and high functioning and have a generally favorable long-term prognosis, the potential exists for such patients to live for decades with the sequelae of treatments. Acute and late toxicity reduction and uncomplicated cure are now the current emphasis in optimal clinical care and the primary end point in numerous ongoing clinical investigations in OPC, generally through treatment deintensification by total radiation therapy dose/volume reduction (e.g., reduced tumor dose), modification of systemic therapy, or both.[23] Proton therapy is another viable approach for treatment deintensification in pharyngeal cancers because it can reduce treatment-related toxicity through delivering a more compact dose distribution around targets, thereby reducing or even eliminating dose to important nontarget normal tissues while maintaining tumor dose. Evidence from initial reports from the MD Anderson

TABLE 13.2 ■ **Studies Evaluating Proton Therapy for Sinonasal Malignancies**

References	Type	Accrual	Pts (*n*)	Technique	Comp photon	CCT (%)	*S* (%)	Histology	Follow-Up (Median)	Outcomes	Late Toxicity
Resto et al.[20]	Retro	1991–2002	102	PSPT	No	4	100	Various	61 mo	5-y LC: 95%, 82%, and 87%; OS 90%, 53%, and 49% for complete resection, partial resection, and biopsy only	NR
Nakamura et al.	Retro	1999–2012	42	PSPT	No	26	0	ENB	69 mo	5-OS/PFS: 100/80% for Kadish A, 86/65% for Kadish B, 76/39% for Kadish C	6 pts with G3–4 (ipsilateral visual impairment, 3; bilateral visual impairment, 1; liquorrhea, 1; cataract, 1)
Russo et al.	Retro	1991–2008	54	PSPT	No	39	69	SCC	82 mo	5-y LRC: 73%; OS: 47%	9 pts with G3 and 6 with G4. Mostly wound site issues (e.g., fistulas). No G5
Dagan et al.	Retro	2007–2013	84	PSPT	No	75	74	Various	32 mo	3-y LC: 83%; NC: 94%; freedom from DM: 73.2%; OS: 68%	G3–5: overall 24%. CNS necrosis: G2 in 11%, G3 in 4%, and G5 in 1 pt. G3–4 bone or soft tissue necrosis in 7 pts. 3 pts died of Tx-related complications (G5)
Nakamura et al.	Pro	2009–2011	26	PSPT	No	100	0	Various	NR	3-y OS: 58%	G4: 2 pts (osteonecrosis, retinopathy); G3: 4 pts (cataract: 2, mucositis/dermatitis: 2)
McDonald et al.	Retro	2010–2014	14 + 26	PSPT	Yes	75	NR	Various	NR	NR	More feeding tubes and more morphine used in IMRT group (but more NPC in IMRT group and more paranasal in proton group)
Zenda et al.	Pro	2008–2012	32	PSPT	No	0	0	Mel	36 mo	1-y LC: 76;3-y OS: 46%; PFS: 36%	No late G3+ toxicity reported

Zenda et al.	Retro	1999–2008	90	PSPT	No	12	18	Various	57 mo	5-y OS: 64%; PFS: 44%	Late toxicity G3 in 17 pts (19%), G4 in 6 pts (7%; encephalomyelitis infection, 2; optic nerve disorder, 4)
Linton et al.	Retro	2004–2012	26	PSPT	No	0	77	ACC	25 mo	2-y LC: 95%; OS: 93% (not previously irradiated)	Late toxicity G3 in 2 pts, G4 in 1, and G5 in 1 (after re-irradiation)
Takagi et al.	Retro	2002–2012	40	PSPT	No	0	0	ACC	38 mo	5-y OS: 63%; PFS: 30%; LC: 76%	36 G3+ events in 21 pts (26%). G+ in 24 pts, mostly osteonecrosis, G4 in 9 pts (mostly vision loss) and G5 in 3 (NP ulcers). Not separated according to proton or carbon ion therapy
Fuji et al.	Retro	2006–2012	20	PSPT	No	0	0	Mel	35 mo	3-y OS: 68%; PFS: 60%	No G3. G4 in 1 pt (optic neuropathy). No G5
Demizu et al.	Retro	2003–2011	33	PSPT	No	0	0	Mel	18 mo	2-y LC: 71%; OS: 44%	G3–4 in 3 pts: 2 G3 (cataract, oral mucositis, and pain); 2 G4 (optic neuropathy and retinopathy)
Patel et al. (meta-analysis)[22]	Retro	1975–2013	286	PSPT + CIT	Yes			Various	38 mo	Pooled OS higher at 5 y for charged particle than for photon therapy (relative risk :1.51; 95% CI: 1.14–1.99; $P = .0038$) and at longest follow-up (1.27; 1.01–1.59; $P = .037$), as well as DFS at 5 y (1·93; 1.36–2.75, $P = .0003$)	

ACC, Adenoid cystic carcinoma; *CCT*, concomitant chemotherapy; *CI*, confidence interval; *CIT*, carbon ion therapy; *Comp*, comparison; *DFS*, disease-free survival; *DM*, distant metastases; *ENB*, esthesioneuroblastoma; *G*, grade; *LC*, local control; *LRC*, locoregional control; *Mel*, melanoma; *Mo*, month; *NR*, nor reported; *NPC*, nasopharyngeal carcinoma; *OC*, oral cancer; *PFS*, progression-free survival; *Pro*, prospective study; *PSPT*, passive scattered proton therapy; *Pts*, patients; *RC*, regional control; *Retro*, retrospective study; *S*, surgery; *SCC*, squamous cell carcinoma; *Tx*, treatment; *y*, year.

From Blanchard P, Gunn GB, Lin A, Foote RL, Lee NY, Frank SJ. Proton therapy for head and neck cancers. *Semin Radiat Oncol.* 2018;28(1):53–63. With permission.

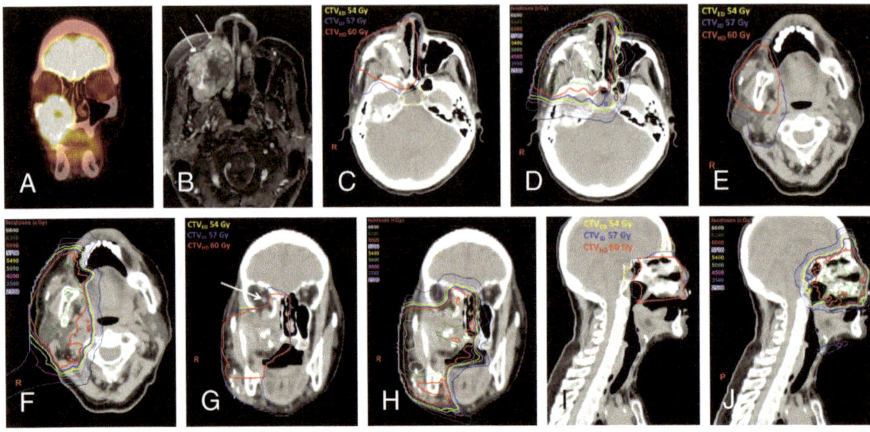

Fig. 13.1 Case study: paranasal sinus tumor. A 61-year-old woman presented with right-sided epiphora and nasal congestion. Imaging revealed a destructive maxillary sinus mass and biopsy showed sarcomatoid squamous cell carcinoma. (A) Coronal projection of staging positron emission tomography/computed tomography showed a hypermetabolic tumor extending through all walls of the maxillary sinus and the floor of the orbit. (B) An axial T1 magnetic resonance image with gadolinium shows the enhancing tumor filling the maxillary sinus with central necrosis and extending anteriorly into soft tissues of the face *(white arrows)* and posterior-laterally into the masticator space. Neither regional nor distant disease was evident on imaging. The patient underwent total maxillectomy and ethmoidectomy with sphenoidotomy and removal of the sphenoid sinus contents, masticator and pterygopalatine space dissection, and resection of involved hard palate. The floor of the orbit was resected, but the globe was preserved. Final pathologic evaluation confirmed poorly differentiated sarcomatoid squamous carcinoma with bone and soft tissue involvement, with final surgical margins free of tumor. The ethmoid sinus specimen contained a tumor, but the sphenoid sinus contents did not. No perineural or lymphovascular invasion was noted. The defect was reconstructed with a free fibula osseocutaneous flap, and the floor of the orbit was also reconstructed with a titanium plate. The patient then received postoperative radiation therapy with active scanning intensity-modulated proton therapy, with treatment simulation and delivery taking place with a mouth-opening and tongue-depressing stent with a bite block. The tumor bed, including the reconstruction flap with margin (high-dose clinical target volume [CTV$_{HD}$]), was treated to 60 Gy (relative biological effectiveness [RBE]), the operative bed (intermediate-dose CTV; CTV$_{ID}$) to 57 Gy (RBE), and the right upper neck levels Ib-II (elective dose to the CTV; CTV$_{ED}$) to 54 Gy (RBE), all given in 30 daily fractions. (C to J) CTVs and dose distributions highlight the conformality of the high-dose regions with limited integral dose to brain, brainstem, and nontarget oral cavity. The maximum dose to the right optic nerve (*white arrow* in G) was limited to 60 Gy (RBE). At 1 year after completing therapy, the patient retained functional vision in both eyes and was free of disease but had low-grade keratopathy and an emerging cataract in the right eye, which was managed conservatively with ocular hydration. (From Garden AS, Beadle BM, Gunn GB. Paranasal sinuses. In: Garden AS, Beadle BM, Gunn GB, eds. *Radiotherapy for Head and Neck Cancers: Indications and Techniques*. 5th ed. New York, NY: Wolters Kluwer; 2017:279-281. With permission.)

and other centers has demonstrated favorable or reduced acute toxicity rates,[24] reduced weight loss and malnutrition, reduced feeding tube placement,[25,26] and reduced osteonecrosis[27] in patients with pharyngeal cancers treated with IMPT as compared with those treated with IMRT.

The first results of the use of proton therapy for pharyngeal cancers were published by Slater et al. in 2005. That study included 29 patients with locally advanced disease treated with a combination of 3D conformal photon therapy with a passive scatter proton concomitant boost. Results were favorable relative to patients treated during the same period and without chemotherapy; at 5 years, the local-regional control rate was 88.0%, and the disease-free survival rate was 65%. The 2-year actuarial incidence of grade 3 (or higher) toxicity was about 16%.[28] Findings from this and more recent reports of proton therapy for OPC, nasopharyngeal carcinoma, and oral cancer are summarized in Table 13.3. Takayama et al. evaluated the use of combination photon-proton therapy with intraarterial chemotherapy as definitive therapy for patients with

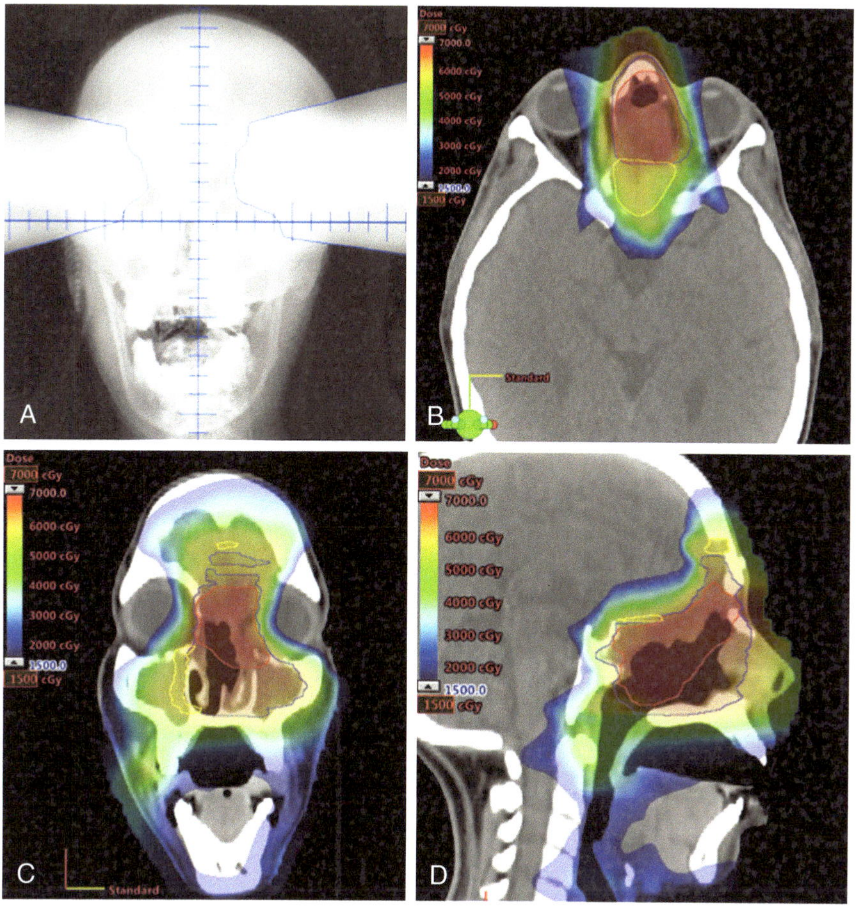

Fig. 13.2 Case study: nasal cavity, anterior skull-base tumor. A 33-year-old woman with esthesioneuroblastoma (Kadish C, Hyams grade 3), with the tumor epicenter in the left nasoethmoid region and extending through the cribriform plate and into the anterior cranial fossa, invading the dura but not the brain, and invading the left lamina papyracea and medial aspect of the left orbit. The patient underwent surgery at an outside facility via a combined endoscopic and open anterior transfacial approach; gross total resection was achieved with numerous positive surgical margins. The patient was given postoperative intensity-modulated proton therapy with concurrent weekly cisplatin. An active (spot) scanning technique was used, with brass apertures for the anterior fields to block the anterior eyes and corneas and to sharpen the lateral penumbra, particularly at the right optic nerve. (B to D) The tumor bed was treated to 64 Gy (relative biological effectiveness [RBE]) (outlined in red), the operative bed to 56 Gy (RBE) (outlined in blue), and elective regions to 54 Gy (RBE) (bilateral facial lymphatics, retropharyngeal nodes, and levels Ib/II nodes) (outlined in yellow), all in a single integrated plan in 32 fractions. (A) anterior oblique field portal image with brass aperture blocking the eyes. Dose distributions in the axial (B), coronal (C), and sagittal (D) planes. The axial (B) and coronal (C) images illustrate sparing of the anterior eye with coverage of the medial aspect of the orbits; the sagittal image (D) illustrates sparing of the brain with coverage of the anterior skull base and dural target.

locally advanced oral cancer who declined surgery. At a median follow-up interval of 43 months, the 3-year rates of local control, regional control, progression-free survival, and overall survival were quite favorable at 87%, 84%, 74%, and 87%, respectively. No grade 3 osteoradionecrosis was observed, although more than one-third of patients experienced dental complications.[29] At MD Anderson, the mainstay of treatment for oral cancer is surgery with postoperative radiation therapy for the presence of adverse pathologic features, with or without chemotherapy.

TABLE 13.3 ■ **Studies Evaluating Proton Therapy for Pharyngeal and Oral Cancers**

References	Subsite	Accrual	Type	Technique (Dose)	Comp IMRT	CCT	Patients (*n*)	Follow-Up (Median)	Outcomes	Toxicity
Slater et al.[28]	OPC	1991–2002	Retro	Cobalt (50.4 Gy), boost PSPT (25.5 Gy)	No	No	29	28 mo	5-y LRC: 88.0%; DFS: 65%	2-y actuarial incidence of G3+ toxicity 16%
Gunn et al.[24]; Blanchard et al.[25]; Sio et al.[30]	OPC	2011–2014	Pro	IMPT (70 Gy)	Yes	Yes	50	30 mo	3-y LRC: 91.0%; OS: 94.3%	Reduced use of gastrostomy tube or severe weight loss at 3 mo and 1 y; less subacute impairment of quality of life
Chan et al.[32]	NPC	2006–2011	Pro	PSPT (70 Gy, upper neck only)	No	Yes	23	28 mo	2-y LRC: 100%; OS: 100%	As expected
Lewis et al.[10]; Holliday et al.[26]	NPC	2011–2013	Pro	IMPT (70 Gy)	Yes	Yes	10	24 mo	2-y LRC: 100%; OS: 88.9%	Less gastrostomy tube in IMPT patients compared with IMRT ($P = .02$)
Takayama et al.[29]	OC	2009–2012	Pro	Photon (36 Gy) and boost PSPT (28.6–39.6 Gy), no surgery	No	IAC	33	43 mo	3-y LC: 86.6%; RC: 83.9%; OS: 87.0%	No grade 3+ osteonecrosis

CCT, Concomitant chemotherapy; *Comp,* comparison; *G*, grade; *IAC,* intraarterial chemotherapy; *IMPT,* intensity-modulated proton therapy; *IMRT,* intensity-modulated (photon) radiation therapy; *LC,* local control; *LRC,* locoregional control; *mo*, month; *NPC,* nasopharyngeal carcinoma; *OC,* oral cancer; *OPC,* oropharyngeal carcinoma; *OS,* overall survival; *Pro,* prospective study; *PSPT,* passive scattered proton therapy; *RC*, regional control; *Retro,* retrospective study; *y,* year.

Note: proton doses are shown in Gy (radiobiologic equivalent [RBE]).

From Blanchard P, Gunn GB, Lin A, Foote RL, Lee NY, Frank SJ. Proton therapy for head and neck cancers. *Semin Radiat Oncol.* 2018;28(1):53–63. With permission.

Oropharyngeal Cancer

Investigators at MD Anderson recently reported a study comparing 50 patients with OPC treated with IMPT who had been matched with 100 contemporary controls treated with IMRT. At a median follow-up time of 32 months, no difference was found in survival rates between the two groups, with 3-year overall survival rates of 94% for the IMPT group and 89% for the IMRT group. However, more patients in the IMRT group had grade 3 weight loss (≥20% from baseline) or required a gastrostomy tube at 3 months after treatment (odds ratio [OR] for IMPT group: 0.44; $P = .05$) and at 1 year after treatment (OR: 0.23; $P = .01$).[25]

A subsequent dosimetric analysis of patterns of local and regional failures among patients given IMPT in the study described above showed no failures within the targeted high-risk volume that would have suggested a geographic target miss; these findings, based on deformable image registration, provided proof of principle of the robustness of these highly modulated IMPT plans. Corresponding details of outcomes in the IMPT group are as follows: median weight loss overall was about 7%, with six patients experiencing loss of more than 10% body weight and one with loss of more than 20%. One patient required a feeding tube before IMPT began, and 11 others required a feeding tube during IMPT; the median interval of feeding tube use after IMPT was 82 days (range: 28–497 days). As for late effects, five patients required a feeding tube for more than 3 months after IMPT, yet only one patient required a feeding tube for more than 1 year; that tube was ultimately removed at 18 months after placement. No patient had persistent grade 3 or higher dysphagia at the most recent follow-up. New-onset aspiration or esophageal stricture after IMPT was not detected in any patient. One patient developed ulceration of the oropharyngeal mucosa at 16 months after treatment completion; the ulcer stabilized and the symptoms improved after hyperbaric oxygen therapy. Some 52% of patients had grade 2+ xerostomia at some time during follow-up, but at the most recent follow-up, among the 48 living patients, only 10 (21%) had grade 2 xerostomia, 32 (67%) had grade 1 xerostomia, and 6 (12%) had grade 0 xerostomia.[24] A longitudinal analysis of patient-reported outcomes reported by Sio et al. showed that IMPT led to fewer occurrences of the 10 most commonly reported symptoms during the subacute or early-recovery phase after IMPT as compared with IMRT, findings that suggest that IMPT may be associated with a more rapid recovery of acute toxicity after therapy than IMRT.[30]

Another comparative analysis from Zhang et al. at MD Anderson evaluated mandibular doses and osteoradionecrosis events after IMPT versus IMRT for OPC. Of 584 patients treated from 2011 through 2014, 50 had received IMPT, and the rest had received IMRT. The median follow-up time was about 33 months, and for those with who experienced osteoradionecrosis, the median time to event was 11.4 months. Overall, aside from maximum point dose (which is driven by the location of the gross tumor volume), the mandibular doses were lower in the IMPT group (e.g., 0.8 Gy versus 7.3 Gy for the minimum dose and 25.6 Gy versus 41.2 Gy for the mean dose; $P < .001$ for both). Both the rate and severity of osteoradionecrosis were lower in the IMPT group: 2% IMPT (grade 1 in 1) versus 7.7% IMRT (grade 4 in 12, grade 3 in 5, grade 2 in 1, and grade 1 in 23).[27]

Given these dosimetric advantages and encouraging early findings on disease control, acute toxicity, and late toxicity, a prospective, multiinstitutional, randomized phase II/III trial was proposed and is currently being conducted to compare IMPT and IMRT for patients with locally advanced OPC (clinicaltrials.gov identifier: NCT01893307). The scientific background, rationale, current status, and considerations in the statistical design of the current primary end point for this trial (noninferiority, progression-free survival), as well as important secondary analyses to quantify the value of proton therapy for OPC, were reported by Frank et al.[31] A prospective, observational study is also being conducted at MD Anderson for patients with earlier-stage or lower-volume OPC dispositioned to single-modality treatment (clinicaltrials.gov identifier: NCT02663583). Patients in the latter study are treated with the current state-of-the-art approach, either IMPT or transoral robotic surgery and neck dissection, and the primary end point is functional outcomes, as measured by patient activity monitoring (using a wearable device) before, during, and after treatment. A case study of a patient who received IMPT for OPC is illustrated in Fig. 13.3.

Nasopharyngeal Carcinoma

IMPT has also been reported to produce excellent outcomes in nasopharyngeal carcinoma. Two single-institution series report excellent 2-year rates of local-regional control (100%) and survival (89%–100%).[10,32] Holiday et al. from MD Anderson also reported clinical outcomes in light of in-depth dosimetric analysis for 30 patients with nasopharyngeal carcinoma, 10 of whom received IMPT and 20 IMRT. By the end of treatment, only 2 patients in the IMPT group (20%) versus 13 in the IMRT group (65%) required a feeding tube ($P = .020$). IMPT led to significantly lower mean doses to the oral cavity, brainstem, whole brain, and mandible, and a higher mean dose to the oral cavity was associated with the need for a feeding tube ($P < .001$). Specifically, no patient who had a mean dose to the oral cavity of less than 26 Gy required a feeding tube, but all patients with a mean oral cavity dose of greater than 41.8 Gy required a tube. Multivariate analysis showed that only a higher mean oral cavity dose was associated with tube placement (OR: 1.31 per 1-Gy excess to the oral cavity; $P = .003$).[26] A case study illustrating the differences in dose distribution for IMPT versus IMRT for nasopharyngeal cancer is shown in Fig. 13.4.

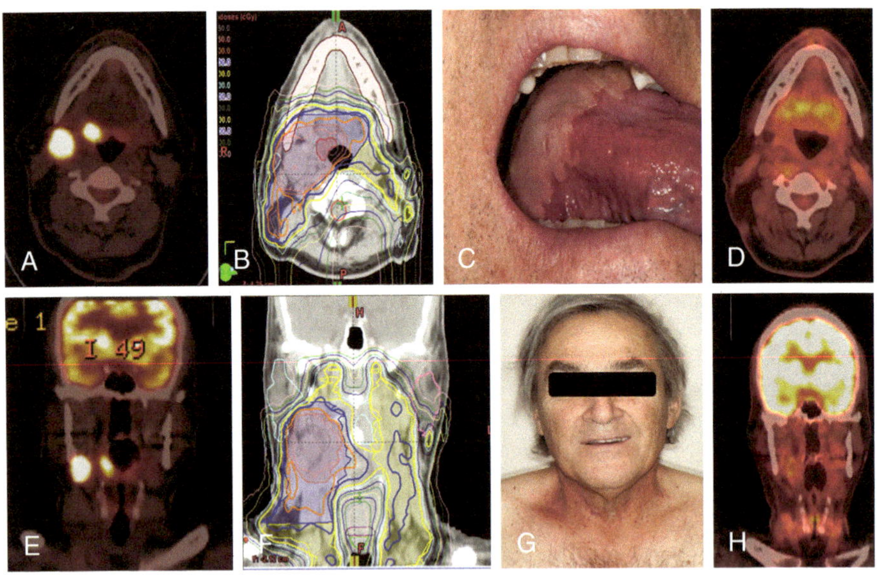

Fig. 13.3 Case study: oropharyngeal cancer. A 67-year-old man with T2N2b (defined per the 7th edition of the American Joint Committee on Cancer staging manual) human papillomavirus–positive squamous cell carcinoma of the right tongue base. (A and E) Positron emission tomography/computed tomography (PET/CT) scans show avid primary tumor and cervical node metastases. (B and F) Isodose lines on multifield optimization intensity-modulated proton therapy treatment plan in the axial (B) and coronal (F) planes. (C and G) Confluent mucositis at the tongue base with no mucositis at the anterior local tongue (C) and grade 2 radiation dermatitis on the neck (G) after receipt of 66 Gy (radiobiologic equivalent [RBE]) with concurrent cetuximab, illustrating treatment reactions consistent with the treatment plan. (D and H) PET/CT scans obtained at 10 weeks after treatment demonstrate complete clinical, metabolic, and radiographic response. The patient remains without evidence of disease at 2.5 years after treatment. (From Frank SJ, Cox JD, Gillin M, et al. Multifield optimization intensity modulated proton therapy for head and neck tumors: a translation to practice. *Int J Radiat Oncol Biol Phys.* 2014;89(4):846-853. With permission.)

Reirradiation of Local-Regional Recurrence

Given the obligation to minimize cumulative radiation doses to avoid severe toxicity, proton therapy is also being considered for retreatment of local-regional recurrence or second primary tumors in HNC. Published outcomes after proton therapy for reirradiation are summarized in Table 13.4, and highlights are presented in the remainder of this section.

One multiinstitutional retrospective analysis of 92 patients who had been reirradiated with passive scatter proton techniques showed that the cumulative incidence of local-regional recurrence was 25% at 1 year after the reirradiation, and the actuarial overall survival rate at that time was 65%.[33] Acute and late toxicity profiles were considered acceptable, with the authors speculating that this resulted from lower doses to surrounding normal tissues when proton therapy was used for reirradiation.

A recent series from MD Anderson published by Phan et al. reported disease control and survival after reirradiation for 60 patients, 15 with passive scatter and 45 with IMPT. At 1 year, both the local-regional failure-free rate (68%) and the overall survival rate (84%) were considered

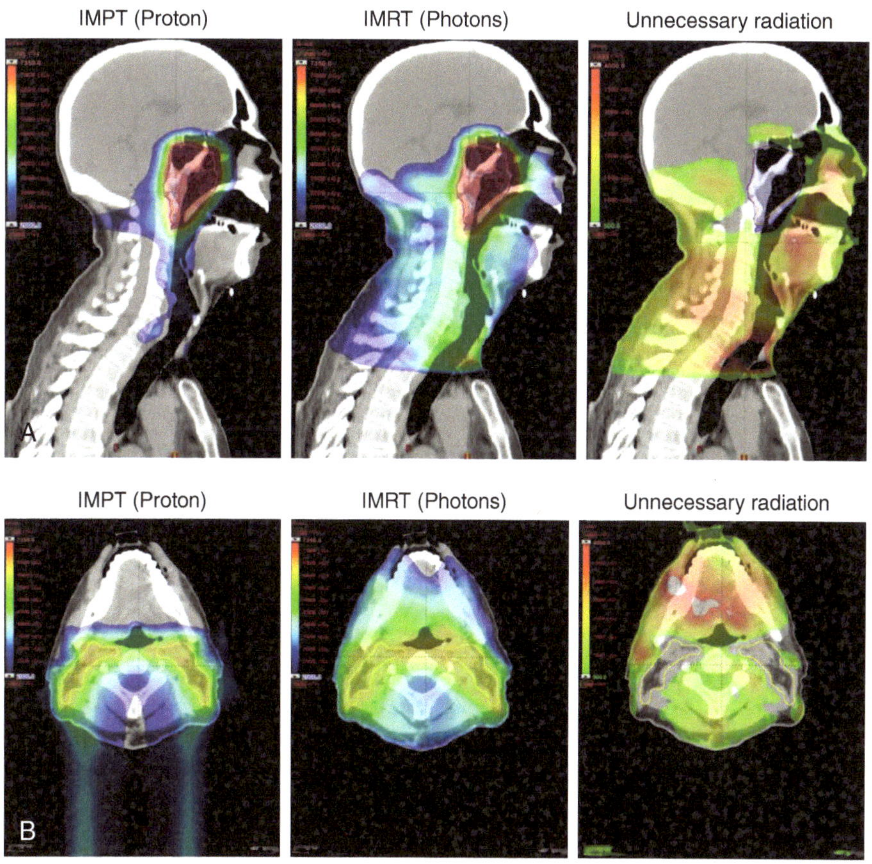

Fig. 13.4 Case study: nasopharyngeal carcinoma (A) Sagittal and (B) axial views of treatment plans for intensity-modulated proton therapy *(IMPT)* or intensity-modulated photon (x-ray) therapy *(IMRT)* for the same patient with nasopharyngeal carcinoma. *Left*, dose distributions on the IMPT plan; *center*, dose distributions on the IMRT plan; *right*, excess unnecessary radiation from IMRT that could be eliminated with IMPT. (From Holliday EB, Garden AS, Rosenthal DI, et al. Proton therapy reduces treatment-related toxicities for patients with nasopharyngeal cancer: a case-match control study of intensity-modulated proton therapy and intensity-modulated photon therapy. *Int J Particle Ther.* 2015;2(1):19-28; distributed under Creative Commons CC-BY. With permission.)

TABLE 13.4 ■ **Studies Evaluating Proton Therapy for Head and Neck Reirradiation**

References	Accrual	Technique	Type	Pts (*n*)	*S* (%)	CCT (%)	Histology (*n*)	Follow-Up (Median)	Outcomes	Toxicity
McDonald et al.	2004–2014	PSPT	Retro	61	47.5	29	SCC (32), other (29)	29 mo	2-y LF: 19.7%; OS: 32.7%	8 G3 (bone and soft tissue necrosis); 3 G4 (2 unilateral blindness, 1 soft tissue necrosis); 3 treatment-related deaths (G5) (1 acute and 2 late)
Phan et al.[34]	2011–2015	PSPT (*n* = 15), IMPT (*n* = 45)	Pro	60	58	73	SCC (40) Other (20)	13.6 mo	1-y LRFFS: 68.4%; OS: 83.8%	Acute G3+ toxicity 30%, including 22% feeding tubes; 1-y G3+ toxicity 16.7%; 3 treatment-related deaths (G5)
Romesser et al.[33]	2011–2014	PSPT	Retro	92	39	39	SCC (52) Other (40)	13.3 mo	1-y LRF: 25.1%; OS: 65.2%	G3+ late toxicity: 6 pts (8.7%) for skin and 4 pts (7.1%) for dysphagia. 1 death during treatment (progression) and 2 G5 late bleeding
Hayashi et al.	2009–2013	PSPT	Pro	25	46	IAC	SCC (25)	24 mo	2-y LF: 30%; OS: 46%	1 pt with late G4. No G5. Patients were a mix of previously irradiated pts and pts with recurrence after single-modality surgery for whom side effects may have been underestimated

CCT, Concomitant chemotherapy; *Comp,* comparison; *G,* grade; *IAC,* intraarterial chemotherapy; *IMPT,* intensity-modulated proton therapy; *LF,* local failure; *LRF,* locoregional failure; *LRFFS,* locoregional failure-free survival; *Mo,* months; *n,* number; *OS,* overall survival; *Pro,* prospective study; *PSPT,* passive scattered proton therapy; pts, patients; *Retro,* retrospective study; *S*, surgery; *SCC,* squamous cell carcinoma; *y,* years.

From Blanchard P, Gunn GB, Lin A, Foote RL, Lee NY, Frank SJ. Proton therapy for head and neck cancers. *Semin Radiat Oncol.* 2018;28(1):53–63. With permission.

quite favorable.[34] Another group at MD Anderson reported clinical outcomes after local-field conformal reirradiation of retropharyngeal nodal metastases in 19 patients who underwent reirradiation to the skull base; no grade 3 (or higher) late toxicity was observed in the 4 patients who had received proton therapy (all of whom were treated with a passive scatter technique).[35]

Regarding the toxicity of reirradiation, the studies in Table 13.4 confirm, as do photon (x-ray) series, that reirradiation to the HN carries an elevated risk of significant and serious toxicity. Seeking to improve on these results, investigators at MD Anderson are conducting a randomized phase II reirradiation study to compare toxicity rates at 2 years for stereotactic ablative radiotherapy versus IMRT or IMPT for previously irradiated patients with inoperable HNC (clinicaltrials.gov identifier: NCT03164460).

Periorbital Tumors

At MD Anderson, selected periorbital tumors are treated with an orbit-sparing, multidisciplinary approach, which has the combined aims of cure, preservation of visual function, and maintenance of facial and orbital cosmesis. Findings were recently reported for 20 patients who received orbit/globe-sparing surgery followed by proton therapy for malignant epithelial tumors of the lacrimal gland (7 patients), nasolacrimal apparatus (10 patients), or eyelid (3 patients); the most common histologic subtypes were adenoid cystic and squamous cell carcinomas. At a median follow-up interval of 27 months, no patient had experienced local recurrence, one had a regional recurrence, and one had a distant recurrence. Major toxic effects were three cases of chronic grade 3 epiphora and three of grade 3 exposure keratopathy. At the most recent follow-up visit, four patients were found to have had decreased visual acuity relative to baseline. Notably, chronic grade 3 toxicity was associated with maximum dose to the cornea: no patient who received less than 36 Gy (RBE) experienced this toxicity, and this threshold has now been implemented as a dose constraint in our current practice.[36] Proton therapy is currently included in the NCCN guidelines as a treatment option for patients with periorbital tumors.[17] Treatment simulation and delivery for patients with medial canthal or nasolacrimal sac tumors include a lateral eye-gaze technique and apertures to sharpen the lateral penumbra to facilitate maximal sparing of the cornea. Attention must be paid during treatment planning to rotation of the optic nerve toward the target volume when an eye-deviation technique is used, and therefore, this technique is not routinely used for lacrimal gland tumors. A case study of proton therapy for a periorbital tumor is illustrated in Fig. 13.5.

Skin, Salivary Gland, and Unilateral Neck Treatment

Adenoid cystic carcinoma arising from the minor salivary glands is discussed separately in the section that follows. Regarding unilateral neck treatment, Kandula et al. compared dosimetric measurements between active (spot) scanning proton therapy and IMRT for five patients who were to undergo unilateral neck radiation. The results showed that proton therapy and IMRT provided equivalent target coverage, but proton therapy led to significantly lower mean doses to the contralateral submandibular and parotid glands, oral cavity, spinal cord, and brainstem.[9] Romesser et al. reported dosimetric results and outcomes for 41 patients after ipsilateral or unilateral neck radiotherapy for major salivary gland malignancies or cutaneous squamous cell carcinoma. That study took place from 2011 through 2014, when the authors' practice was shifting away from the routine use of IMRT and toward the use of proton therapy for such cases. Twenty-three patients (56%) were treated with IMRT, and 18 (44%) received proton therapy. Compared with the proton plans, the IMRT plans led to higher median maximum brainstem dose (29.7 Gy vs. 0.62 Gy [RBE]; $P < .001$), maximum spinal cord dose (36.3 Gy vs. 1.88 Gy [RBE]; $P < .001$), mean oral cavity dose (20.6 Gy vs. 0.94 Gy [RBE]; $P < .001$), mean contralateral parotid dose (1.4 Gy vs. 0.0 Gy [RBE]; $P < .001$), and mean contralateral submandibular gland dose (4.1 Gy vs. 0.0 Gy

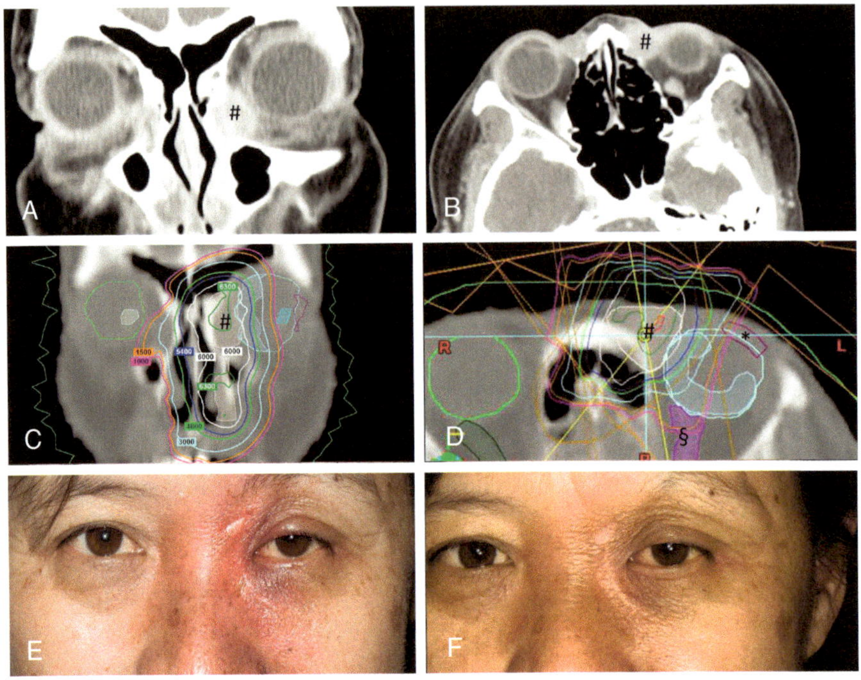

Fig. 13.5 Case study: periorbital tumor. Preoperative coronal (A) and axial (B) computed tomography scans of a patient with squamous cell carcinoma of the left nasolacrimal duct *(#)* treated with orbit-sparing surgery followed by proton therapy, during which eye deviation was used. (C) Coronal and (D) axial treatment plans show 60 Gy(relative biological effectiveness) to be delivered to the tumor cavity (#) with avoidance of the cornea *(*)* and optic nerve *(§)*. Photographs obtained at the end of treatment (E) and at 6 months' follow-up (F) show resolution of radiation dermatitis in the treatment field. This patient remained free of disease at 7 years after treatment, with visual acuity maintained at pretreatment levels with no significant ocular toxicity. (From Holliday EB, Esmaeli B, Pinckard J, et al. A multidisciplinary orbit-sparing treatment approach that includes proton therapy for epithelial tumors of the orbit and ocular adnexa. *Int J Radiat Oncol Biol Phys.* 2016;95(1):344-352. With permission.)

[RBE]; $P < .001$). Notably, patients given proton therapy also had lower rates of grade 2 (or higher) acute dysgeusia (5.6% vs. 65.2%; $P < .001$), mucositis (16.7% vs. 52.2%; $P = .019$), and nausea (11.1% vs. 56.5%; $P = .003$).[37] This study provides proof of principle of clinical benefit from proton therapy for other tumor sites that are amenable to unilateral radiotherapy, such as well-lateralized carcinomas of the tonsillar fossa, a case study of which is given in Fig. 13.6.

Adenoid Cystic Carcinoma

The choice of proton or photon therapy for individual patients must consider not only anatomic tumor site but also tumor histology; adenoid cystic carcinomas have been of particular interest given their general resistance to traditional radiation therapy. These tumors arise from major and minor salivary glands, and primary surgical treatment is preferred, generally with postoperative radiation. Unresectable adenoid cystic carcinomas, which often arise from the nasopharynx or involve the base of skull, are treated with definitive radiation therapy or concurrent chemoradiation. A small series of nine patients treated at MD Anderson was reported by Bhattasali et al. All nine patients had unresectable adenoid cystic carcinoma of the HN (five nasopharynx, two paranasal sinus, one oropharynx, and one larynx); all received definitive proton therapy (one passive scatter and eight IMPT) to a dose of 70 Gy (RBE) with concurrent weekly cisplatin. At a median follow-up time of 27 months, four of the nine patients had achieved complete response, another four had stable disease, and one had disease progression, for a

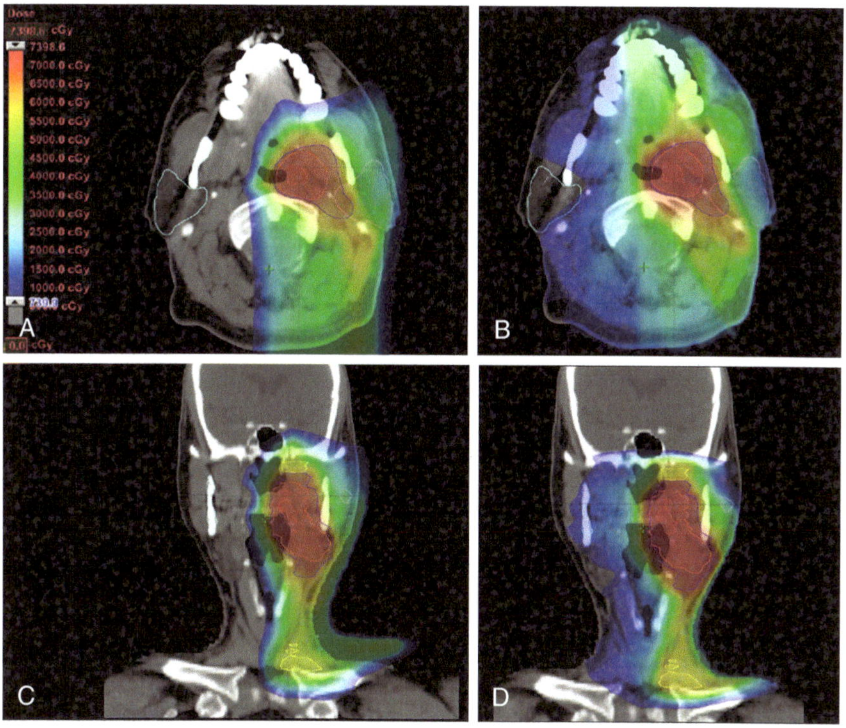

Fig. 13.6 Case study: unilateral tonsil tumor. Representative axial and coronal views of intensity-modulated radiation therapy (B and D) and active-scanning proton therapy (A and C) plans for the same patient demonstrate similar conformality but less integral dose with proton therapy. (From Kandula S, Zhu X, Garden AS, et al. Spot-scanning beam proton therapy vs intensity-modulated radiation therapy for ipsilateral head and neck malignancies: a treatment planning comparison. *Med Dosim.* 2013;38(4):390-394. With permission.)

crude local progression rate of 11%. Regarding toxicity, four patients experienced five grade 3 acute events, and one patient developed a chronic G4 optic nerve disorder (an anticipated event given the tumor location and dose required for local control).[38] Pommier et al. also reported favorable control rates for adenoid cystic carcinoma at the base of skull after treatment incorporating proton therapy with dose escalation (median dose: 76 Gy [RBE]) without concurrent chemotherapy. In that 23-patient study, all but 3 patients were treated with gross disease (either after biopsy or subtotal resection), and at a median follow-up time in excess of 5 years, the 5-year local control rate was 93%.[39] To our knowledge, these are the best long-term results published for unresectable adenoid cystic carcinoma.

In a smaller study, Holliday et al. reported outcomes for 16 patients with adenoid cystic carcinoma of the HN treated with surgery and postoperative IMPT to a median dose of 60 Gy (RBE); 12 patients also received concurrent platinum-based chemotherapy. The median follow-up time was >24 months. At the most recent follow-up, all patients but one were alive without evidence of disease. These results demonstrated evidence of the robustness and effectiveness of IMPT plans designed to account for tissue inhomogeneity within the postoperative paranasal sinus region.[40]

Conclusions

Proton therapy, and IMPT in particular, is currently considered a standard form of highly conformal radiotherapy for HNC, and its safety and clinical efficacy in terms of both tumor control and toxicity reduction have been demonstrated in numerous single-institution reports. Current clinical indications for proton therapy in HNC are given in our standard guidelines (Table 13.5).

TABLE 13.5 ■ **Summary of Current Clinical Indications for Proton Therapy for Head and Neck Cancer at the University of Texas MD Anderson Cancer Center**

Location/ Disease	Common Histologies (Including, But Not Limited To)	Clinical and Pathologic Indications for PT	ClinicalTrials.gov Identifier(s), Current PT Studies at MD Anderson[a]
Nasal cavity (NC)/ paranasal sinus (PNS)	SCC, SNUC, ACC, MEC, NECs, ENB, melanoma	Definitive: inoperable/unresectable; postoperative: T3/4, PNI, bone invasion, PSM, lymph node+, ECE; doses to critical and avoidance structures exceed tolerance with photon therapy and may lead to toxicity (brain, brainstem, optic structures, cornea, mucosa, bone, nerves, etc.) Cavernous sinus involvement via direct tumor extension or neural/ perineural spread for which irradiation of cavernous sinus or skull-base foramen is required (e.g., foramen rotundum, foramen ovale, stylomastoid foramen, etc.) To facilitate preservation of orbit/eye, functional vision, and cosmetic outcome	NCT01627093 NCT00707473
Base of skull	Chordoma, chondrosarcoma, SCC, SNUC, ACC, MEC, ENB, melanoma		
Periorbital	SCC, ACC, MEC; tumors of the lacrimal sac/duct, lacrimal gland, eyelid		
Nasopharynx	NPC (keratinizing and nonkeratinizing SCC and undifferentiated carcinoma), ACC	NPC: definitive; ACC: definitive (as commonly unresectable); postoperative: T3/4, PNI, bone invasion, PSM, lymph node+, ECE	NCT01627093
Oropharynx	SCC, ACC, MEC	SCC: definitive; postoperative: T3/4, PNI, bone invasion, PSM, lymph node+, ECE; T0 (unknown primary) when pharyngeal source is suspected; ACC/ MEC as per NC/PNS; retropharyngeal nodal target at skull-base/jugular foramen; unilateral neck RT volume	NCT01627093 NCT01893307 NCT02663583
Larynx/hypopharynx	SCC, ACC, MEC	For stage I/II glottic SCC, PT is increasingly considered for maximal carotid artery sparing beyond that achievable with IMRT to reduce late vascular sequelae (e.g., stroke); for other larynx sites/stages and hypopharynx, selection of PT is individualized	NCT01627093
Thyroid	Differentiated, undifferentiated, and medullary thyroid carcinomas	Selection of PT is individualized and considered when normal tissue constraints cannot be sufficiently met with photon-based approaches	NCT01627093

TABLE 13.5 ■ **Summary of Current Clinical Indications for Proton Therapy for Head and Neck Cancer at the University of Texas MD Anderson Cancer Center** (Continued)

Location/ Disease	Common Histologies (Including, But Not Limited To)	Clinical and Pathologic Indications for PT	ClinicalTrials. gov Identifier(s), Current PT Studies at MD Anderson[a]
Salivary gland (major and minor)	ACC, MEC, salivary duct carcinoma, carcinoma ex-PA, acinic cell carcinoma, SCC involving the parotid	As per NC/PNS/base of skull/periorbital; unilateral neck RT volume	NCT01627093
Skin (scalp, face, eyelids/canthi, neck)	SCC, BCC, MCC, melanoma	Definitive or postoperative when target volume tracks toward or involves skull base (e.g., neural/perineural spread), periorbital location, or target overlies critical/avoidance structure(s) (e.g., partial or total scalp RT with underlying brain); unilateral neck RT volume	NCT01627093
Oral cavity	SCC, ACC, MEC	As per NC/PNS/base of skull/periorbital; unilateral neck RT volume	NCT01627093
Local-regional recurrence/reirradiation	SCC, SNUC, NPC, ACC, MEC, ENB	Definitive/salvage: unresectable/inoperable; postoperative: considered for higher-risk features (e.g., PNI, ECE, PSM). Note: Given the potential for serious toxicity, the risk:benefit of reirradiation to the head and neck must be carefully considered, and patients should be evaluated/managed at specialty centers with sufficient expertise	NCT01627093 NCT03164460
Benign tumors	Paraganglioma (glomus tumor) at skull base (e.g., jugulare/tympanicum) and neck (e.g., vagale/carotid body), PA	Progressive or symptomatic paraganglioma (or for prevention of symptoms) dispositioned to definitive RT; multiply recurrent or multifocal PA dispositioned to postoperative RT or definitive RT for unresectable disease	NCT01627093

Lymphomas, sarcomas, and pediatric tumors of the head and neck are discussed in separate chapters.
[a]All patients with head and neck cancer treated with proton therapy at our center are eligible to participate in Data Collection of Normal Tissue Toxicity for Proton Therapy (clinicaltrials.gov identifier: NCT00991094).
ACC, Adenoid cystic carcinoma; *BCC,* basal cell carcinoma; *ECE,* extracapsular extension; *ENB,* esthesioneuroblastoma; *IMRT,* intensity-modulated radiation therapy; *MCC,* Merkel cell carcinoma; *MEC,* mucoepidermoid carcinoma; *NECs,* neuroendocrine carcinomas (including small cell carcinoma); *NPC,* nasopharyngeal carcinoma; *PA,* pleomorphic adenoma; *PNI,* perineural invasion; *PSM,* positive surgical margin; *PT*, proton therapy; *RT,* radiation therapy; *SCC,* squamous cell carcinoma; *SNUC,* sinonasal undifferentiated carcinoma; *UC,* undifferentiated carcinoma.

Continued technical advances in proton therapy planning and delivery and in modeling its biophysical properties will allow the full potential of proton therapy to be realized. Several clinical trials are underway to more fully quantify the clinical benefits and define the value of proton therapy for HNC.

References Available Online.

CHAPTER 14

Proton Therapy for Hematologic Malignancies

Jillian R. Gunther ■ Bouthaina S. Dabaja

Introduction

As early as the 1970s, proton therapy was considered a promising treatment for hematologic malignancies, specifically for use in total nodal irradiation, the historic standard of care treatment for Hodgkin lymphoma (HL).[1] In one report, it was recognized that patients treated with 4000 to 4400 rad to the mantle and inverted Y fields experienced considerable morbidity when treated with standard photons, including, but not limited to, nausea, vomiting, hair loss, and decreased blood counts. The authors suggested that this treatment could be delivered by using proton irradiation, which would not only decrease treatment toxicity but also treatment length because both fields could be treated simultaneously. They also recognized the value in sparing bone marrow, as lymphoma patients often depend on marrow reserves to tolerate chemotherapy. Interestingly, this publication focused on acute toxicities of treatment, as the authors admitted that the time required for documentation of late toxicities had not yet elapsed, although hepatic, cardiac, and pulmonary changes had been documented. They concluded that "the improved dose distribution should be manifested by increased local control of irradiated cancer, as well as by decreased patient morbidity."[1]

The treatment paradigm for HL and other hematologic malignancies has certainly evolved since those times, with chemotherapy replacing radiation as the primary therapy and the overall focus shifting to de-escalation of treatment, given the excellent treatment outcomes.[2–6] Because such patients tend to receive treatment at a young age and long life expectancies are anticipated, they must be spared the late toxicities that can manifest decades later.[7–11] Both chemotherapy and radiation therapy (RT) have been progressively deintensified and optimized; research efforts have focused on identifying the minimum treatment necessary to maintain these excellent outcomes.[12,13]

Proton therapy has, in more recent years, been highlighted once again as a mode of radiation delivery ideal for this patient population. Radiation field sizes and doses have been decreased markedly from the days of total nodal irradiation, and the current standard of care uses a technique called involved-site RT,[14] in which only initial sites of disease are treated, with no elective nodal irradiation performed. Some institutions with workflows that allow prechemotherapy positron emission tomography-computed tomography imaging while the patient is in the radiation treatment position can even achieve involved-node RT,[14] a technique that results in the smallest treatment fields used thus far. With these decreased field sizes and decreased radiation doses, the acute toxicities of treatment are typically not the primary concern. The patient age at treatment, long life expectancy, and close proximity of critical structures (e.g., heart and lungs) necessitate careful consideration of late toxicities of radiation before treatment is prescribed. Therefore, it is imperative that techniques be used to reduce the dose to normal tissues as much as possible. Technology has improved dose distributions of photon treatment and spared normal tissue via implementation of inverse planning with intensity-modulated

RT (IMRT). Other modifications of the treatment setup and delivery, including the use of deep inspiration breathhold (DIBH), have strikingly improved the total radiation dose delivered to the heart and lungs. Although these advances are notable, the distinct physical properties of photon treatment that result in exit dose to normal tissues cannot be modified, and many have pointed toward particle therapy with protons as a revolutionary method of radiation treatment delivery for this unique patient population. The unique absence of exit dose achieved with proton therapy (see Chapter 2) allows not only decreased dose to specific critical structures but also decreased total body radiation dose (integral dose), which is exceedingly important for patients in whom secondary malignancy is a primary concern.

DOSIMETRIC ADVANTAGE OF PROTONS COMPARED WITH PHOTON-BASED THREE-DIMENSIONAL CONFORMAL AND INTENSITY-MODULATED RADIATION THERAPY

More recent investigations of the value of proton therapy for patients with lymphoma have compared the dosimetric advantages of delivering proton therapy versus more conventional RT techniques (e.g., three-dimensional [3D] conformal, IMRT). These reports have usually focused on patients with the most common disease site presentation, the mediastinum. Early comparisons of conventional photon RT with 3D proton treatment for patients with HL confirmed that proton therapy reduced the doses to the heart, lungs, esophagus, and coronary arteries.[15] One report by Chera et al. reproduced treatment plans with 3D conformal RT (CRT), IMRT, and 3D proton therapy for nine patients with early-stage HL without disease involving or below the hila. They concluded that, although IMRT, produced the most conformal high-dose distributions, proton therapy afforded the lowest mean doses to nontarget tissues including breast, lung, and total body.[16] In a similar study comparing 3D CRT, IMRT, and proton therapy for early-stage HL using involved-node techniques, Hoppe et al. concluded that the dose to cardiac substructures (chambers, valves, and vessels) was significantly decreased with proton therapy, and this should translate to a decrease in cardiac toxicity.[17] Proton therapy, when used with involved-node techniques, has been shown to give less dose to the carotid arteries compared with volumetric-modulated arc therapy and mantle field radiation (but not 3D CRT),[18] potential improvements in head and neck treatment delivery for some patients,[19] and the lowest-risk estimates (based on dosimetry) of nearly all esophageal complications when compared with photon-based treatments.[20] A study of pediatric patients with HL determined that proton therapy, when compared with 3D CRT, allowed the reduction of unnecessary breast dose by as much as 80%,[21] and another comparison of passive scatter proton therapy to tomotherapy and 3D CRT also confirmed the advantage of proton therapy for better sparing breast tissue.[22]

Advances in proton therapy, including pencil beam scanning, have allowed additional comparisons. Ten patients with mediastinal lymphoma had RT treatment plans designed for 3D CRT, IMRT, pencil beam scanning (PBS) proton therapy, and proton double-scattering techniques. Authors concluded that PBS significantly decreased the mean lung and mean heart doses compared with the other modalities. They also measured deviations from planned dose and determined that PBS plan robustness can be maintained with repainting or large spot sizes.[23] Although these studies provided valuable information, they did not take advantage of treatment delivery techniques such as DIBH that are known to significantly reduce dose to critical structures such as the heart and lungs.[24,25] A more recent publication describing involved-node techniques compared IMRT to PBS proton therapy, each planned using both free-breathing and DIBH planning scans, and estimated the risk of late effects and life years lost for these young patients. Interestingly, IMRT free-breathing plans were inferior to all others, but IMRT DIBH plans were not significantly different from proton free-breathing plans. The lowest number of life-years lost was achieved with proton therapy DIBH plans, although the authors cautioned that this combination is rarely available, and the most likely treatment alternatives will be IMRT DIBH or free-breathing proton therapy.[26] A report by Moreno et al. from MD Anderson similarly concluded that proton therapy is advantageous in the setting of DIBH. IMRT plans using breath hold were comparable in terms of dose to heart, breasts, and coronary arteries when compared with proton free-breathing plans.[27]

PROTON THERAPY FOR HEMATOLOGIC MALIGNANCIES OUTSIDE THE MEDIASTINUM

In HL patients presenting with subdiaphragmatic disease, proton therapy has also been compared with 3D CRT and IMRT and found to provide significant reductions in dose to structures such as the stomach, liver, pancreas, bowel, and kidneys.[28] For patients with central nervous system (CNS) involvement of leukemia and lymphoma, proton therapy has been implemented to deliver craniospinal irradiation (CSI) before stem cell transplantation. In that work, both photon and proton therapy offered excellent local control, and acute mucositis occurred less often with proton CSI.[29]

POTENTIAL FOR DECREASED LATE EFFECTS WITH PROTON THERAPY

With all emerging modern technologies that reduce the dose to normal tissues, there are predictions of decreased late toxicity, especially important in this young and favorable-risk patient population. Unfortunately, many late effects of treatment develop decades later, and these findings are not available to inform treatment decisions today. In the absence of this information, practitioners must rely on "worst-case scenario" results from radiation treatments delivered using larger fields, higher doses, and more intensive combination chemotherapy regimens. Alternatively, models may allow prediction of toxicities that patients will experience after these more gentle treatment regimens. An early publication used the International Commission on Radiological Protection calculation scheme to calculate cancer incidence from dose distributions and found that proton treatment would result in lower cancer incidence than photon treatment.[30] In the report by Rechner et al. described above, the authors used dose-effect models based on epidemiological data to estimate the risk of late effects from the compared treatments and to confirm the benefit of proton therapy for long-term patient outcomes. Admittedly, models introduce uncertainty to any conclusions, but the results, especially when used comparatively across different treatments, can allow tentative conclusions to be drawn. That study used normal tissue doses to estimate the incidence of various late effects and to convert those events into number of life years lost, thus taking into account the severity of different late toxicities.[26] A separate study by Maraldo et al. compared proton therapy with photon-based techniques, including mantle field radiation, and confirmed that modern RT provides decreased dose to normal tissues, and proton therapy was superior in terms of life-years lost.[31] Another study of 20 patients with intrathoracic HL compared radiation treatment plans generated for 3D CRT, IMRT (as helical tomotherapy), and IMPT. They estimated IMPT neutron dose from published measurements and used the relative seriality model to predict excess cardiac mortality risk. Excess absolute risk of lung cancer and breast cancer induction was predicted by using a modified linear-quadratic model and with parameters derived from published data. Although no significant difference in predicted excess cardiac risk was found, IMPT decreased the risk of secondary lung cancer and breast cancer when compared with 3D CRT.[32] Another comparison of photon radiation techniques with proton therapy concluded that advanced RT techniques adequately spare normal tissues; however, only proton therapy reduced the risk of secondary malignant neoplasms (estimated via the organ equivalent dose model) compared with 3D CRT and IMRT and tomotherapy increased the risk of secondary breast and lung cancers.[33] These studies provide additional evidence of the benefits of proton therapy for long-term patient outcomes.

OTHER CONSIDERATIONS FOR USING PROTON THERAPY FOR LYMPHOMA

Management of Tumor Motion

Again, because the most common disease presentation for lymphoma patients involves the mediastinum/thorax, it is imperative that motion management be considered in the simulation and treatment planning process. Although techniques such as DIBH have remarkably improved photon-based treatment plans, this technology is often not available in combination with proton radiation.[26] Without motion management, larger margins must be applied to free-breathing imaging, and these larger margins reduce the benefit of proton therapy in terms of decreased dose to surrounding normal tissues. Studies have shown comparable dosimetric results in terms of proton therapy–delivered free-breathing compared with photon-based IMRT treatments delivered with the breath hold technique.[26,27] The density dependence of proton linear energy transfer (see Chapter 2) also requires that tumor and normal tissue motion be restricted or carefully accounted for during the treatment planning process. The advantages and limitations of the available technologies must be considered when recommending the best treatment for each patient.

Mediastinal Anatomy

The anatomy of the mediastinum/thorax includes numerous critical structures, including the lungs, heart (coronary arteries, valves), esophagus, and brachial plexus. Proton treatment plans should use beam angles that place the distal edge of the Bragg peak in noncritical structures; damage to serial structures such as nerves or vessels from dose underestimation can have devastating consequences. The interface between soft tissue and air or bone (and the displacement of this interface with breathing motion) must also be carefully taken into consideration. The complexities of proton treatment in the mediastinum must not be minimized, and proton treatment should only be delivered by experts who understand these nuances; otherwise, the potential advantage of protons is certainly lost.

Craniospinal Irradiation

Proton therapy provides a unique advantage for CSI, as it allows near-complete sparing of organs that lie anterior to the spinal cord, a feat that is impossible to accomplish with photon treatment. Protons have been often implemented for pediatric CSI treatment (see Chapter 15), but the benefit has also been shown in adults.[29] However, patients with hematologic malignancies requiring CSI have often received multiple regimens of chemotherapy, usually with CNS-directed or intrathecal treatments, and radiation treatment carries a high risk of CNS toxicity.[34] In these situations, we typically recommend that an additional margin is added anteriorly beyond the spinal cord to avoid the possibility that the distal end of the Bragg peak (with the associated uncertainty and potential high relative biological effectiveness) would overlap with the spinal cord. For patients such as these, bone marrow sparing is also a consideration, and part of the vertebral body can be blocked to allow this, but first and foremost, we must avoid potentially catastrophic side effects of treatment.

Indications

Protons provide a distinct advantage for patients with hematologic malignancies based on their young age at treatment and expected long life expectancy. The potential for decreased dose to normal structures and decreased integral dose should afford lower long-term complication rates, including cardiac and pulmonary disease, as well as lower rates of secondary malignancy. However, depending upon the specific disease presentation within the mediastinum, the use of proton therapy for lymphoma may not provide a distinct advantage when compared with carefully planned and delivered photon treatments.[35] For example, patients with disease involvement that is fully superior to the heart can likely be treated safely with photon-based treatments (Fig. 14.1). Similarly, patients with disease on only one side of the mediastinum and far from the coronary arteries (right-sided disease) can often be treated with favorable photon-based plans, although protons may offer some advantages (Fig. 14.2). However, patients with disease on both the right and left sides of the heart

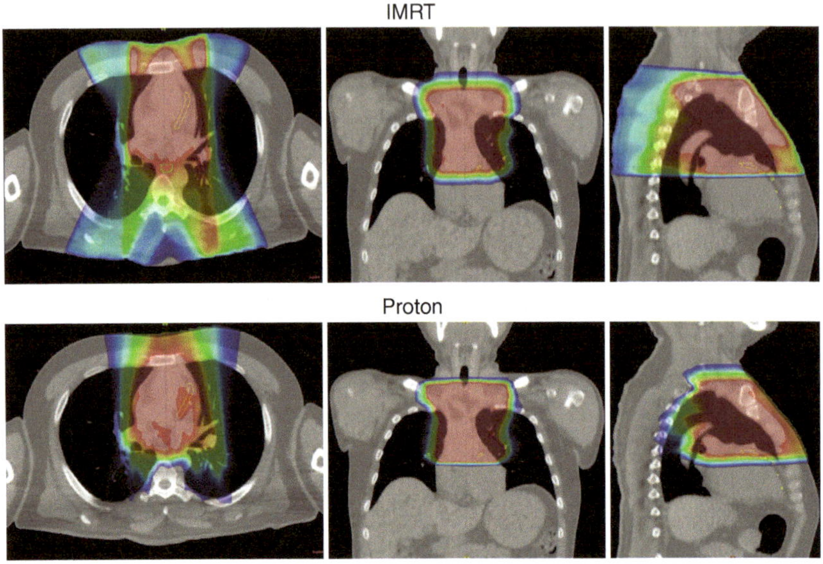

Fig. 14.1 For patients with disease ending above the cardiac structures, photon *(top panel)* and proton *(bottom panel)* plans are often comparable. *IMRT,* Intensity-modulated radiation therapy.

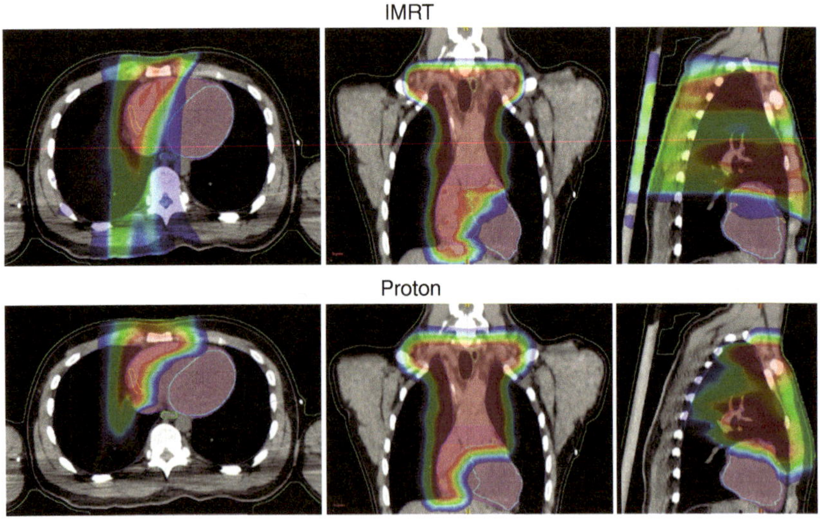

Fig. 14.2 This patient had disease on the right side of the heart only. In these situations, protons *(bottom panel)* can sometimes deliver decreased dose to the heart and lung compared with photon *(top panel)* plans, but each case should be carefully reviewed and comparison plans generated before a final treatment plan is decided upon. *IMRT,* Intensity-modulated radiation therapy.

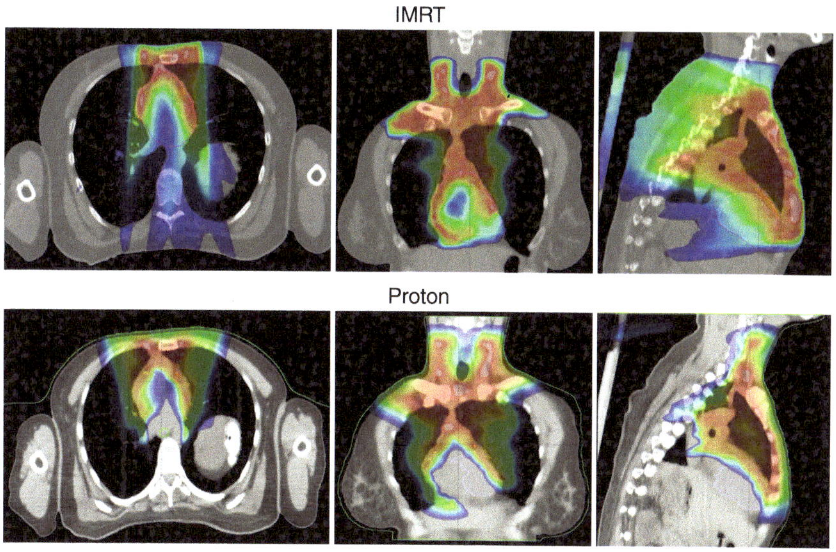

Fig. 14.3 A patient with disease positioned anterior to the heart on both right and left sides, extending all the way to the diaphragm. In these situations, proton therapy *(bottom panel)* can deliver a clearly superior plan, sparing the cardiac structures. *IMRT,* Intensity-modulated radiation therapy.

are the ones who most benefit from the use of protons in treatment planning (Fig. 14.3). Also, patients with axillary disease can be treated with posterior proton beams, therefore allowing breast sparing in female patients. Regardless of the clinical characteristics, proton therapy should not be recommended without excellent knowledge of the complexities of treatment so that RT can be delivered safely and effectively.

Although traditionally proton radiation has been considered for the most favorable subset of lymphoma patients, i.e., those with HL, a second population of patients with hematologic malignancy, those with relapsed/refractory disease, also gain significant benefit from the reduced doses to normal tissues that proton therapy affords. Unfortunately, these patients have often received many and varied chemotherapy and immunotherapy regimens, each with its own associated toxicity. Stem cell transplantation will be recommended to some of these patients in the hope of addressing aggressive disease, and this procedure carries it is own associated toxicities and risks. Patients with relapsed disease have sometimes received prior radiation to the same or neighboring structures. Because these patients are at high risk of complications from any additional therapy, proton therapy is often the best choice to deliver RT with the lowest risk profile.

As investigations continue to confirm that smaller radiation fields confer the same local control benefit with decreased toxicity, these techniques will be more widely adopted. Fortunately, proton therapy also seems to be equally effective as photon therapy when used with smaller involved-node approaches[36]; this lends confidence that these smaller treatment fields do not produce inferior results when combined with the sharp dose fall-off characteristic of proton therapy. Hopefully, the continued advancements in technology, combined with a better understanding of the treatment needs of patients with hematologic malignancy, will result in improved treatment efficacy with markedly reduced toxicities. The unique advantages that proton therapy offers align with the goals for treatment of this population and will certainly ensure a continued role of this modality in the treatment of lymphoma.

References Available Online.

CHAPTER 15

Pediatric Considerations for Proton Therapy

Arnold C. Paulino

Introduction

Approximately 10,500 cases of childhood cancer are diagnosed each year, which represent about 1% of all new cancers in the United States. Nearly 45% of these cancers will either be acute lymphoblastic leukemia or brain and other central nervous system (CNS) tumors. More than 80% of patients afflicted with childhood cancer will be alive at 5 years from initial diagnosis. In 2014, an estimated 1350 deaths occurred secondary to cancer in children 14 years of age or younger.[1] About 25% of deaths in children who survive at least 5 years from their diagnosis die of treatment-related complications.[2] Many of the late effects of treatment can be linked to the use of radiotherapy (RT). The reduction of RT dose has been implicated in the corresponding reduction in late toxicities, including secondary neoplasms.[3–6]

Proton therapy has the potential to reduce complications in children because of the reduction of integral dose to normal tissues when compared with photons. The ability of protons to spare normal tissues beyond a specified depth can be advantageous to the somatic and function of the organ or tissue beyond the target and may result in the reduction of secondary neoplasms.

Unique Problems in Children

The late effects of RT in children can be different from those in adults. Although the predominant manifestation of radiation injury in the adult will usually be fibrogenic or inflammatory, which contributes to loss of organ function, in children, there is an added clinical manifestation of growth delay and impaired maturation of the organ.[7] Young children under 7 years of age are particularly vulnerable if the brain and musculoskeletal organs are irradiated because this is the time when these organ systems are growing and developing. Teenagers are particularly vulnerable to secondary neoplasms when the breast tissue is irradiated during puberty, resulting in a higher incidence of secondary breast cancer compared with irradiation of a young child or adult.[8] Hence, strategies to eliminate or reduce RT during these vulnerable periods have been used. For children under 3 years of age with brain tumors, adjuvant chemotherapy has been used to delay the start of RT until the child is 3 years old. In ependymoma, for example, only 40% and 20% of children are progression-free at 2 years and 5 years, respectively, with this approach.[9,10] This dogma has been challenged by researchers from St. Jude Children's Research Hospital, who have shown a 3-year progression-free survival (PFS) rate of 74.7% in 88 children with a median age of 2.9 years; neurocognitive testing showed stable cognitive findings, with more than half of the children tested at 2 years after RT.[11] Currently, many young children with brain tumors to be treated with RT are referred for proton therapy to minimize late effects.

Proton Therapy Literature on Children

Although the theoretical benefit of proton therapy is obvious, many in the pediatric oncology community have questioned whether protons have the same tumor control efficacy as photons.[12–14] Others have questioned whether the reduction of integral dose will have a clinically significant effect on long-term toxicity when compared with very sophisticated photon plans possible using intensity-modulated radiation therapy (IMRT), volumetric arc therapy, and tomotherapy. Although few publications deal with protons and their effectiveness for tumor control, the current literature suggests that protons are equivalent to photons with regard to local control of tumors. Furthermore, literature is evolving to suggest that some acute and late effects can be minimized by using proton therapy.

MEDULLOBLASTOMA

Patients with medulloblastoma have a lot to gain by not receiving radiation doses to organs anterior to the spine during the craniospinal portion of the treatment. Structures such as the thyroid gland and breast tissue are particularly prone to developing secondary cancers. Cardiovascular late effects after RT have also been reported for patients with medulloblastoma.[15] Craniospinal doses for patients with average-risk and standard-risk disease are 23.4 and 36 Gy. The tumor bed is given an additional RT boost dose to a total dose of 54 to 55.8 Gy.

In a multiinstitution study of 88 patients with standard-risk medulloblastoma given chemotherapy and proton (n = 45) or photon (n = 43) therapy, the 6-year relapse-free survival rates were 78.8% and 76.5%, repectively, whereas the 6-year overall survival (OS) rates were 82.0% and 87.6% for protons and photons, respectively. Patterns of failure were similar among both groups.[16] At MD Anderson, the 3-year event-free survival (EFS) rates were 77.0% and 53.0%, whereas the 3-year OS rates were 90.7% and 73.4% for standard (n = 63) and high-risk (n = 33) groups, respectively, which was similar to the historical photon literature.[17]

A comparison of adult medulloblastoma patients treated with protons (n = 19) or photons (n = 21) revealed that the proportions of patients with more than 5% body weight loss (P = .004), grade 2 nausea and vomiting (P = .004), medical management of esophagitis ($P < .001$), reduction of white count (P = .04), reduction of hemoglobin (P = .009), and reduction of platelets (P = .05) were smaller with protons compared with photons.[18]

A recent phase II trial of 59 patients treated with proton therapy for medulloblastoma revealed that the cumulative incidence of Pediatric Oncology Group (POG) grade 3 to 4 ototoxicity was 16% at 5 years. The full-scale intelligence quotient decreased by 1.5 points per year without a change in perceptual reasoning index and working memory. The cumulative index of any neuroendocrine deficit at 5 years was 55%.[19] A recent comparison of grade 3 to 4 ototoxicity that used three different ototoxicity scales (POG, Brock, and International Society of Pediatric Oncology [SIOP – Boston]) showed essentially the same proportions of proton and photon patients developing hearing loss.[20] Although protons led to a reduction in the RT dose to the cochlea relative to photons, this did not translate into hearing preservation, probably because patients also received cisplatin.

Hypothyroidism has also been shown to be less common among children receiving proton craniospinal irradiation (CSI).[21] A retrospective comparison of standard-risk medulloblastoma patients treated with protons versus photons showed that the hypothyroidism rate was reduced from 69% to 23% with protons ($P < .001$). Use of photons for CSI was also associated with a greater risk of sex hormone deficiency (19%–3%; P = .025), a requirement for any endocrine replacement therapy (78%–55%; P = .030), and a greater height standard deviation score difference compared with proton CSI. No differences were found in the incidence of growth hormone deficiency, adrenal insufficiency, or precocious puberty.

EPENDYMOMA

As mentioned, RT is now routinely used to treat young children with ependymoma. Children who are at least 1 year old receive adjuvant RT to the tumor bed. The only exception for postoperative RT is for a child with a grade II supratentorial tumor that has undergone gross total resection. Investigators from Boston have reported comparable local control and PFS with protons compared with other photon series. The 3-year PFS rates were 88% and 54% for gross total and subtotally resected disease from using protons, respectively,[22] and compares well with the St. Jude 5-year PFS rates of 91.5% and 41% for gross total and subtotally resected disease in children, respectively.[11] At the Texas Children's Hospital and the MD Anderson Proton Center, investigators compared the 3-year PFS rates for children with ependymoma treated with both RT modalities. The 3-year PFS rates were 82% and 60% for proton and photon patients, respectively ($P = .031$); however, gross total resection was more common in the proton group than in the photon group (93% vs. 76%, respectively; $P = .043$).[23]

CRANIOPHARYNGIOMA

In a retrospective comparison of 52 children with craniopharyngioma treated with protons and photons, researchers from the MD Anderson and the Texas Children's Hospital showed no difference in cystic failure-free, nodular failure-free, and OS rates between the two groups. The 3-year cystic failure-free and nodular failure-free survival rates were 75.5% (67% protons, 76.8% photons) and 95% (91.7% protons, 96.4% photons), respectively.[24]

INTRACRANIAL GERM CELL TUMORS

At the Massachusetts General Hospital, the 3-year local control, PFS, and OS rates for 22 patients with intracranial CNS germ cell tumors were 100%, 95%, and 100%, respectively.[25] At the MD Anderson Proton Center, the 5-year local control, PFS, and OS rates for germinoma and nongerminomatous germ cell tumor (NGGCT) were 89%, 89%, and 100% for germinoma and 82%, 82%, and 82% for NGGCT, respectively.[26] The above reports indicate that proton therapy does not compromise local control or PFS in intracranial germ cell tumors.

LOW-GRADE GLIOMA

At the Massachusetts General Hospital, 32 pediatric patients received proton therapy for low-grade glioma of the brain or spinal cord.[27] The 6- and 8-year PFS rates were 89.7% and 82.8% with an 8-year OS rate of 100%, respectively. Some decline in neurocognitive function was seen in children irradiated when they were younger than 7 years. A higher dose to the left temporal lobe and hippocampus was also implicated in cognitive decline. The incidence of endocrinopathy was higher among those receiving more than 40 Gy (relative biological effectiveness [RBE]) to the hypothalamus, pituitary, or optic chiasm. The progression-free and OS rates above are similar to those in a series of 39 patients with low-grade glioma treated with IMRT, with 8-year PFS and OS rates of 78.2% and 93.7%, respectively.[28]

ATYPICAL TERATOID/RHABDOID TUMOR

At the MD Anderson Proton Center, 31 children received proton therapy for atypical teratoid/rhabdoid tumor. [29] The median age at the time of rhabdoid tumor was 24 months, with 17 receiving radiation to the primary site and 14 receiving CSI followed by primary site irradiation. With a median follow-up time of 2 years, the median PFS time was 20.8 months, and the median OS time was 34.3 months, which is comparable to the historical photon series.[30,31]

RETINOBLASTOMA

Proton therapy might be beneficial for children with retinoblastoma, as they are often very young; some with hereditary disease have a high chance of developing secondary tumors. In a retrospective analysis of 49 patients with retinoblastoma (84% with bilateral disease), the local control rates with proton therapy were high.[32] The enucleation rate was 11% for International Classification for Intraocular Retinoblastoma (ICIR) stage A to B disease and 23% for ICIR stage C to D disease. In a prospective study of 12 children with bilateral retinoblastoma treated with protons, none of the patients had hormonal deficiencies. Facial hypoplasia was less common after proton therapy relative to after enucleation.[33] Patient and parent-proxy quality of life were not severely affected by proton therapy. An analysis of proton- versus photon-treated children with retinoblastoma found that none of the patients who received protons had an in-field secondary malignancy, whereas 14% of patients treated with photons developed in-field tumors ($P = .015$).[34] The 10-year cumulative incidence rates of secondary tumors (in-field and out of field) were 5% for protons and 14% for photons ($P = .12$).

RHABDOMYOSARCOMA

In a phase II study from researchers at the Massachusetts General Hospital and the MD Anderson Cancer Center, 57 children with low- and intermediate-risk rhabdomyosarcoma received proton therapy. The 5-year local control, event-free, and OS rates were 81%, 69%, and 78%, respectively.[35] At the University of Florida, 66 children with rhabdomyosarcoma received proton therapy with a 2-year local control rate of 88%. All of the local failures were within the 95% isodose line.[36] Several dosimetric studies of rhabdomyosarcoma at various body sites have shown a theoretical benefit from protons by reduction of doses to surrounding normal tissues.[37–39] To date, however, no clinical findings have been reported to confirm improvements in toxicity from protons.

EWING SARCOMA

A retrospective review of 30 patients with Ewing sarcoma treated with proton therapy at Massachusetts General Hospital revealed a 3-year local control, EFS, and OS of 86%, 60%, and 89%, respectively.[40] The 3-year actuarial rates of EFS, local control, and OS were 60%, 86%, and 89%, respectively.

CHORDOMA/CHONDROSARCOMA

Although protons have been used to treat chordomas and chondrosarcomas with excellent results, most studies have included mostly adults, with only two publications including primarily children. At the Paul Scherrer Institute, 19 patients with chordoma and 7 with chondrosarcoma received proton therapy, with 5-year local control rates of 81% and 80%, respectively.[41] At the Institut Curie Proton Center in Orsay, 26 children with skull-base and cervical chordoma received proton therapy, with a 5-year local control rate of 81%.[42]

NEUROBLASTOMA

Proton therapy was given to 21 sites in 14 patients with advanced neuroblastoma at the University of Tsukuba. The 3-year locoregional control rate was 82%.[43] At the University of Pennsylvania, 13 patients underwent proton therapy, with 5 patients receiving treatment to more than 2 sites. At a median follow-up time of 16 months, there were no local failures at irradiated sites.[44] At the Massachusetts General Hospital, nine children with high-risk neuroblastoma received proton therapy. At a median follow-up time of 38 months, there were no locoregional failures.[45] These results compare favorably with locoregional control rates reported after photon therapy.[46–48]

WILMS TUMOR

A dosimetric study comparing protons to the tumor bed only versus photons given in parallel opposed anteroposterior/posteroanterior fields showed more sparing of normal tissues with the approach using protons.[49] However, because the target volumes were much smaller in the proton patients, this finding is expected. If the tumor bed alone is considered the target, then proton beam therapy will have an advantage in reducing the dose to normal tissues anterior to the tumor bed.

Patient Selection for Proton Therapy

Which pediatric patients are best suited for treatment with proton therapy? In general, patients who are most likely to gain from proton therapy are those with curable tumors and with tumors that are near critical structures that are not part of the target volume. Children with localized tumors will probably have more benefits relative to children with metastatic disease. A consensus conference on proton therapy for children was recently held in Stockholm and identified the following tumors as being the best candidates for proton therapy: low-grade glioma, optic pathway tumors, intracranial germ cell tumors, medulloblastoma, ependymoma, craniopharyngioma, pineal tumors, chordoma/chondrosarcoma, rhabdomyosarcoma, Ewing sarcoma, and retinoblastoma.[50] For neuroblastoma and lymphoma, the experts were noncommittal for either modality, whereas for high-grade glioma of brain and brainstem and Wilms tumor, most favored photon therapy. The expert participants also questioned the value of proton therapy for cases requiring total body, whole abdominal, whole lung, and whole brain RT. Neutron contamination generated by proton scatter, which may result in a higher rate of secondary neoplasms, was not considered a major barrier to the use of proton therapy.[51]

The magnitude of benefit for proton therapy should also be considered when proton centers prioritize cases. Children receiving CSI will likely have more benefit with protons because of the sparing of heart, lungs, thyroid gland, abdominal organs, and gonads from the exit dose of the photon spinal field. For other patients, the magnitude of benefit may be weighed against the cost of treatment, including the patient's family moving for 2 months to cities where proton therapy is available. Proton therapy is still a scarce commodity in the United States and worldwide; it not uncommon for patients to travel across state lines or to different countries to receive protons.[52–54]

With the number of proton centers in the United States increasing from 2004 to 2013, the number of children treated with proton therapy have followed the same trend. Currently, about 17.5% of children requiring RT receive proton therapy. A recent study of the National Cancer Database found that children receiving protons tend to be younger, have insurance, and have higher median household income and higher levels of education.[54]

Summary

Proton therapy is a good option for the radiotherapeutic management of many curable types of childhood cancer. The current data suggest equivalence in local control, progression-free, and OS for many childhood tumors. Based on single-institution prospective and retrospective studies, proton therapy may be able to reduce certain acute and late toxicities of RT. In a group of patients likely to survive the disease, the reduction of late effects is paramount for maintaining a good quality of life.

References Available Online.

CHAPTER 16

Proton Therapy and Sarcomas

Andrew J. Bishop ■ Stephen M. Hahn

Introduction

Sarcomas are a rare and heterogenous group of malignant tumors that arise from soft tissues or bone.[1] They constitute less than 1% of all adult malignancies and approximately 12% of pediatric cancers.[2–4] Approximately 80% to 84% of sarcomas originate from soft tissues, and the rest originate from bone.[3,5] Given the histopathologic spectrum and ability of sarcomas to arise anywhere in the body, treatment paradigms are often dictated by the histology, grade, site of origin, stage, and age of the patient.

Surgical resection remains the mainstay of treatment when possible. For soft tissue sarcomas, radiation therapy (RT) has an integral role in the treatment approach. The combination of RT and a wide local excision (limb-sparing surgery) leads to better local control (LC) than does either modality alone for most soft tissue sarcomas.[6–8] This was demonstrated in two randomized trials, both of which showed that combined-modality therapy resulted in a reduced risk of local recurrence by approximately 20% to 25%. RT can be administered preoperatively or postoperatively, and both have their advantages.[9] Our practice consistently uses preoperative RT, which is endorsed by our multidisciplinary teams because of the lower rates of radiation-related late toxicities.

The use of RT for bone sarcomas depends strongly on the histology and resectability of the tumor. For bone sarcomas that are unresectable, primary RT is commonly used to achieve LC, with varying degrees of success; one study showed a 5-year LC rate of 56% among patients with nonmetastatic extremity osteosarcoma who refused resection.[10] Postoperative radiation may also be used for sarcomas originating in bone, depending on the margin status and response of the tumor to chemotherapy.

Although the list of sarcoma histologies is too exhaustive to review in this chapter, readers should be aware of several of the more common types. Some of the most common types of soft tissue sarcomas include undifferentiated pleomorphic sarcoma (historically called malignant fibrous histiocytoma), liposarcoma, leiomyosarcoma, and synovial sarcoma. Unusual but important subtypes also include desmoid tumors and dermatofibrosarcoma protuberans, both of which can be locally aggressive. Several of the more common bone sarcomas include osteosarcoma, Ewing sarcoma, and chondrosarcoma.

Much of the treatment paradigm, consisting of surgery and RT, with or without chemotherapy, is based on histology. However, the anatomic site of origin is also a critical factor to consider, particularly for the choice of local therapy. For instance, the strategy to treat a sarcoma in the distal leg is often different than that for a sarcoma that arises in the base of skull or retroperitoneum. Not only does the site of origin matter from a surgical standpoint, but also it factors into the approach taken by the radiation oncologist. Different anatomic sites require thoughtful radiation planning because of treatment volumes, neighboring critical structures, and toxicity considerations.

One radiation modalities with increasing applicability for the treatment of sarcomas is proton beam radiation. The goal of this chapter is to provide some perspective on the use of proton beam RT and summarize the available data supporting its use in the treatment of sarcomas.

SARCOMAS AND PROTON BEAM RADIATION

Both access to and justification for the use of proton beam therapy (PBT) for treatment of various malignancies is increasing. However, debate still exists among the wider health care community regarding its value. Contextually, it is important to understand that protons were initially developed during the era of two-dimensional (2D) photon therapy. Therefore, PBT provided, at one time, a way to deliver more conformal and often higher doses of radiation than could be achieved with photons. Yet with the development of intensity-modulated RT (IMRT), photons gained the capability of highly conformal dose-escalated distributions as well. The disadvantage of IMRT is its higher integral dose; PBT delivers 50% to 60% less integral dose to the rest of the body at the same or higher doses.[11,12]

In a joint phase II study by the MD Anderson Cancer Center and the Massachusetts General Hospital, pediatric patients with rhabdomyosarcoma were treated with PBT from 2005 through 2012.[13] A secondary objective of the study involved generating comparison IMRT plans for each patient. The authors observed a statistically higher integral dose for IMRT plans for treating tumors of the head and neck (1.8× higher), genitourinary system (1.8× higher), trunk and extremities (2.0× higher), and orbit (3.5× higher).[14] The main concern related to higher integral doses is that they may influence the risk of secondary malignancies, which was observed in a study by Chung and colleagues.[15] They reported that patients treated at Harvard with PBT had an observed 6.9 cancers per 1000 person-years compared with 10.3 cancers per 1000 person-years in matched patients from the Surveillance, Epidemiology, and End Results (SEER) registry receiving photon-based radiation. The higher integral dose of IMRT and the potential difference in late toxicities make PBT particularly enticing for patients with sarcoma. Sarcomas disproportionately affect younger patients than do other common types of cancers, which makes these concerns particularly relevant[16]; sarcomas affect 1% to 2% of adults with cancer worldwide, compared with 11% of adolescents and young adults (15–29 years old) and 6% to 15% of pediatric children (<15 years old).[17] Also, sarcomas are also commonly quite large, meaning that higher integral doses are needed to achieve comparable coverage. Finally, as previously mentioned, sarcomas occur throughout the body. For certain cancers arising at various anatomic sites (e.g., head and neck cancers; gastrointestinal cancers), growing bodies of literature support the benefit of PBT in sparing late toxicities; these findings may be extrapolated to sarcomas arising at the same anatomic sites.

CHORDOMAS AND CHONDROSARCOMAS

Sarcomas of the skull base, vertebral column, and sacrum are uncommon and pose particular management challenges. Given the anatomic locations, negative margin resections are difficult to achieve without significant morbidity, and radiation doses are limited by nearby critical structures. Chordomas and chondrosarcomas are the most common types of sarcomas to arise in these locations. Because of their similar behavior and central axis involvement, they are often described together.

Chordomas are rare tumors of bone that arise from notochordal remnants. Approximately 50% of chordomas are found in the sacrococcygeal region, whereas 35% occur in the base of skull and 15% within the vertebral column.[18] Chondrosarcomas are a heterogenous group of bone sarcomas that arise from cartilaginous elements; with several subtypes of various biology and behavior, chondrosarcomas are the second-most-common primary bone sarcoma after osteosarcoma, and they are generally thought to have a better prognosis than chordomas. However, survival rates for both chordomas and chondrosarcomas have improved over the past two decades, with expected 5-year overall survival (OS) of about 80%.[19–22]

The clinical presentation for both tumor types is similar and often is compressive in nature, with patients commonly experiencing pain or symptoms related to nerve dysfunction.

Chordomas and chondrosarcomas are both locally aggressive tumors that pose challenges for management. Resection, if possible, is the treatment of choice. However, negative margins are difficult to achieve, and the rate of local recurrence is high. Therefore, radiation was integrated into the treatment approach as a way to improve outcomes. Notably, however, both histologies are considered quite radioresistant, requiring high doses of radiation to achieve disease control.

The radiation doses required for maximum tumor control often in excess of 70 Gy, exceed the tolerances of nearby structures[23,24]; because of this small therapeutic ratio, chordomas and chondrosarcomas were some of the first tumors to be successfully treated by PBT, as it provided a way to deliver more precise radiation than was possible with its 2D/three-dimensional (3D) photon counterparts, thereby allowing the therapeutic ratio to be widened. One early study reported in 1982 by Suit and colleagues reported that doses of up to 76 cGE were delivered using PBT without significant morbidity.[25] Several subsequent studies helped to establish the dose-response relationship of chordomas and chondrosarcomas. Rich and colleagues reported on 48 patients with chordoma treated at the Massachusetts General Hospital, of whom 32 received postoperative RT. In that study, none of the patients (n = 18) receiving less than 60 Gy had no evidence of disease (NED), whereas 64% of the patients (n = 14) who received greater than 60 Gy did achieve NED status.[26] In a similar report Pearlman and Friedman, LC rates of 80% were achieved by using doses of 80 Gy compared with a 20% after doses of up to 60 Gy were delivered.[27,28] Finally, Keisch and colleagues reported on 12 patients treated with doses from 35 Gy to 70 Gy; all patients experienced relapse.[29]

Since these early experiences with using PBT to treat chordomas and chondrosarcomas, doses have been increased, with noticeable corresponding gains in LC. A large retrospective review by Munzenrider and Liebsch of more than 600 patients with chordoma and chondrosarcoma of the base of skull and spine treated with PBT with doses ranging between 66 to 83 cGE revealed 5-year LC rates of 73% for skull base chordomas and 98% for chondrosarcomas.[30] In a separate report on untreated spine chordomas receiving definitive mixed proton/photon RT to a median dose of 77.4 Gy, the 5-year LC rate was 80%.[31]

Significant amounts of retrospective evidence of favorable LC are available for chordomas and chondrosarcomas after dose-escalated PBT; however, prospective findings remain rare. One of the few prospective studies done to date was reported by Delaney and colleagues, who undertook a phase II trial for patients with spine and paraspinal sarcomas. Fifty patients were treated with pre- or postoperative proton/photon RT, with or without resection. Twenty-five patients received less than 73 Gy, and the other half received 76.6 to 77.4 cGE. The 5-year LC rates were 94% for patients with de novo presentations compared with 81% for the entire cohort.[32,33]

These findings, considered in their entirety, tell an interesting story. Chordomas and chondrosarcomas are relatively radioresistant tumors that are locally aggressive after surgery or moderate doses of radiation. However, higher doses of PBT can overcome this radioresistance and provide durable LC for tumors in some of the most anatomically difficult places to treat; for these tumor types, PBT is considered the standard of care.

RHABDOMYOSARCOMA

Another type of malignant soft tissue tumor is rhabdomyosarcoma, for which outcomes data after PBT are increasing. These tumors originate from skeletal muscle progenitor cells and are more common in children and adolescents or young adults than in older patients. Outcomes over the past few decades have improved with the increasing use of a multimodality approach to care, including radiation, which as noted earlier has an important role in LC. Because of its tendency to occur in younger patients, there is significant interest in using PBT to minimize late toxicity.

One of the first studies to report proton-associated outcomes in the treatment of rhabdomyosarcomas was published in 2005. The authors reported favorable tumor control outcomes for seven children with orbital rhabdomyosarcomas treated with PBT and chemotherapy, with excellent orbit function.[34] When comparing conformal 3D photon plans to the delivered PBT plans, Yock and colleagues showed that PBT reduced the average radiation dose to all the orbital and central nervous system structures, with the largest reductions observed for the optic nerve (95%), pituitary (94%), orbital bone (93%), retina (91%), and chiasm (90%). A similar study by Cotter and colleagues evaluated outcomes in seven children treated with PBT for bladder/prostate rhabdomyosarcomas; five patients remained NED at last follow-up with acceptable toxicities. Dosimetric comparisons of the PBT plans with those generated for IMRT revealed that PBT provided significantly lower mean organ doses to the bladder, testes, femoral heads, growth plates, and pelvic bones.[35]

These preliminary reports provided enough evidence to prompt a phase II study to prospectively evaluate PBT for patients with rhabdomyosarcoma. That trial enrolled 57 patients aged up to 21 years with rhabdomyosarcomas primarily classified as parameningeal (n = 27) or orbital (n = 13) to a median dose of 50.4 Gy (radiobiological effectiveness [RBE]) (range 36–50.4). After a median follow-up interval of 47 months (range 14–102), the 5-year event-free survival, OS, and LC rates were 69%, 78%, and 81%, with 5-year LC rates of 93% for low-risk disease and 77% for intermediate-risk disease. Eleven patients (13%) had a grade 3 acute toxicity attributable to RT, mostly odynophagia and dermatitis. Only three patients (7%) had a grade 3 late toxicity (cataract, chronic otitis, and retinopathy).[13] The authors concluded that these findings indicated that PBT had a favorable toxicity profile compared with photons, while acknowledging the lack of a modern prospective IMRT cohort for comparison.

A subsequent study reported the comparison IMRT plans that were generated as part of the phase II prospective proton trial for patients with rhabdomyosarcoma.[14] Although the target coverage (mean clinical target volume [CTV]: V_{95}) was similar between the PBT and the IMRT plans (P = .82), the IMRT plans delivered a significantly higher integral dose regardless of the tumor site, with as much as a 3.5-fold increase for tumors in the orbit. The PBT plans also delivered significantly lower doses to 26 of the 30 critical structures evaluated.[14] It will be interesting to determine if these dosimetric advantages translate into reductions in late toxicities when the long-term follow-up data have matured.

The role of radiation for pediatric patients with rhabdomyosarcomas is well defined, and for those who are to receive radiation, we consider PBT the standard modality. PBT should be given careful consideration when RT is recommended for adolescents and young adults. Importantly, though, practices vary in the use of radiation for rhabdomyosarcoma for older adult patients. We commonly treat rhabdomyosarcomas in such patients like other soft tissue sarcomas, delivering preoperative radiation in combination with surgery for improved LC. PBT should be considered for young patients in light of its dosimetric advantages.

RETROPERITONEAL SARCOMAS

Retroperitoneal sarcomas are often discussed together despite their heterogeneity because of the shared intraabdominal anatomic considerations. Retroperitoneal sarcomas constitute about 10% to 15% of all soft tissue sarcomas, with the most common histologies in adults being liposarcomas and leiomyosarcomas. Their management is somewhat controversial because of varying management practices, limited high-quality data, and high rates of tumor recurrence. Most series report 5-year LC rates of around 50%, which is why many practitioners advocate a combined-modality approach with the goal of improving outcomes.[36–39] However, the role of radiation is controversial. No prospective, randomized data are available to compare the role of radiation and surgery versus surgery alone. Because of this lack of prospectively defined benefit, some question the utility of radiation, given its risk of toxicity.

When radiation is incorporated into the treatment approach for retroperitoneal sarcomas, most, if not all, multidisciplinary high-volume sarcoma groups advocate preoperative treatment.[38,39] Several advantages exist when radiation is delivered preoperatively, including: (1) the target delineation is clear, (2) normal tissues and bowel are displaced, (3) treatment may increase the probability of a negative resection margin, and (4) cytoreduction of the tumor may occur. Therefore, when radiation is used in combination with surgery, it should ideally occur preoperatively, and in the absence of prospective data showing improved outcomes with combination therapy, patient selection is important to minimize toxicity. The properties that make PBT an enticing tool may improve the therapeutic ratio, particularly for sarcomas in the retroperitoneum (Fig. 16.1).

One study by Swanson and colleagues provided dosimetric data favoring PBT over conformal 3D photon RT and IMRT for eight patients with intraabdominal or retroperitoneal sarcomas; the mean integral dose was significantly lower for PBT than for either IMRT (P = .01) or 3D photon RT (P = .01).[40] Regarding organ-specific doses, PBT also had an advantage over IMRT in several measures, including the V15 to the small bowel (P = .0005), the mean (P = .03) and V5 (P = .049) to the contralateral kidney, and the mean liver dose (P = .02).[40] These findings provide dosimetric support for using PBT to treat tumors within the retroperitoneum, but the clinical benefit of these low-dose parameters is poorly defined.

The early experience and associated clinical outcomes treating 28 patients with retroperitoneal sarcomas with PBT or IMRT were reported by Yoon and colleagues.[41] The 3-year

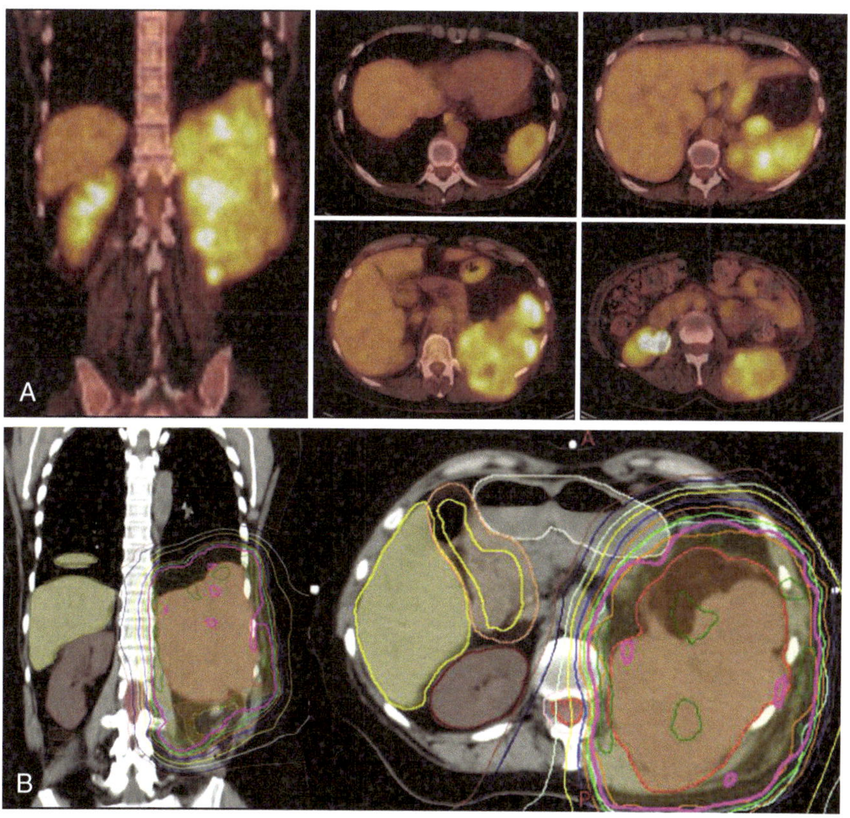

Fig. 16.1 Positron emission tomography and computed tomography scans of a 49-year-old woman with a multiply recurrent retroperitoneal liposarcoma who received preoperative proton radiation to a dose of 50.4 cGE followed by surgical resection.

recurrence-free survival rate was 90% for patients with de novo tumors and 30% for those with recurrent tumors. Four patients (14%) had complications associated with radiation, which was considered a favorable proportion. Interestingly, however, despite the use of RT, several patients in their series had an R1 or R2 resection (58%), which is one of the challenges for resecting tumors at this anatomic location.[41]

In an attempt to improve outcomes related to margin status, a phase I/II multiinstitutional trial is underway for patients with retroperitoneal sarcomas in which the dose is escalated to areas at risk of positive margins. The preliminary results of the phase I dose-escalation component using PBT were recently reported. The PBT was delivered in 28 fractions, and the dose to the area at risk was escalated from 60.2 GyRBE to 63 GyRBE. No acute dose-limiting toxicities were observed.[42] The PBT phase II component is now accruing and the dose is being escalated to 63 GyRBE. As additional findings emerge, PBT may be seen to improve the therapeutic ratio for treating retroperitoneal sarcomas, thereby making the use of preoperative RT more favorable.

We do not routinely recommend combined-modality therapy for all patients with retroperitoneal sarcomas. The decision to use preoperative RT should involve a multidisciplinary discussion to weigh the benefits against the possible risks. Several factors that should influence the decision include the intraabdominal location, tumor histology, tumor size, timing of presentation (de novo vs. recurrent tumor), and proximity to kidney or other organs at risk (i.e., volume of nearby bowel). When radiation is used preoperatively, the delivery method is critically assessed to weigh the advantages and disadvantages of both PBT and IMRT. Anecdotally, we find that patients tolerate preoperative PBT for retroperitoneal sarcomas better than expected. As more data emerge and PBT delivery becomes further refined, we expect it to have an increasing role for these soft tissue sarcomas.

SARCOMAS OF THE EXTREMITIES AND SUPERFICIAL TRUNK

The most common locations for sarcomas to arise are in the extremities and superficial trunk.[43] As is true for tumors at other anatomic locations, radiation is incorporated into the treatment approach in combination with surgery to improve LC while also attempting to maximize functional outcomes and to minimize toxicity.[7–9] Unfortunately, information is limited on the use of PBT for sarcomas in the extremities/superficial trunk, largely tumors in these locations are adequately treated with 3D conformal photon radiation, without much clear gain from PBT. PBT may have some benefit in terms of preventing the exit dose associated with photon RT for patients with large, superficial trunk tumors. However, the dosimetric benefits of PBT must always be weighed against the higher skin doses for patients for whom wound complications and wound healing are important considerations.

Reirradiation can be considered for patients who develop a local recurrence after previous combined-modality therapy, there is often discussion about the role of reirradiation. These clinical scenarios pose a challenge with regard to balancing optimal tumor control against the morbidity of treatment. A small prospective study recently enrolled patients with soft tissue sarcomas in previously irradiated fields.[44] Some 23 patients received PBT for reirradiation, although its timing in relation to surgery varied. The authors of that study recommended delineation of a more conformal target (i.e., CTV expansion of only 5–10 mm compared with the 3–4 cm recommended in the de novo setting), given the increased risks of retreatment toxicity. About half of the patients ($n = 12$) experienced local failure at a median interval of 10 months, and the other 11 patients had local tumor control at death or last follow-up. Surprisingly, only three patients had grade 3 late toxicities, and none had grade 4 or 5 toxicity. The authors concluded that proton reirradiation was well tolerated among patients with recurrent or secondary sarcomas, but acknowledged that longer follow-up is needed.[44]

Although these findings provide a starting point for discussion of reirradiation for patients with locally recurrent sarcomas, we recommend individualized treatment decisions that include the patient and multidisciplinary providers. The relative unresponsiveness of gross tumors in patients with sarcoma makes reirradiation less enticing than for other more radiosensitive tumor histologies, particularly because the radioresistance of previously irradiated tumors is known in advance. Also, other salvage therapies for recurrent disease may have less risk. Although our standard practice does not involve reirradiation, when reirradiation is to be considered, repeat PBT seems to be well tolerated.

Conclusion

Sarcomas represent a heterogenous group of tumors that arise throughout the body, and radiation has an integral part in their treatment to improve LC. Few outcomes studies are available for PBT in these rare tumors. Therefore the data that are available must be combined with other anatomic site-specific data for different tumor types to guide the choice of radiation modality. Strong data support the use of PBT for chordomas and chondrosarcomas of the axial skeleton, and evidence regarding the use of PBT the treatment of rhabdomyosarcomas and retroperitoneal sarcomas, and perhaps for reirradiation, is increasing. Patients diagnosed with sarcomas need prompt referral to a high-volume sarcoma center where expert multidisciplinary care can be provided and the potential benefits of PBT identified.

References Available Online.

CHAPTER 17

Esophagus Cancer

Steven H. Lin ■ Heng Li ■ Daniel R. Gomez

Introduction

Esophageal cancer (EC) is the sixth leading cause of cancer death worldwide and is responsible for 400,000 new cases (4.9% of all cancers) cancer deaths annually.[1] The incidence of EC differs greatly according to geographic region, with the highest incidence in Asian and Middle Eastern countries.[2] In most Western countries, such as the United States, adenocarcinoma has eclipsed squamous cell carcinoma as the predominant histologic type, and it usually afflicts white men. In contrast, squamous cell carcinoma is mostly related to smoking and alcohol consumption in Asia and Middle Eastern countries. Adenocarcinoma is also closely linked with obesity, which, with the associated reflux esophagitis and Barrett preneoplasia, are becoming epidemic in the West and in developed countries.[3]

Historically, the previous standard treatment approach, surgical resection with or without adjuvant therapy, produced cure rates of only about 20%; thus, the addition of preoperative chemoradiation is increasingly being adopted, given the evidence that this approach improves overall survival (OS) relative to surgery alone. The largest of the randomized trials performed in the modern era was a phase III randomized study from a Dutch group, in which 366 evaluable patients were randomized to surgery versus preoperative chemoradiation to 41.4 Gy with carboplatin and paclitaxel.[4] The preoperative chemoradiation substantially improved the median OS time (49.4 months vs. 24.0 months in the surgery-only group). The pathologic complete response rate in the preoperative chemoradiation group was 29% and was higher among patients with squamous cell carcinoma than those with adenocarcinoma (49% vs. 23%; $P = .008$), which also translated to improved OS from chemoradiation relative to surgery alone for squamous tumors relative to adenocarcinomas (adjusted hazard ratio: 0.42 [95% confidence interval (CI): 0.23–0.79] vs. 0.74 [95% CI: 0.54–1.02]).

Because of the location of the esophagus, mid- and distal esophageal tumors span posteriorly across the heart and are in very close proximity to the left atrium and anteriorly to the thoracic vertebrae. Proton beam therapy (PBT) is therefore ideal for the treatment of EC, given the tight dose conformality it provides. Comparisons of PBT with three-dimensional (3D) conformal therapy and intensity-modulated (photon) radiation therapy (IMRT) are described in further detail later in this chapter. The following sections describe procedures for treatment simulation, radiation dose and fractionation, target delineation, and treatment verification when using PBT for esophageal tumors, followed by descriptions of aspects of treatment planning that are specific to the two major types of PBT: passive scattering or intensity-modulated proton therapy (IMPT).

Treatment Simulation

For treatment simulation, patients with cervical tumors should be supine and immobilized with a five-point mask, with indexed head, neck, and shoulder stabilization. Patients with thoracic or gastroesophageal junction tumors are also positioned supine and immobilized with the use of an indexed upper Vac-Loc/alpha cradle, with both arms up; potential deflation of the cradle must be monitored. The isocenter is placed at the carina. Respiratory motion should be assessed by four-dimensional (4D) scanning, as the esophagus and surrounding structures can move substantially with respiratory motion, particularly at the gastroesophageal junction. Simulation should ideally take place with the patient's arms above their head to maximize the number of beam arrangements that can be used. To improve reproducibility, patients should be advised to consume nothing by mouth for at least 3 hours before the simulation and before each daily treatment.

Radiation Dose and Fractionation, Target Delineation, and Treatment Verification

A summary of these topics, discussed in further detail below, is provided in Table 17.1.

RADIATION DOSE AND FRACTIONATION

Because tumors of the upper esophagus are less likely to be excised surgically, escalation of dose beyond 50.4 Gy can be considered (e.g., 50.4–60 Gy in 1.8- to 2.0-Gy fractions). For tumors of the lower esophagus, the standard dose remains 40 to 50.4 Gy in 1.8- to 2.0-Gy fractions. Dose escalation for lower esophagus tumors can be considered in the context of a clinical trial.

TARGET DELINEATION

Target delineation differs depending on the location of the tumor within the esophagus. Upper esophagus tumors are defined as those within the cervical and upper thoracic regions, and lower esophagus tumors are in the mid- and distal esophagus, including those at the gastroesophageal junction. Target delineation of Siewert type III gastroesophageal junction tumors should be similar to that of gastric cancers.

TABLE 17.1 ■ **Key Definitions and Recommendations for Using Proton Beam Therapy to Treat Upper and Lower Esophagus Cancer**

	Upper Esophagus Tumors	Lower Esophagus Tumors
GTV (with internal motion)	Gross tumor	Gross tumor
CTV	Cervical: superior to cricoid cartilage, inferior 3.5 cm, lateral 1 cm (respecting anatomic boundaries), bilateral SCV fossa Upper thoracic: superior-inferior 3.5 cm, lateral 1 cm (respecting anatomic boundaries)	Middle esophagus: Superior-inferior 3.5 cm, lateral 1 cm (respecting anatomical boundaries), left gastric and celiac lymph nodes not considered unless involved. Distal esophagus/GEJ (Siewert I/II): superior-inferior 3.5 cm, lateral 1 cm (respecting anatomic boundaries), routinely electively cover left gastric lymph nodes, celiac nodes in node-positive disease Siewert type III: treat like gastric cancer
Patient setup margin	0.5–1.0 cm; 0.5 cm if daily kV IGRT is used	0.5–1.0 cm; 0.5 cm if daily kV IGRT used
Prescription dose	50.4–60 Gy (RBE) in 1.8–2.0 Gy (RBE) fractions	40–50.4 Gy (RBE) in 1.8–2.0 Gy (RBE) fractions

CTV, clinical target volume; *GEJ,* gastroesophageal junction; *GTV,* Gross tumor volume; *IGRT,* image-guided radiation therapy, *RBE,* radiobiological effectiveness; *SCV,* supraclavicular.

For upper esophagus tumors, the gross tumor volume (GTV) encompasses the gross tumor. The clinical target volume (CTV) consists of a 3.5-cm margin superiorly-inferiorly and a 1-cm margin laterally, but not crossing anatomic boundaries (or modified for boundaries such as vessels or bone). However, for cervical esophagus lesions, the upper margin should be the inferior border of the cricoid cartilage. The CTV should also include elective treatment of the supraclavicular fossa bilaterally, even in the absence of involvement.

For lower esophagus tumors, the GTV and CTV are similar to those for upper esophagus tumors, that is, the GTV covers the gross tumor, and the CTV consists of a 3.5-cm margin superiorly-inferiorly and a 1-cm margin laterally, but not crossing anatomic boundaries (or modified for boundaries such as vessels or bone). For lower esophagus tumors, the CTV should also include the left gastric lymph nodes for patients with distal esophagus or gastroesophageal junction tumors (Siewert type I/II disease). For patients with node-positive disease, the celiac axis should also be electively covered, even in the absence of involvement.

For particle therapy, a planning target volume (PTV) is used only for recording and reporting purposes.[5] In practice, the PTV is generated by expanding the CTV with the patient setup margin, which ranges from 0.5 to 1.0 cm based on the image guidance that is available. At MD Anderson, we use daily kV imaging and thus a 0.5-cm PTV margin.

In addition to the PTV, a dosimetric margin is also needed for particle therapy to account for beam range uncertainties and modulations of beams, as described in further detail in the section Treatment Planning.

TREATMENT VERIFICATION

For daily treatment verification, patients are positioned as described for treatment simulation, that is, supine and immobilized with either a five-point mask or a Vac-Loc cradle, with the isocenter placed at the carina. Daily kV imaging should be used for all patients. If in-room volumetric imaging (e.g., cone-beam computed tomography [CT] or CT-on-rails) is available, scans can be obtained weekly.

Breathhold and gating techniques are not typically used during the treatment of esophageal tumors, although they can be used for target motion management.

Substantial changes in anatomy or tumor size over the course of treatment are rare, and thus, adaptive simulations are not routinely scheduled. However, if daily or weekly imaging shows changes in normal tissues or tumor, or if the patient undergoes a prolonged treatment break, then we recommend that a verification CT scan be obtained as soon as possible.

Treatment Planning

PASSIVE SCATTERING PROTON BEAM THERAPY

Typically, the beam arrangement for distal tumors is most commonly posteroanterior (PA) and left lateral oblique. However, optimal beam arrangements are determined on a case-by-case basis, and alternative beam arrangements can be used. For proximal to midesophagus tumors, an anteroposterior (AP) and PA beam arrangement could be considered, although caution should be used in the AP direction because beam range uncertainty may lead to irradiation of the spinal cord.

For free-breathing treatments, target coverage during all breathing phases is ensured by creating a planning diaphragm structure from the T0 and T50 phases of the 4D CT scan. The density of the diaphragm is then overridden by using the average Hounsfield units of the maximum-intensity projection scan generated from the 4D CT scans. The treatment plan is then designed with the overridden average CT. This technique ensures adequate coverage to the

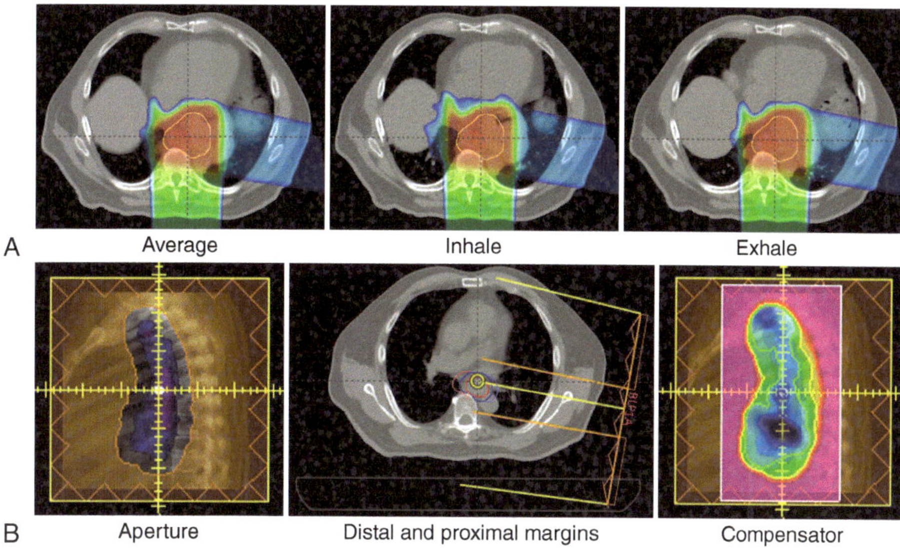

Fig. 17.1 Overriding the diaphragm in treatment for esophageal cancer. (A) *Left:* plan dose calculated on average computed tomography with diaphragm override; middle: dose calculated on T0; *right:* dose calculated on T50. (B) *Left:* aperture design with lateral margin consists of setup margin and dosimetric margin to account for beam penumbra; middle: distal *(red)* and proximal *(blue)* margins; *right:* compensator design with smearing.

distal end of the target even with respiratory motion, as shown in Fig. 17.1A. Aperture design with setup margin and dosimetric margin, beamline design that includes distal and proximal margins based on beam range to account for range uncertainties, and compensator design with smear margin to ensure distal target coverage[6] are illustrated in Fig. 17.1B.

INTENSITY-MODULATED PROTON THERAPY

IMPT offers superior dose conformity compared with passive scattering proton therapy, and it delivers less integral dose than IMRT. However, IMPT is more sensitive to respiratory motion than passive scattering proton therapy, posing an even greater challenge for implementing this technique, particularly for distal esophageal tumors.

One way to assess the impact of respiratory motion is to assess the changes in water-equivalent thickness (WET) of the proton beam. One group showed that the change in WET is correlated with respiratory motion, which generates dose uncertainty in distal esophageal treatment plans.[7] The same study also established that for tumors in the distal esophagus, the optimal beam angles range between 150 and 210 degrees to avoid diaphragm motion in the beam path. Typically, two to three beams could be used for plans in this range (Fig. 17.2).

Both single-field optimization (SFO), in which each field is optimized to deliver the prescribed target dose to the target volume,[8] and IMPT, in which all spots from all fields are optimized simultaneously, can be used for planning pencil beam scanning treatments. In general, IMPT offers more flexibility with more degrees of freedom and could result in more conformal dose distribution, but IMPT plans are also less robust than SFO plans, owing to the complex dose distribution in each field. For esophageal tumors, either SFO or IMPT plans could be used, although the dose to the spinal cord would be slightly higher in the SFO plans, within 45 to 50 Gy (radiobiological effectiveness [RBE]). Indeed, 4D treatment planning and robustness optimization could further reduce the influence of

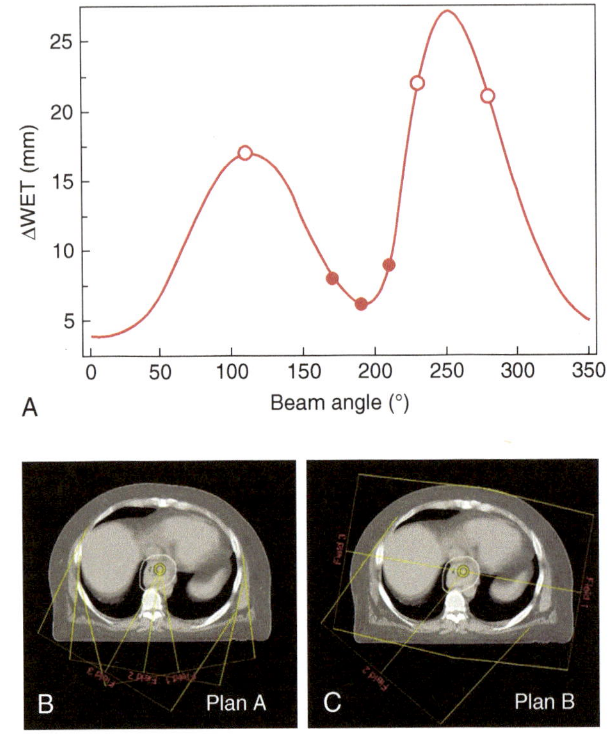

Fig. 17.2 Identifying optimal beam angles for intensity-modulated proton therapy. (A) An example of a change in water-equivalent thickness *(ΔWET)* curve created by plotting ΔWET value against beam angle. The solid circles indicate the three beam angles that are in the approximate range of the minimum ΔWET. These are the beam angles used in plan A. The open circles correspond to the three beam angles around the maximum ΔWET, which are the beam angles used in plan B. (B) Beam arrangement for plan A. (C) Beam arrangement for plan B. The contour is the internal clinical target volume (ICTV). (From Yu J, Zhang X, Liao L, et al. Motion-robust intensity-modulated proton therapy for distal esophageal cancer. *Med Phys.* 2016;43(3):1111.)

respiratory motion on the dose distribution, but these techniques may not be readily available.[7] However, active target motion management techniques such as breath hold can be used instead.

Dosimetric and Toxicity Comparisons of Proton Versus Photon Therapy

Use of 3D conformal radiation therapy to treat EC involves relatively high radiation doses to the heart, especially when an AP beam is used. By contrast, use of IMRT can reduce high-dose scatter across the heart by placing the entrance dose posteriorly, thereby subjecting the heart and lung dose to low exit doses. PBT further improves the dosimetric variables because the Bragg peak involves virtually no exit dose. Therefore even using only two beams in passive scattering proton therapy leads to a substantial reduction in dose to the lung and heart (Fig. 17.3). Numerous dosimetric planning studies have been done to compare dose distributions from PBT with photon modalities. In one such study comparing photons versus protons, both with 3D planning techniques, for five patients, the passive scattering proton therapy plan led to improved dosing to the spinal cord, lung, heart, and kidneys relative to the 3D conformal photon plan, with the best proton plan improving the tumor control probability by 2% units to 23% units (mean: 20%).[8,9]

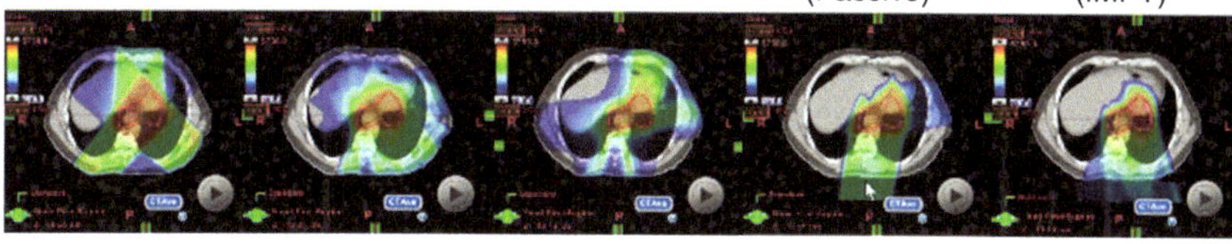

Fig. 17.3 Dosimetric comparisons of the lung, heart, and liver of photon (three-dimensional conformal radiation therapy *[3D-CRT]*, intensity-modulated radiation therapy *[IMRT]*, or volumetric arc therapy *[VMAT]*) and proton (passive scattering or intensity-modulated proton therapy *[IMPT]*) plans for a distal esophageal tumor.

Dosimetric benefits are also observed when plans for passive scattering proton therapy are compared with IMRT plans. In one such study, IMRT was compared with two-field AP/PA or three-field AP/two posterior obliques passive scattering proton therapy field arrangements in 15 patients.[10] Although proton therapy led to substantial reductions in lung V5 to V20, mean lung dose, and spinal cord dose, no dose-sparing effect was observed for the heart. This discrepancy is likely the result of suboptimal beam arrangements in these early studies. To address this point, we compared plans for passive scattering proton therapy with those for IMRT in 55 patients with mid- to distal EC to identify dosimetric or anatomic factors that led to suboptimal proton dose distribution.[11] Specifically, we identified patients whose proton plans had "suboptimal" dosimetry relative to IMRT plans and then attempted to determine whether the dosimetric characteristics could be improved with alternative approaches. We found that the primary reasons for suboptimal dosimetry were: (1) nonstandard beam arrangements such as AP/PA or AP/PA/left lateral approach, (2) 1:1 beam weighting of the left lateral/PA beam, and (3) unique patient anatomic features such as a CTV that wrapped around the heart.

Investigators at MD Anderson have also compared toxicity after proton versus photon techniques for EC, both dosimetrically and in terms of clinical outcomes. In one such study, plans were evaluated for 444 patients with EC treated with 3D conformal radiation therapy (n = 208), IMRT (n = 164), or PBT (n = 72), each with concurrent preoperative chemotherapy, from 1998 through 2011.[12] Significant differences in mean lung dose and mean heart dose were evident among the three modalities, particularly for PBT compared with the two other photon modalities. That study also evaluated the rates of postoperative pulmonary, cardiac, wound, and gastrointestinal complications in those patients according to treatment modality. On univariate analysis, several factors predicted adverse events, but radiation modality was associated only with pulmonary and gastrointestinal complications. On multivariate analysis, only radiation modality and preradiation diffusion capacity of the lung for carbon monoxide (D_{LCO}) were independently associated with pulmonary complications. Radiation modality, that is, proton therapy, seemed to be associated with fewer gastrointestinal complications as well, although that apparent difference was not statistically significant. Comparisons among the three radiation modalities showed significant increases in pulmonary complications for 3D conformal versus IMRT (odds ratio [OR]: 4.10; 95% CI: 1.37–12.29) and 3D conformal versus proton therapy (OR: 9.13; 95% CI: 1.83–45.42), but no difference in pulmonary complications were found between IMRT and PBT after adjustment for the preradiation D_{LCO} level; rather, only mean lung dose predicted pulmonary complications.[12]

Investigators from the University of Pennsylvania recently published a prospective study of 14 patients given passive scattering proton therapy for recurrent EC over a 15-year period, with the goals of assessing outcomes and toxicity. The two cases of grade 5 toxicity (one acute, from an esophagopleural fistula, and another late, from an esophageal ulcer) were thought to be related to tumor progression rather than treatment. Although no patients had acute grade 4 toxicity, late grade 3 toxicities experienced were heart failure, esophageal stricture, esophageal ulceration, and dependence on a percutaneous endoscopic gastrostomy tube. The median OS time was 14 months, leading the authors to conclude that this approach was associated with "encouraging" symptom control and "favorable" survival.[13]

At this time, the relative value of PBT (passive scattering or IMPT) versus photon (IMRT) techniques for treating EC should be evaluated further in prospective randomized trials. MD Anderson is currently leading a phase IIB randomized study comparing proton therapy with IMRT (NCT01512589), with the coprimary end points being total toxicity burden and disease-free survival. Anticipated accrual is 180 patients, and over 50% of evaluable patients had accrued when this chapter was written.

Conclusions and Future Directions

Substantial progress has been made in the use of proton therapy for esophagus cancer over the past decade. Proton dosimetry has been compared with that of IMRT and 3D conformal radiation therapy; optimal beam arrangements have been defined, planning techniques have been refined, IMPT has been implemented, and comparativeness effectiveness studies initiated. The next 10 to 20 years will likely involve further refinements of IMPT for EC, along with standardization of planning approaches. Ways of identifying patients who would benefit from proton therapy (as opposed to IMRT) are also critical needs, and one substantial benefit from the completion of ongoing randomized studies will be the ability to identify subsets of patients who derive the greatest clinical benefit from the use of proton therapy. Ideally, proton therapy will be possible for an increasing number of patients with limited treatment options, such as those with in-field local failures. Finally, increasingly sophisticated imaging techniques will deepen our understanding of the differences between proton and photon therapies in terms of both tumor response and toxicity. The use of radiomics in combination with sensitive imaging or functional imaging modalities such as magnetic resonance imaging or positron emission tomography will further extend our comprehension of the early responses to protons and whether such responses can be predictive and prognostic of ultimate outcomes.

Acknowledgments

Portions of this chapter appear in Lee N, Leeman JE, Jiang G, Lu JJ, Sine K, Both K, eds. *Target Volume Delineation and Treatment Planning for Particle Therapy*. Basel, Switzerland: Springer International Publishing; 2018.

References Available Online.

CHAPTER 18

Lung Cancer

Daniel R. Gomez ■ Heng Li ■ Xiaodong Zhang ■ Joe Y. Chang ■ Zhongxing Liao ■ Steven H. Lin

Introduction

Lung cancer is one of the most common malignancies, accounting for approximately 234,000 new cases and 160,000 deaths per year in the United States.[1] Treatment for lung cancer depends on the disease stage at presentation, with disease at early stages treated by surgery or radiation alone and more advanced tumors receiving bi- or trimodality therapy.

Several studies have shown dosimetric benefits from particle therapy over intensity-modulated radiation therapy (IMRT) for some patients with lung cancer.[2–4] This dosimetric superiority has been demonstrated for both early-stage and locally advanced disease and when three-dimensional (3D) conformal therapy and IMRT are compared with proton beam therapy (PBT). Notably, improvements in normal tissue dose have been noted mostly in low-dose regions, such as the volumes receiving 5 Gy (relative biological effectiveness [RBE]) (V5) or 10 Gy (RBE) (V10). This selective benefit results from the sharp dose buildup and abrupt dose drop beyond the target possible with PBT. This is particularly important for lung cancer, given the proximity of the lungs, heart, esophagus, major airways, large blood vessels, and spinal cord. The benefits in terms of reducing or eliminating the so-called *low-dose bath* with PBT cannot be accomplished at present with advanced photon techniques.

Clinical outcomes after particle therapy have been reported for both early-stage and locally advanced nonsmall cell lung cancer (NSCLC).[5–9] The outcomes in these studies seem to be similar to or improved over those obtained with advanced photon modalities such as IMRT or volumetric modulated arc therapy. When this chapter was written, only one randomized trial that directly compared particle therapy with photons for locally advanced NSCLC had been reported. In that randomized phase II study, toxicity (pneumonitis) and local disease control were evaluated after patients received IMRT or passive scattered PBT, and no statistical differences in these end points were found between the two modalities.[10] Future analyses from this study focus on comparisons of imaging data, blood samples, additional toxicity end points, and quality of life to assess how these factors may influence outcomes.

To summarize, proton therapy seems to have dosimetric benefits over various forms of photon therapy in some clinical situations, but thus far, no strong evidence has been found that "all comers," that is, anyone with lung cancer, would benefit from PBT over advanced photon techniques. Thus, indications for PBT and criteria with which to select patients for PBT are of critical importance, particularly when passive scattering techniques are used.

Small cell lung cancer (SCLC) nearly always presents as locally advanced or metastatic disease, and therefore principles for PBT simulation, target delineation, and treatment planning are similar for locally advanced NSCLC and SCLC. However, experience with using PBT for SCLC is very limited. In one report of six patients with a median follow-up time of 12 months, 1-year overall survival (OS) and progression-free survival (PFS) rates were 83% and 66%, respectively.[11] Thus although much of the discussion on NSCLC with regard to particle therapy techniques can be extrapolated to SCLC, additional investigation is needed regarding outcomes after PBT, including rates of local control and the benefit of such modalities as intensity-modulated proton therapy (IMPT).

Patient Selection Criteria

PASSIVE SCATTERING PROTON THERAPY

Appropriate criteria for identifying patients who may benefit from passive scattering PBT are important because in some cases, the treatment plans are better for advanced conformal techniques, such as IMRT, for the following reasons. First, passive scattering PBT involves some limitations in beam angles because of dose uncertainties in the beam path. Second, passive scattering PBT requires a "backstop" to provide much of the sharp dose falloff, which can be difficult in the context of early-stage lung parenchymal tumors. When no high-density tissue is present distal to the target, dose "spikes" can occur that substantially affect the dosimetry and contribute to more dose being delivered to the normal tissues than necessary, thereby leading to toxicity.

With these limitations in mind, from a dosimetric standpoint, the following patients are good candidates for passive scattering PBT rather than IMRT: (1) those with tumors located in tissue that can provide a suitable backstop to exploit the dose falloff properties of proton therapy, (2) those for whom IMRT is not feasible because of the inability to meet low dose constraints (e.g., V5, V10, or V20), and (3) those with anterior mediastinal tumors in that are proximal to the heart, lung, spinal cord, and esophagus.

INTENSITY-MODULATED PROTON THERAPY

IMPT offers the following benefits over passive scattering proton therapy: (1) improved conformality and (2) lesser influence of beam placement because the dose can be supplemented where necessary through "patching," which also can reduce the magnitude of hotspots. IMPT can also be suitable for simultaneous integrated boost (SIB) regimens because, by placing the proton Bragg peak in the target, the target dose can be escalated while contributing very little dose to normal tissue. A comparative clinical trial is ongoing at MD Anderson to evaluate IMPT and IMRT for SIB.

Limitations of IMPT include (1) its greater sensitivity of dose to changes in anatomy and tumor size because of the lower number of beams used and its very high conformality, and (2) risk of reduced local control when spot scanning delivery interacts with respiratory motion, leading to targets being missed during certain phases of the respiratory cycle. Two specific scenarios in which dose to the lung cancer target has been reduced are in the development (or reduction of) atelectasis (Fig. 18.1) and changes in tumor size during treatment.

IMPT has often been used for (1) mediastinal but laterally displaced tumors, in which dose distribution is improved to the lung and esophagus; (2) extremely challenging cases in which dose constraints cannot be met with other techniques (e.g., large bilateral mediastinal masses); and (3) reirradiation, in which the goal is to almost completely avoid dose to one or more normal structures. As both the availability of and experience with IMPT increase, more patients have been selected for this approach, particularly those with locally advanced lung cancer. Several trials are ongoing to examine the safety and efficacy of IMPT for lung tumors, with particular attention being paid to local control given the concerns with respiratory motion interplay.

Treatment Simulation

Treatment simulation should take place while patients have their arms over their heads; the selection of beam arrangement resembles that for photon techniques. Immobilization of the upper body should be used in conjunction with four-dimensional (4D) image acquisition to capture respiratory motion. If patients cannot raise their arms above their heads, the simulation can be done with their arms at their sides, although this setup can markedly limit the potential for dosimetric benefit, particularly if passive scattering PBT is being used.

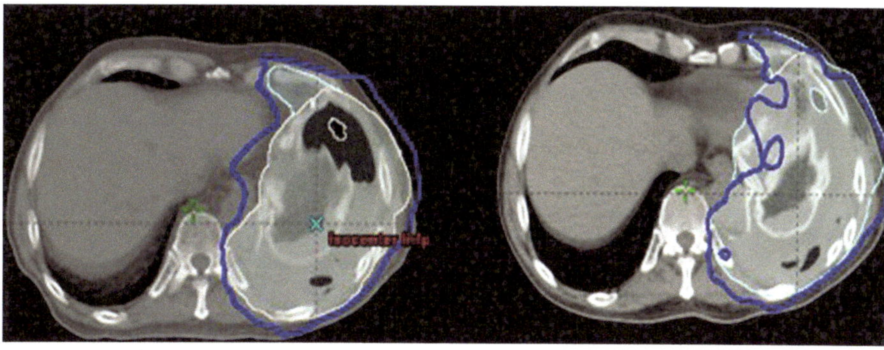

Fig. 18.1 Target dose is reduced to reflect changes in lung volume occurring midway through a 5-week course of radiation therapy to the lung.

Radiation Dose and Fractionation, Target Delineation, and Treatment Verification

A summary of these topics, discussed in further detail later, is provided in Table 18.1.

RADIATION DOSE AND FRACTIONATION

Several 1- to 10-fraction dose regimens are used for PBT. At MD Anderson, all proton prescription doses are reported with a constant RBE value of 1.1; we routinely use a dose of 50 Gy in 4 fractions for peripheral disease and 70 Gy (RBE) in 10 fractions for central disease.[12–14] For locally advanced NSCLC that is to be treated with chemotherapy and radiation, the standard dose is 60 Gy (RBE) in 30 fractions, based on the recently published Radiation Therapy Oncology Group (RTOG) 0617 trial demonstrating no benefit from dose escalation to 74 Gy.[15] For SCLC, the standard dose regimen remains 45 Gy (RBE) in 30 fractions delivered twice daily, based on the results of a randomized trial comparing once-daily to twice-daily radiation.[16] However, the recently published phase III randomized Concurrent ONce-daily VErsus twice-daily RadioTherapy (CONVERT) study, which enrolled 547 patients, demonstrated equivalence in a cohort of patients with limited-stage SCLC when comparing 45 Gy in 30 fractions to 66 Gy in 33 fractions. The authors note that because the trial was designed to demonstrate the superiority of once-daily radiation and wasn't powered to show equivalence, twice-daily regimens should continue to be considered the standard of care for such patients.[17]

SIB regimens have also been used in the treatment of lung cancer with either photons or protons,[18–21] and numerous studies are ongoing to evaluate the safety and efficacy of this approach.

TARGET DELINEATION

Involved-field techniques with 4D computed tomography (CT)–based planning are used for both node-negative and node-positive disease, regardless of whether the treatment technique involves photons or protons. The gross tumor volume (GTV) is contoured on a CT scan of the chest with contrast with positron emission tomography scans used for guidance; histologic findings from mediastinoscopy or endobronchial ultrasonography are also used when available.

Two potential approaches can be used to expand the GTV to capture both internal motion and microscopic disease. The first involves expanding the GTV to the clinical target volume

TABLE 18.1 ■ **Key Definitions and Recommendations for Using Proton Beam Therapy to Treat Locally Advanced Non-small Cell Lung Cancer and Small Cell Lung Cancer**

	Proton Beam Therapy	Locally Advanced Non-Small Cell Lung Cancer	Small Cell Lung Cancer
Prescribed dose and number of fractions	Many 1–10 fractionation schedules in use. At MD Anderson, peripheral disease is treated with 12.5 Gy (RBE) × 4 fractions, and central disease with 7 Gy (RBE) × 10 fractions	Standard regimen: 60 Gy (RBE) in 30 once-daily fractions with concurrent chemotherapy	Standard regimen: 45 Gy (RBE) in 30 twice-daily fractions with concurrent chemotherapy
iGTV to CTV margin	0 cm	0.6–0.8 cm	0.6–0.8 cm
CTV to PTV setup margin	0.5 cm (GTV to PTV) if daily CT available. If not available, 0.5–1.0 cm, ideally with fiducial placement	1.0–1.5 cm without daily IGRT 0.5 cm with daily kV imaging 0.3 cm with daily CBCT	1.0–1.5 cm without daily IGRT 0.5 cm with daily kV imaging 0.3 cm with daily CBCT
Daily treatment verification	CT scanning (e.g., CBCT, CT-on-rails) if available and strongly recommended. If not available, strongly consider fiducial placement and then daily kV imaging with 0.5- to 1.0-cm setup margin	Daily kV imaging, weekly CBCT if available.	Twice-daily kV imaging (with each fraction), weekly CBCT if available
Verification simulation		At least once during treatment (week 3–4), more often if significant tumor changes are observed	Consider after first week of treatment for bulky disease

CBCT, Cone-beam computed tomography; *CTV,* clinical target volume; *GTV,* gross tumor volume; *IGRT,* image-guided radiation therapy; *iGTV,* internal gross tumor volume; *PTV,* planning target volume; *RBE,* relative biological effectiveness.

(CTV), followed by a further expansion to the internal target volume (ITV) to account for internal motion, followed by an expansion to the planning target volume (PTV) to cover daily variations in patient position and movement. The second approach, often used at MD Anderson, is to delineate the GTV, assess its internal motion, and create an "envelope" structure called the iGTV, which is then expanded to create the iCTV (which is very similar to the ITV).

The advantage of the latter approach is its assessment of the internal motion of gross disease, which may be easier to delineate.

For early-stage lung cancer, per RTOG standards, no distinct CTV margin is included, and only a PTV is delineated. For locally advanced disease, standard GTV-to-CTV treatment margins (from the GTV [or iGTV] to the CTV) are 0.6 to 0.8 cm to cover microscopic disease, as defined in prior pathologic studies.[22]

With regard to expansion to a PTV for proton therapy, there is no standard uniform PTV akin to that used in photon planning to cover errors in patient setup (typically fixed at 0.5–1.0 cm). Rather, the PTV for proton therapy includes two components: (1) the *setup margin*, which accounts for day-to-day setup errors and depends on the image-guided radiation therapy (IGRT) method used, and (2) the *dosimetric margin*, which is field-specific and encompasses proximal, distal, and lateral margins for that particular field (to account for dose uncertainty in the beam path).

The CTV-to-PTV setup margin for PBT corresponds to the 0.5 cm used for photon techniques and is an extension directly from the GTV. However, this setup margin presumes that cone-beam CT (CBCT) is available for daily localization. If daily CT imaging is not available, we strongly recommend considering fiducial placement, with daily kV imaging during treatment and a 0.5- to 1.0-cm PTV setup margin.

For locally advanced lung cancer, the following PTV margins are used: 1.0 to 1.5 cm without daily IGRT (e.g., kV imaging or CBCT); 0.5–1.0 cm for either 4D CT planning or CBCT, but not both; 0.5 cm for 4D CT planning and daily kV imaging; or 0.3 cm for 4D CT planning and CBCT guidance.

The field-specific dosimetric margin depends on the water-equivalent range relative to the most proximal and distal points of the CTV from a specific beam angle; these margins typically range from approximately 0.5 to 1.0 cm.

As an alternative to a geometric PTV, physicists at MD Anderson are exploring the use of beam-specific PTVs for passive scatter proton therapy planned with single-field optimization.[23] This method provides significant advantages over the conventional method using a single PTV for all beams because the magnitude of each margin can be individualized for each field to account for tissue misalignment (patient setup error) and tissue heterogeneity without the use of a physical compensator.[24]

TREATMENT VERIFICATION

For daily treatment verification, most patients undergo daily kV imaging and at least one verification simulation to ensure that no substantial changes have taken place in tumor volume or other aspects of patient anatomy that would warrant repeat treatment planning. Use of midtreatment verification is particularly important for particle therapy, where seemingly minor changes in these factors can have pronounced dosimetric effects. If in-room CT capability is present, we recommend weekly CBCT scans in addition to the midtreatment verification scan.

Dose Constraints

PBT involves several dose constraints, based in part on the number of fractions being delivered. These dose constraints are derived from those for photon therapy established in the National Comprehensive Cancer Network guidelines (www.nccn.org). Our institutional dose constraints for standard-fractionation, once-daily proton therapy are given in Table 18.2. For twice-daily regimens, such as those given for SCLC, constraints are similar except for the dose to the spinal cord, which should be limited to a maximum dose of less than 40 Gy (RBE).

TABLE 18.2 ■ **Dosimetric Constraints for Proton Beam Therapy Given in Standard Once-Daily Fractions**

Normal Structure	Dose Constraint
Spinal cord	Maximum dose ≤45 Gy
Heart	V30 ≤ 45 Gy (RBE), mean dose <26 Gy (RBE)
Esophagus	Mean dose <34 Gy (RBE), V50 < 50%
Total lung	Mean dose <20 Gy (RBE), V20 <35%
Kidney	20 Gy (RBE) <33% of each kidney
Liver	V30 ≤ 40%

RBE, Relative biological effectiveness.

Treatment Planning

PASSIVE SCATTERING PROTON BEAM THERAPY

The process for planning passive scattering proton therapy at MD Anderson is as follows. First, the physician contours the GTV and CTV and specifies the setup margin that should be used for the PTV. Second, to adequately cover the target, all iGTV contours that overlap with lung parenchyma are overridden to represent solid tissue. If this is not done, the proton beam may "undershoot" the intended target. However, this practice also creates the dosimetric disadvantage of potentially "overshooting" the tumor during certain phases of the respiratory cycle.[25] Third, the tissue in the diaphragm is overridden so that the diaphragm does not enter the treatment field, producing an inadequate distal margin (again with the risk of overshooting the target in specific cycles).

The fourth step is the selection of beams. Beams that traverse through breast tissue are generally avoided to maximize reproducibility and stability. For similar reasons, beams also are not placed through the edge of the couch or into the spinal cord. At MD Anderson, we typically use at least one beam that is off-cord. Finally, a beam is selected that minimizes the aperture size to reduce the dose to normal tissues.

After beam selection, the compensator and aperture are edited to optimize the plan. Then, the weighting of the beam is adjusted as needed to further improve target and normal structure dose. Finally, the robustness of the plan is verified on both the T0 and T50 breathing phases. This verification is again particularly important in proton therapy because the dose is sensitive to variations in spatial density from tissue heterogeneity.[25]

If dose constraints cannot be met at the desired dose with either photon techniques or passive scattering PBT, IMPT (also called pencil beam scanning proton therapy) can be considered instead.

INTENSITY-MODULATED PROTON THERAPY

Treatment planning for IMPT differs substantially from that for passive scattering PBT in several ways. First, beam selection is based largely on the minimal excursion of the proton beam path length covering the target throughout the respiratory cycle. Second, 4D treatment planning, in which multiple phases of the 4D CT scan instead of the averaged CT are used for planning, can further reduce the influence of respiratory motion. Third, given that IMPT is sensitive to changes in anatomy and tumor size between fractions, robustness optimization is often used to reduce this sensitivity. Finally, evaluation of the robustness of the treatment plan ensures that the dose distribution and doses to both the target and organs at risk remain acceptable, and setup and range uncertainties are considered.

An example in which beam angles are selected by analyzing the change in water-equivalent thickness (WET) between the T0 and T50 phases of the 4D CT scan is shown in Fig. 18.2. A beam angle of 160 degrees was selected for this patient based on the small WET change at that angle (indicating less influence from respiratory motion) in addition to other considerations such as anatomy and tumor location (not shown). The use of 4D CT-based treatment planning,[26] along with fractionation and delivery techniques such as rescanning and optimization of the delivery sequence,[27] can be used to reduce the impact of intrafractional respiratory motion in IMPT. Robustness optimization can reduce the sensitivity of the dose distribution to uncertainties associated with interfractional setup and proton beam range or changes in anatomy, and can be combined with 4D treatment planning.[26] Finally, evaluation of plan robustness is crucial to IMPT planning. For lung cancer cases, we consider a difference of 5% or less between the worst-case dose distribution and the nominal dose to be acceptable.[28] If a plan was found to be not robust (i.e., characterized by a difference of >5%), then the plans are typically reoptimized.

A flowchart summarizing the workflow for quality assurance in IMPT treatment planning is shown in Fig. 18.3.[28]

Clinical Outcomes After Proton Beam Therapy for Lung Cancer

Several retrospective and single-arm prospective studies have reported outcomes from PBT for lung cancer. With regard to early-stage cancer, several studies have demonstrated results analogous to those after stereotactic ablative photon radiation therapy (SABR), with high rates of local control and low toxicity.[5,29–31] In one study, investigators from Loma Linda examined outcomes

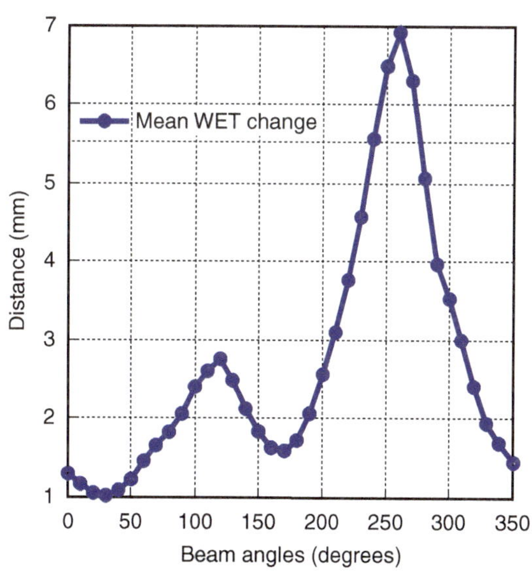

Fig. 18.2 Change in water-equivalent thickness *(WET)* required to cover the target volume between T0 and T50 as a function of beam angle. (From Chang JY, Li H, Zhu XR, et al. Clinical implementation of intensity modulated proton therapy for thoracic malignancies. *Int J Rad Oncol Biol Phys.* 2014;90(4):809-818.)

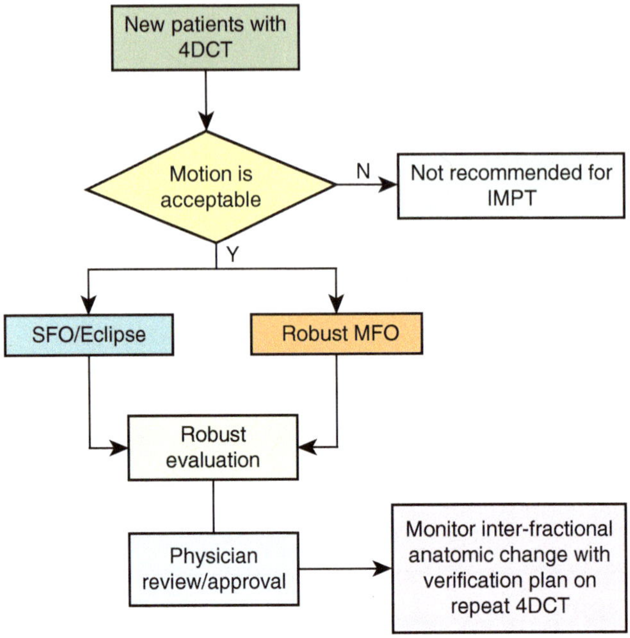

Fig. 18.3 Procedural flowchart for intensity-modulated proton therapy *(IMPT)* quality assurance. *MFO,* Multifield optimization; *SFO,* single-field optimization; *4DCT,* four-dimensional computed tomography. (From Chang JY, Li H, Zhu XR, et al. Clinical implementation of intensity modulated proton therapy for thoracic malignancies. *Int J Radiat Oncol Biol Phys.* 2014;90(4):809-818.)

after hypofractionated PBT to doses of 51 to 70 Gy (RBE), given in 10 fractions over 2 weeks, for stage T1/T2N0M0 biopsy-proven NSCLC. At 4 years, the disease-specific survival rate was 88%, and the OS rate was 60%. None of the 111 patients reported required steroids for radiation pneumonitis, and central versus peripheral tumor location did not correlate with survival outcomes. These investigators concluded that this regimen produced excellent outcomes that may warrant exploration of further dose escalation.[31] Of course, the primary obstacle for using PBT to treat early-stage disease is that baseline toxicity rates are low and local control rates high with photon-based SABR techniques, which can make physicians and patients reluctant to enroll in comparative effectiveness studies. Indeed, one recent trial from MD Anderson that attempted to compare these two techniques for centrally located tumors was closed early for poor accrual. However, the results were published earlier this year, and of the 21 patients who were enrolled, the 3-year local control rate was 87.5%, with a 3-year regional control rate of 90%. One patient in the proton therapy group developed grade 3 skin toxicity, and no patient had a grade 4/5 toxicity. The study concluded that the poor accrual was secondary to several factors, including the lack of volumetric imaging and difficulties with insurance coverage.[32]

Use of PBT for locally advanced lung cancer has achieved more momentum given the high local failure rates and the common difficulty of achieving dose constraints in such cases. Of the published analyses of clinical outcomes after PBT for locally advanced NSCLC,[33–38] the single-arm and retrospective analyses suggest great promise for PBT in terms of improving the standard of care in definitive treatment. One group from Japan retrospectively studied 57 patients with stage III NSCLC treated with PBT to a median dose of 74 Gy (RBE) (range: 50–85 Gy [RBE]) in 2-Gy (RBE) fractions (range: 2–6.6 Gy [RBE]), none with concurrent chemotherapy.[39] The OS rates were 65.5% at 1 year and 39.4% at 2 years. At a median follow-up interval of 22 months (for surviving patients), the 2-year rates of PFS and local control were 24.9% and 64.1%. Distant metastasis was the most common site of initial recurrence. A phase II study conducted at MD Anderson evaluated outcomes after passive scattering PBT and concomitant weekly carboplatin-paclitaxel chemotherapy for patients with unresectable stage III NSCLC. In the preliminary analysis of 44 patients, overall and PFS rates at 1 year were 86% and 63%, and the median OS time was 29.4 months. In that trial, the most common sites of recurrence were distant (19 patients; 43%) and isolated local (4 patients; 9.1%).[40] Final results for this study were published in 2017. With a median follow-up time of 27.3 months for all 64 patients, the 5-year PFS rate was 22%, with a 5-year locoregional recurrence rate of 28% and a distant metastasis rate of 54%. There was an 8% rate of grade 3 esophagitis and one episode of grade 4 esophagitis. The rates of grade 2 and 3 pneumonitis were 16% and 12%, respectively, and two patients developed a grade 2 bronchial stricture. Overall, the authors concluded that concurrent chemotherapy with PBT offered "promising clinical outcomes and rates of toxic effects compared with historical photon therapy data." The investigators emphasized that further optimization with IMPT was needed.[41]

These outcomes compare favorably with prior studies of concurrent chemoradiation for locally advanced NSCLC, particularly the OS interval of nearly 30 months. Possible reasons for these excellent outcomes include improved patient selection, use of higher tumor doses leading to improved disease control, and a direct correlation of reduced normal tissue dose and decreased toxicity. However, the premise of clinical superiority with PBT versus photon techniques requires rigorous testing through randomized trials directly comparing the two modalities. The only such trial published to date was a phase II Bayesian randomized study conducted by MD Anderson and the Massachusetts General Hospital to compare IMRT with passive scattering PBT for locally advanced lung cancer. In that trial, 149 patients with locally advanced disease were randomized to undergo either IMRT or PBT to a dose of 60 to 74 Gy (RBE), and every patient received the highest dose level that could be achieved within this range without exceeding critical dose constraints. No difference was found between modalities in terms of the joint primary end points of local recurrence and severe radiation pneumonitis.[10] Proton and photon treatments are currently being tested in RTOG 1308 (NCT01993810), a larger phase III study in which OS is the primary end point.

Conclusions and Future Directions

Motion management in IMPT for lung cancer is crucial because of the sensitivity of the proton beam to both the path length change induced by respiratory motion and changes in anatomy over time. Currently, in most cases, IMPT is delivered while the patients are free breathing. However, concerns over motion-induced uncertainties usually limit the range of "acceptable" respiratory motion, with one group limiting that range to less than 5 mm.[25,28] Advanced motion management techniques are being developed to make IMPT available to more patients. For example, real-time gated PBT was recently developed in an effort to efficiently deliver gated treatment.[42] Another major concern regarding the use of IMPT for lung cancer is anatomic changes over time, which prompt the need for adaptive therapy in a large proportion of such cases, even when robustness optimization is used, and therefore, repeat imaging and adaptive therapy must be considered mandatory.[28,43,44] Techniques that reduce the need for, or improve the efficiency of, adaptive therapy for IMPT are highly desirable.

From the standpoint of clinical outcomes, prior studies have demonstrated the feasibility of PBT producing similar, if not improved, results in comparison with photon-based techniques. The most promising outcomes seem to be in locally advanced disease, where dose constraints are more difficult to meet and rates of local-regional failure can reach 50%. Disappointingly, after the apparent superiority of PBT over 3D conformal photon radiation therapy had been shown in dosimetric, retrospective, and prospective trials, the only prospective randomized comparative effectiveness trial reported to date demonstrated no difference between treatment modalities in either toxicity or local control. The investigators of that trial have proposed several potential reasons for this lack of benefit, including that treatment was based, in all cases, on 3D planning techniques and that adequate proton delivery probably requires a learning curve, a premise that was supported by the results of this trial. This concept is being further tested in an ongoing cooperative group trial in which OS is the primary end point. However, given these negative results, it is clear that the threshold for justifying PBT "for all comers" has been elevated. Therefore, future trials are likely to focus on criteria for optimal patient selection and novel delivery techniques such as spot-scanning proton arc therapy[45] or dynamic collimation[46] that can offer robust delivery with further reductions in dose to organs at risk.

Acknowledgments

Portions of this chapter appear in Mehta M, ed. *Principles and Practice of Clinical Proton Therapy*. Middleton, WI: Advanced Medical Publishing; in press; and Lee N, Leeman JE, Jiang G, Lu JJ, Sine K, Both K, eds. *Target Volume Delineation and Treatment Planning for Particle Therapy*. Basel, Switzerland: Springer International Publishing; 2018.

References Available Online.

SECTION IV

Future Outcomes and Advancements

CHAPTER 19

Technological Advancements and Outlook in Proton Therapy

X. Ronald Zhu ■ Xiaodong Zhang ■ Matthew Palmer ■ Steven J. Frank

Introduction

Intensity-modulated proton therapy (IMPT) using pencil beam scanning (PBS) technology has revolutionized the practice of particle therapy in recent years.[1,2] In PBS delivery, a particle pencil beam is magnetically scanned in the plane transverse to the beam direction, creating a large field without requiring scattering elements in the beam paths. Monoenergetic pencil beams with different energies from an accelerator are stacked to create the desired dose distribution along the beam direction.[3,4] Neither an aperture nor a compensator is required, although external collimation could be beneficial for reducing the penumbra of low-energy beams.

The desired dose distribution over the clinical target volumes can be achieved by optimizing the weights of individual pencil beams with different energies by using an inverse planning process. Two general approaches have been used to optimize a scanning beam plan. The first is called multifield optimization (MFO), which simultaneously optimizes all spots from all fields.[5–9] The second approach is single-field optimization (SFO),[10,11] in which each field is optimized individually to deliver a fraction of the prescribed dose to the entire target volume(s). The single-field uniform dose (SFUD)[5,10,12,13] is the most common application of SFO to produce a uniform dose over the entire target volume by each field. The single-field integrated boost (SFIB) is another application of the SFO technique reported by Zhu et al.[11] The SFIB technique optimizes the plan with dose constraints to create the desired coverage of different target volumes by different dose levels. Clinically, MFO and SFO techniques have been applied to various disease sites.[14–21] IMPT is one of the most advanced forms of radiation therapy available to date. Despite its superior dosimetric advantages, various challenges limit the realization of its full potential. Various technologies have been advanced and will continue to be advanced to meet these challenges.

Accelerator and Beam Delivery Technologies

Traditionally, the most common configuration of a proton therapy facility consists of an accelerator with three to five treatment rooms. The accelerator, either cyclotron or synchrotron, has standard sizes and requires a fairly large room to host it. The standard gantry is also large and can weigh as much as 200 tons. Superconducting-based cyclotrons and compact synchrotrons have become available commercially in recent years that allow smaller-footprint accelerator rooms. All proton therapy system vendors offer single-room configurations at this time. These efforts have reduced the cost and made proton systems more affordable to more clinics. One vendor is offering a superconducting gantry, which not only reduces the weight of the gantry but also opens up more space for new and innovative imaging technologies to provide better imaging guidance. We expect that proton therapy delivery systems will be further miniaturized in the coming years.

The most common delivery method for PBS is spot scanning, which is a discrete step-and-shoot approach to beam delivery.[3] The major advantage of the approach is that it is safe and reliable for delivering each spot. The main disadvantage is that it is less efficient owing to the "dead time" between the spots. Raster scanning is similar to spot scanning except that the beam is not switched off when moving to the next spot.[3,22,23] This causes a small amount of transient dose that is delivered during the move. The transient dose should be included and modeled correctly by the treatment planning system (TPS). This technique is faster than spot scanning for treatment delivery because the dead time is reduced to the time required to travel to the next position. In continuous line scanning, the beam is continuously scanned, normally along the axes in the plane of constant energy.[24,25] The beam is switched off only when the energy is changed. Continuous line scanning is technically more challenging than either spot scanning or raster scanning,[24] but it can deliver a beam very quickly and can be useful for repainting. Although spot scanning technology is the current standard in delivery technology, raster scanning (also called dose-driven continuous scanning) and continuous line scanning are becoming available commercially. These technologies improve the delivery efficiency and make layering and volumetric repainting more practical for motion mitigation.

Delivery of IMPT using PBS technology requires a switch to a different, usually lower, energy after completing a given energy layer. The energy switch time has been reduced for cyclotron- and synchrotron-based systems in recent years. For synchrotrons, the typical time required to change energy is on the order of 1 to 2 seconds.[26,27] This is the time required to deaccelerate the remaining protons with the previous energy in the synchrotrons and accelerate a new spill of protons with the new desired energy. The time needed for the adjustment of the beam transport line is similar between the two types of accelerator. For cyclotrons, the additional time is determined by how fast the energy selection system can be adjusted for the next energy. The energy change can be as fast as less than 0.1 second when an energy selection system is used,[24] although most systems in clinical use would take approximately 1 to 2 seconds. For synchrotrons, the energy switching time is expected to be reduced significantly with a new technology called "multiple energy extraction,"[28] which is currently being developed and implemented for commercial accelerator systems.

Proton arc therapy was proposed by Sandison et al.[29] to reduce the lung dose relative to electron arc therapy. For men with prostate cancer, Rechner et al.[30,31] showed that the risk of second cancers using proton arc therapy is less or equal to that of photon volumetric modulated arc therapy (VMAT). Seco et al.[32] proposed that proton arc therapy could reduce the range uncertainty effects and spare the healthy lung relative to photon VMAT for lung stereo tactic body radiation therapy. Proton arc therapy using spot scanning[33] could be promising for further improving the dosimetric results for patients with locally advanced stage nonsmall cell lung cancer.[34] We expect that the advantages of proton arc therapy will be further explored for possible clinical advantages in the near future.

Range Uncertainty

Although it can be accurately measured in water, the proton beam range in a patient has an uncertainty, typically 3.5% of the range in current clinical practices.[35,36] Without any physiological variation, the range uncertainty in patients originates from (1) uncertainties in the Hounsfield units (HUs) of computed tomography (CT) images, (2) the conversion of HUs to proton stopping powers, and (3) the uncertainty of the stopping powers primarily from the mean excitation energy (*I*-value).[37] These uncertainties have the potential to alter the proton range and dose distribution, which would result in underdosing the target volume or overdosing critical structures. Additional uncertainties from setup could result in a combined effect of range uncertainties in inhomogenous tissues of a patient, which can also alter the ranges of protons and influence dose distribution. Range uncertainty is one of the fundamental physical limitations of particle therapy. Research efforts to directly reduce the range uncertainties and minimize the impact of range uncertainty are described further below.

Reduce the range uncertainty. Dual-energy CT (DECT) using kV x-rays has the potential to reduce uncertainties in stopping power ratios (SPRs) and therefore the uncertainties in the proton beam ranges over the single-energy CT (SECT).[38] The DECT approach combines information from two images with different x-ray energies to resolve the ambiguities in the HUs-to-SPR conversion.[39] Although it is generally agreed that there are improvements in determining SPRs with DECT over SECT, the reported reduction of uncertainties of SPRs varies from study to study, ranging from approximately 0.4% to 1.5%.[37,40,41] One of the reasons preventing DECT from gaining larger benefits over SECT is high-level noise on DECT images.[42] Comprehensive uncertainty analysis by Li et al. showed that the DECT method could reduce the overall range uncertainty to approximately 2.2% (2σ) in clinical settings.[43]

Proton radiography (pRG) and proton CT (pCT)[39,44] provide direct measurements of proton SPRs and therefore more accurate estimates of proton beam ranges. pRG would allow direct range verification as well as image guidance.[44] pCT does not suffer from metal artifacts as do kV x-ray CT images. However, many technical challenges remain to be solved before pCT imaging becomes routine practice in proton clinics around the world. One of the fundamental limitations is lateral straggling of the proton beam, which limits the spatial resolution of pRG and pCT and also results in image artifacts.[44] One promising design is proton tracking, which is best able to handle the problem of multiple scattering of protons for pRG and pCT.[39,44]

Minimize the impact of range uncertainty. One effective method to minimize the impact of range uncertainty is the use of robust optimization that incorporates setup and range uncertainties.[45,46] The robustness of a treatment plan can be assessed by using robust evaluation. A more difficult question is: What is clinically acceptable robustness? In an attempt to answer this question, Li et al. studied a group of patients with oropharynx cancer who received IMPT for possible correlation between local control and the robustness of the target volume coverage.[47,48]

Monitoring the proton beam range in patients. In vivo monitoring of the proton beam range in patients would provide direct information about where the proton beam is stopped. Methods being developed include proton-induced positron-emission tomography,[49–51] prompt gamma,[52,53] and proton-induced acoustics.[54,55]

Treatment Plans and Dose Calculations

The quality of an IMPT treatment plan depends on an effective planning process, particularly a good optimization. The current optimization process with commercial TPSs involves an iterative process to refine the optimization parameters. It is a trial-and-error process that can be time-consuming. Automatic treatment planning and optimization based on prior knowledge, machine learning, and artificial intelligence have the potential to generate the best possible plan for each patient.[56]

Accuracy of dose calculation is critical to clinical implementation of IMPT. It was suggested recently that analytical dose calculation algorithms may not have sufficient accuracy for highly inhomogenous tissues such as lung.[57] Monte Carlo simulation–based dose calculation is more desirable.[58]

Motion Interplay Effect

When PBS technology is used to treat moving tumors, the dynamic pencil beam and target motion can lead to interference caused by similarities in the time scale involved in beam delivery and target motion; in other words, the motion of the target can result in misplacement of the individual pencil beam spots. This phenomenon, also referred to as the motion interplay effect, can cause additional degradation of the delivered dose distribution, potentially manifesting as extreme local tumor underdosage and normal structure overdosage.[8,59–61] A guideline for treating moving targets recently published by the Particle Therapy Co-Operative Group Thoracic Subcommittee[62] recommends assessing the motion for each patient and using different motion mitigation strategies, including beam angle and scanning direction selection, four-dimensional (4D) robust optimization, layer or volume repainting, breath hold and gating based on the motion analysis, and 4D dynamic doses, as necessary.

Biological Uncertainties

The relative biological effectiveness (RBE) of protons is defined as the ratio of the absorbed doses that produce the same biological effect or clinical end point between a high-energy photon and proton beam irradiation under the same conditions.[63] Proton therapy treatments are currently planned assuming a constant proton RBE relative to high-energy photons of 1.1.[64] The actual RBE of protons is a complex function of numerous factors such as treatment technique, dose, depth, cell type, oxygenation, intrinsic radiosensitivity, and the biological or clinical end point of interest.[63] Different RBE models may predict different results. Linear energy transfer (LET) may in fact be a better surrogate for biological effects because it is a physical quantity, independent of models.[64] By optimizing the plan such that the higher LET is in the target volume and the lower LET is in the critical normal structures,[64–66] it may be possible to improve the tumor control probability and reduce the normal tissue complication probability (NTCP).

Variation of Anatomy

An important source of uncertainty comes from changes in the patient's anatomy, including weight loss, tumor shrinkage, and opening or blocking airways, which can significantly change the proton stopping power distribution along the path of the beam. The influence of these uncertainties becomes more significant in IMPT plans because the individual fields can be highly modulated, and steep dose gradients can be located in the middle of the target.[67] A recent retrospective study showed that robust optimization using both original planning CT and adaptive CT image sets could improve the IMPT plan's robustness with respect to anatomic changes in eight patients with lung cancer.[68] By including synthetic CTs with varying nasal cavity filling in their robust optimization, van de Water et al.[69] concluded that anatomic robust optimization effectively accounted for changes in nasal cavity filling during IMPT, providing substantially improved clinical target volume and organs-at-risk doses compared with conventional SFUD optimization.

Online adaptive planning for each fraction will be the ultimate adaptive strategy in radiation oncology. Recently, Bernatowicz et al.[70] studied the feasibility of online IMPT adaptation by using fast, automatic, and robust dose restoration. The essential requirements for online adaptation include diagnostic-quality images with the patient in the treatment position for every fraction, automatic contouring, fast optimization, dose calculation, and online quality assurance for each adaptive plan. With recent advances in artificial intelligence and machine learning and fast dose calculation and optimization, online adaptive planning for patients undergoing IMPT will be come practical in the near future.

Cone-beam CT (CBCT) equipment has become standard in modern proton gantries.[71] CBCT installed in proton treatment rooms typically has flat panels mounted on the gantry and x-ray tubes installed on the floor. A new design of the CBCT system involves its to the treatment couch with a ring. In general, CBCT image quality suffers from scatter and results in CT numbers that are not sufficiently accurate for proton dose calculation. One approach to improve the CT numbers of CBCT is to deform the planning CT scan onto the CBCT scan.[71,72] Alternatively, some proton therapy centers have installed CT-on-rails, which has diagnostic image quality and DECT capability. Integrating a magnetic resonance imaging scanner with proton treatment delivery is also being investigated by researchers and manufacturers.

Response of Proton Therapy

The superior physical dose distributions of IMPT have shown promising clinical advantages in some clinical scenarios.[73–82] For example, an analysis with 50:100 (1:2) matching of IMPT to IMRT for patients with oropharyngeal carcinoma found that that IMPT was associated with reduced rates of feeding tube dependency and severe weight loss.[73] The oncologic, toxicity, and functional outcomes after IMPT for such patients are encouraging.[82] In a series of patients treated with IMPT for definitive reirradiation of thoracic cancers, Ho et al. concluded that that IMPT provided durable local control with minimal toxicity and suggested that higher doses may improve outcomes.[77]

NTCP and tumor control probability after radiation therapy are multifactorial and complex functions of physical, biological, and clinical conditions. Machine learning has promise for navigating the complex nature of the problem.[56] Applications of machine learning and artificial intelligence[56,83] could provide stronger evidence of the clinical advantages of IMPT.

Summary

IMPT is the most advanced radiation therapy modality available to date. With reduced physical and biological uncertainties, advanced imaging guidance, online adaptation, and better understanding of the outcomes, the full potential of IMPT can be realized in the near future.

References Available Online.

APPENDIX 1

The University of Texas MD Anderson Cancer Center's Recommended Proton Therapy Indications

Recommended Breast Cancer Proton Therapy Indications

INDICATIONS

1) **Accelerated partial breast irradiation**
   - The safety and efficacy of proton partial breast irradiation (PBI) is established for early-stage breast cancer. Proton PBI provides a more homogeneous dose distribution and reduction in exposure to the normal breast, heart, and lung compared with photon and brachytherapy PBI techniques and has been associated with excellent local control and reduced toxicity.[35] We are investigating a 10-fraction hypofractionated proton regimen, which may be more cost-effective and also improve the therapeutic ratio.
   - **Inclusion criteria**
     i. The patient must have stage 0, I, or II breast cancer. If stage II, the tumor size must be 3 cm or less.
     ii. On histological examination, the tumor must be ductal carcinoma in situ (DCIS) or invasive adenocarcinoma of the breast.
     iii. Surgical treatment of the breast must have been lumpectomy. The margins of the resected specimen must be histologically free of tumor (DCIS and invasive). Reexcision of surgical margins is permitted.
     iv. Gross disease must be unifocal with pathologic (invasive and/or DCIS) tumor size 3 cm or less. (Patients with microscopic multifocality are eligible as long as total pathologic tumor size is $\leq$3 cm.)
     v. The target lumpectomy cavity must be clearly delineated, and the target lumpectomy cavity/whole breast reference volume must be less than or equal to 30% based on the postoperative/preenrollment computed tomography (CT) scan.
   - **Exclusion criteria:**
     i. Men are not eligible.
     ii. T2 (>3 cm), T3, stage III, or stage IV breast cancer.
     iii. More than three histologically positive axillary nodes.
     iv. Axillary nodes with definite evidence of microscopic or macroscopic extracapsular extension.
     v. Palpable or radiographically suspicious ipsilateral or contralateral axillary, supraclavicular, infraclavicular, or internal mammary nodes at time of enrollment unless there is histologic confirmation that these nodes are negative for tumor.
     vi. Suspicious microcalcifications or densities (in the ipsilateral or contralateral breast as documented on mammogram or breast ultrasound) unless biopsied and found to be benign.

vii. Nonepithelial breast malignancies such as sarcoma or lymphoma.
viii. Proven multicentric carcinoma (invasive cancer or DCIS) in more than one quadrant or separated by 4 or more centimeters.
ix. Paget disease of the nipple.
x. Surgical margins that cannot be microscopically assessed or are positive at pathologic evaluation. (If surgical margins are rendered free of disease by re-excision, the patient is eligible.)
xi. Clear delineation of the extent of the target lumpectomy cavity not possible.
xii. Treatment plan that includes regional nodal irradiation.
xiii. Prior radiation to the index breast.
xiv. Documented diagnosis of collagen vascular disease, specifically dermatomyositis with a creatine phosphokinase level above normal or with an active skin rash, systemic lupus erythematosus, or scleroderma.
xv. Pregnancy or lactation at enrollment.
xvi. Women of reproductive potential must agree to use an effective nonhormonal method of contraception during therapy.

2) **Left or right-sided early or locoregionally advanced breast cancer** requiring breast or chest wall plus regional nodal irradiation (i.e., lymph node-positive disease, advanced T stage, and/or medial tumor location)

- Adjuvant radiotherapy improves survival in breast cancer patients, suggesting that persistence of locoregional tumor is associated with an increased risk of developing metastases and death. Results of modern randomized controlled clinical trials highlight the importance of regional nodal irradiation in reducing distant events in this population.[27,39] Targeting of the regional lymphatics results in lung and heart doses associated with increased major cardiac events, cardiac deaths, lung cancer, and lung cancer deaths in a patient population where advances in systemic therapy and other multidisciplinary care has resulted in decreasing breast cancer-specific mortality. Proton radiotherapy improves coverage of the regional lymphatics while substantially reducing mean lung and mean heart doses (MHDs) to levels significantly correlated with reduced cardiac events, lung cancer, and symptomatic pneumonitis.[39] We are currently enrolling patients in the national RADCOMP trial (NCT02603341) that is randomizing patients who receive regional nodal irradiation between proton and photon radiation.
- **Inclusion criteria**
  i. Age 18 years or older.
  ii. Histologic confirmation of breast cancer resected by lumpectomy or mastectomy with or without immediate reconstruction and whole breast/chest wall and regional nodal irradiation planned with or without a boost to the lumpectomy cavity/chest wall.
  iii. The axilla must be staged by sentinel node biopsy alone, sentinel node biopsy followed by axillary node dissection, or axillary lymph node dissection alone.
  iv. pStage T1-T4N0-N3M0 or ypStage T0-4N0-N3M0.
  v. Indications for regional nodal irradiation per treating physician (lymph node–positive disease, T3 to T4, medial tumor location).
  vi. Breast implants and expanders allowed.
- **Exclusion criteria**
  i. Medical contraindication to receipt of radiotherapy.
  ii. Severe, active comorbid systemic illnesses or other severe concurrent disease that, in the judgment of the investigator, would make the patient inappropriate for entry into this study or interfere significantly with the proper assessment of safety and toxicity of the prescribed regimens.

iii. Active systemic lupus or scleroderma.
iv. Pregnancy or women of childbearing potential who are sexually active and not willing/able to use medically acceptable forms of contraception.

SCIENTIFIC EVIDENCE

1. Ares C, Khan S, Macartain AM, et al. Postoperative proton radiotherapy for localized and locoregional breast cancer: potential for clinically relevant improvements? *Int J Radiat Oncol Biol Phys.* 2010;76:685-697.
2. Bradley JA, Dagan R, Ho MW, et al. Initial report of a prospective dosimetric and clinical feasibility trial demonstrates the potential of protons to increase the therapeutic ratio in breast cancer compared with photons. *Int J Radiol Oncol Biol Phys.* 2016;95(1):411-421.
3. Bush DA, Do S, Lum S, et al. Partial breast radiation therapy with proton beam: 5-year results with cosmetic outcomes. *Int J Radiat Oncol Biol Phys.* 2014;90(3):501-505.
4. Bush DA, Slater JD, Garberoglio C, Do S, Lum S, Slater JM. Partial breast irradiation delivered with proton beam: results of a phase II trial. *Clin Breast Cancer.* 2011;11(4):241-245.
5. Chang JH, Lee NK, Kim JY, et al. Phase II trial of proton beam accelerated partial breast irradiation in breast cancer. *Radiother Oncol.* 2013;108(2):209-214.
6. Clarke M, Collins R, Darby S, et al. Effects of radiotherapy and of differences in the extent of surgery for early breast cancer on local recurrence and 15-year survival: an overview of the randomised trials. *Lancet.* 2005;366(9503):2087-2106.
7. Darby SC, McGale P, Taylor CW, Peto R. Long-term mortality from heart disease and lung cancer after radiotherapy for early breast cancer: prospective cohort study of about 300,000 women in US SEER cancer registries. *Lancet Oncol.* 2005;6(8):557-565.
8. Darby SC, Ewertz M, McGale P, et al. Risk of ischemic heart disease in women after radiotherapy for breast cancer. *N Engl J Med.* 2013;368(11):987-998.
9. Darby S, McGale P, Correa C, et al. Effect of radiotherapy after breast-conserving surgery on 10-year recurrence and 15-year breast cancer death: meta-analysis of individual patient data for 10,801 women in 17 randomised trials. *Lancet.* 2011;378(9804):1707-1716.
10. Depauw N, Batin E, Daartz J, et al. A novel approach to postmastectomy radiation therapy using scanned proton beams. *Int J Radiat Oncol Biol Phys.* 2015;91(2):427-434.
11. Doyen J, Falk AT, Floquet V, et al. Proton beams in cancer treatments: clinical outcomes and dosimetric comparisons with photon therapy. *Cancer Treat Rev.* 2016;43:104-112.
12. EBCTCG (Early Breast Cancer Trialists' Collaborative Group), McGale P, Taylor C, et al. Effect of radiotherapy after mastectomy and axillary surgery on 10-year recurrence and 20-year breast cancer mortality: meta-analysis of individual patient data for 8135 women in 22 randomised trials. *Lancet.* 2014;383(9935):2127-2135.
13. Galland-Girodet S, Pashtan I, MacDonald SM, et al. Long-term cosmetic outcomes and toxicities of proton beam therapy compared with photon-based 3-dimensional conformal accelerated partial-breast irradiation: a phase 1 trial. *Int J Radiat Oncol Biol Phys.* 2014;90(3):493-500.
14. Haviland JS, Owen JR, Dewar JA, et al. The UK Standardisation of Breast Radiotherapy (START) trials of radiotherapy hypofractionation for treatment of early breast cancer: 10-year follow-up results of two randomised controlled trials. *Lancet Oncol.* 2013;14(11):1086-1094.

15. Johansson J, Isacsson U, Lindman H, Montelius A, Glimelius B. Node-positive left-sided breast cancer patients after breast-conserving surgery: potential outcomes of radiotherapy modalities and techniques. *Radiother Oncol.* 2002;65(2):89-98.
16. Overgaard M, Jensen MB, Overgaard J, et al. Postoperative radiotherapy in high-risk postmenopausal breast-cancer patients given adjuvant tamoxifen: Danish Breast Cancer Cooperative Group DBCG 82c randomised trial. *Lancet.* 1999;353(9165):1641-1648.
17. MacDonald SM, Patel SA, Hickey S, et al. Proton therapy for breast cancer after mastectomy: early outcomes of a prospective clinical trial. *Int J Radiat Oncol Biol Phys.* 2013;86(3):484-490.
18. MacDonald SM, Jimenez R, Paetzold P, et al. Proton radiotherapy for chest wall and regional lymphatic radiation; dose comparisons and treatment delivery. *Radiat Oncol.* 2013;8:71.
19. Mast ME, Vredeveld EJ, Credoe HM, et al. Whole breast proton irradiation for maximal reduction of heart dose in breast cancer patients. *Breast Cancer Res Treat.* 2014;148(1):33-39.
20. McGee LA, Iftekaruddin Z, Chang JHC, et al. Postmastectomy chest wall reirradiation with proton therapy for breast cancer. *Int J Radiat Oncol Biol Phys.* 2017;99(2):E34-E35.
21. Moon SH, Shin KH, Kim TH, et al. Dosimetric comparison of four different external beam partial breast irradiation techniques: three-dimensional conformal radiotherapy, intensity-modulated radiotherapy, helical tomotherapy, and proton beam therapy. *Radiother Oncol.* 2009;90(1):66-73.
22. Plastaras JP, Berman AT, Freedman GM. Special cases for proton beam radiotherapy: re-irradiation, lymphoma, and breast cancer. *Semin Oncol.* 2014;41(6):807-819.
23. Olivotto IA, Whelan TJ, Parpia S, et al. Interim cosmetic and toxicity results from RAPID: a randomized trial of accelerated partial breast irradiation using three-dimensional conformal external beam radiation therapy. *J Clin Oncol.* 2013;31(32):4038-4045.
24. Ovalle V, Strom EA, Shaitelman S, et al. Proton partial breast irradiation: detailed description of acute clinico-radiologic effects. *Cancers (Basel).* 2018;10(4).
25. Ovalle V, Strom EA, Godby J, et al. Proton partial-breast irradiation for early-stage cancer: is it really so costly? *Int J Radiat Oncol Biol Phys.* 2016;95(1):49-51.
26 Patel SA, Tan T, Chin Y, et al. Assessment of cardiac function following proton radiation in a cohort of post mastectomy patients with locally advanced breast cancer. *Int J Radiat Oncol Biol Phys.* 2015;93(3 Suppl):e52.
27. Poortsman PM, Collette S, Kirkove C, et al. Internal mammary and mediastinal supraclavicular irradiation in breast cancer. *N Engl J Med.* 2015;373(4):317-327.
28. Presley CJ, Soulos PR, Herrin J, et al. Patterns of use and short-term complications of breast brachytherapy in the national Medicare population from 2008–2009. *J Clin Oncol.* 2012;30(35):4302-4307.
29. Ragaz J, Jackson SM, Le N, et al. Adjuvant radiotherapy and chemotherapy in node-positive premenopausal women with breast cancer. *N Engl J Med.* 1997;337(14):956-962.
30. Shah C, Badiyan S, Berry S, et al. Cardiac dose sparing and avoidance techniques in breast cancer radiotherapy. *Radiother Oncol.* 2014;112(1):9-16.
31. Stick LB, Yu Jen, Maraldo MV, et al. Joint estimation of cardiac toxicity and recurrence risks after comprehensive nodal photon versus proton therapy for breast cancer. *Int J Radiat Oncol Biol Phys.* 2017;97(4):754-761.
32. Strom EA, Amos R, Shaitelman SF, et al. Proton partial breast irradiation in the supine position: treatment description and reproducibility of a multibeam technique. *Pract Radiat Oncol.* 2015;5(4):e283-e290.
33. Strom EA, Ovalle V. Initial clinical experience using protons for accelerated partial-breast irradiation: longer-term results. *Int J Radiat Oncol Biol Phys.* 2014;90(3):506-508.

34. Taylor CW, Wang Z, Macaulay E, et al. Exposure of the heart in breast cancer radiation therapy: a systematic review of heart doses published during 2003 to 2013. *Int J Radiat Oncol Biol Phys*. 2015;93(4):845-853.
35. Verma V, Shah C, Mehta M. Clinical outcomes and toxicity of proton radiotherapy for breast cancer. *Clin Breast Cancer*. 2016;16(3):145-154.
36. Verma V, Iftekaruddin Z, Badar N, et al. Proton beam radiotherapy as part of comprehensive nodal irradiation for locally advanced breast cancer. *Radiother Oncol*. 2017;123(2):294-298.
37. Wang X, Zhang X, Li X, et al. Accelerated partial-breast irradiation using intensity-modulated proton radiotherapy: do uncertainties outweigh potential benefits? *Br J Radiol*. 2013;86(1029):20130176.
38. Wang X, Amos RA, Zhang X, et al. External-beam accelerated partial breast irradiation using multiple proton beam configurations. *Int J Radiat Oncol Biol Phys*. 2011;80(5):1464-1472.
39. Whelan TJ, Olivotto I, Parulekar WR, et al. Regional nodal irradiation in early-stage breast cancer. *N Eng J Med*. 2015;373(4):307-316.
40. Xu N, Ho MW, Li Z, Morris CG, Mendenhall NP. Can proton therapy improve the therapeutic ratio in breast cancer patients at risk for nodal disease? *Am J Clin Oncol*. 2014;37:568-574.

Recommended Central Nervous System Proton Therapy Indications

INDICATIONS

1. **Adult craniospinal radiotherapy**: primary central nervous system (CNS) tumors
   a. Decrease acute toxicity
      i. Reduce weight loss, hydration issues, nausea, vomiting[3]
      ii. Minimize treatment breaks that affect disease control[3]
      iii. Improve chemotherapy tolerance
   b. Reduce late toxicities
   c. Improve quality of life and symptom burden
2. **Adult low-grade glioma** and **anaplastic oligodendroglioma** in whom long-term survival is expected[12,13]
   a. Decrease neuroendocrine and auditory toxicity
   b. Decrease neurocognitive deficits[1]
   c. Improve quality of life and symptom burden
3. **Selected meningiomas** and **Sellar tumors:** large tumors, young patients, other comorbidities (neurofibromatosis, Li-Fraumeni, etc.)
   a. Evidence of better survival in aggressive meningioma with higher dose possible with proton radiation therapy[11]
   b. Long-term survival expectation
   c. Decrease neuroendocrine, auditory toxicity
   d. Decrease neurocognitive deficits
   e. Improve quality of life and symptom burden
4. **Recurrent, previously irradiated tumors in the brain, thorax, or abdomen:** proton therapy will decrease the risk of overlap in normal organs during treatment planning for recurrent disease.
5. **Intensity-modulated proton therapy** is indicated for intracranial brain tumors and tumors near the skull base, such as chordoma[10]

SCIENTIFIC EVIDENCE

1. Shih HA, Sherman JC, Nachtigall LB, et al. Proton therapy for low-grade gliomas: results from a prospective trial. *Cancer.* 2015 121(10):1712-1719.
2. Douw L, Klein M, Fagel SS, et al. Cognitive and radiological effects of radiotherapy in patients with low-grade glioma: long-term follow-up. *Lancet Neurol.* 2009;8(9):810-818.
3. Brown AP, Barney CL, Grosshans DR, et al. Proton beam craniospinal irradiation reduces acute toxicity for adults with medulloblastoma. *Int J Radiat Oncol Biol Phys.* 2013;86(2):277-284.
4. Farnia B, Allen PK, Brown PD, et al. Clinical outcomes and patterns of failure in pineoblastoma: a 30-year, single-institution retrospective review. *World Neurosurg.* 2014; 82(6):1232-1241.
5. Barney CL, Brown AP, Grosshans DR, et al. Technique, outcomes, and acute toxicities in adults treated with proton beam craniospinal irradiation. *Neuro Oncol.* 2014;16(2):303-309.
6. Arvold ND, Lessell S, Bussiere M, et al. Visual outcome and tumor control after conformal radiotherapy for patients with optic nerve sheath meningioma. *Int J Radiat Oncol Biol Phys.* 2009;75(4):1166-1172.
7. Hug EB, Devries A, Thornton AF, et al. Management of atypical and malignant meningiomas: role of high-dose, 3D-conformal radiation therapy. *J Neurooncol.* 2000;48(2):151-160.
8. Speirs CK, Simpson JR, Robinson CG, et al. Impact of 1p/19q codeletion and histology on outcomes of anaplastic gliomas treated with radiation therapy and temozolomide. *Int J Radiat Oncol Biol Phys.* 2015;91(2):268-276.
9. Brown AP, Barney CL, Grosshans DR, et al. Proton beam craniospinal irradiation reduces acute toxicity for adults with medulloblastoma. *Int J Radiat Oncol Biol Phys.* 2013;86(2):277-284.
10. Kabolizadeh P, Chen YL, Liebsch N, et al. Updated outcome and analysis of tumor response in mobile spine and sacral chordoma treated with definitive high-dose photon/proton radiation therapy. *Int J Radiat Oncol Biol Phys.* 2017;97(2):254-262.
11. Weber DC, Ares C, Villa S, et al. Adjuvant postoperative high-dose radiotherapy for atypical and malignant meningioma: a phase-II parallel non-randomized and observation study (EORTC 22042-26042). *Radiother Oncol.* 2018;128(2):260-265.
12. Cairncross G, Wang M, Jenkins R, et al. Phase III trial of chemoradiotherapy for anaplastic oligodendroglioma: long-term results of RTOG 9402. *J Clin Oncol.* 2013;31(3): 337-343.
13. Buckner JC, Shaw EG, Pugh SL, et al. Radiation plus procarbazine, CCNU, and vincristine in low-grade glioma. *N Engl J Med.* 2016;374:1344-1355.
14. Moeller BJ, Chintagumpapa M, Philip JJ, et al. Low early ototoxicity rates for pediatric medulloblastoma patients treated with proton radiotherapy. *Radiat Oncol.* 2011;6:58.

Recommended Esophagus Cancer Proton Therapy Indications

INDICATIONS

1) Stage I–III esophageal cancer

- Proton therapy had clinical benefit in terms of postoperative morbidity and hospitalization in a multinational study comparing protons and intensity-modulated photon therapy for esophageal cancer after accounting for patient, tumor, and treatment factors.[1]
  i. Postoperative overall complications reduced by 40%.

ii. Postoperative pulmonary complications reduced by 47%.
iii. Postoperative cardiac complications reduced by 48%.
iv. Postoperative wound complications reduced by 75%.
v. Postoperative length of hospitalization reduced from a mean of 12.4 days (photons) to 9.2 days (proton).
vi. Postoperative 90-day mortality: 4.3% (photon) versus 0.9% (proton).

- The relative benefits of proton therapy compared with the best intensity-modulated radiation therapy (IMRT) plans are based on the following systematic evaluation of a 55-patient cohort study[15]:
  i. Mean lung dose reduced by at least 30%.
  ii. Lung volume of 5 Gy reduced by 45%, volume of 10 Gy reduced by 30%, and volume of 20 Gy reduced by 20% to 5%.
  iii. Mean heart dose reduced by at least 35%.
  iv. Mean liver dose reduced by 70% (for mid to distal esophageal tumors).
  v. Maximum spinal cord hot spot dose reduced by 20%.
- Proton therapy significantly spares heart and cardiac substructures in a large cohort of esophageal cancer[2]
  i. Compared with IMRT, proton beam therapy (PBT) resulted in significantly lower mean heart dose (MHD) and heart V5, V10, V20, V30, and V40, along with lower radiation exposure to the four chambers and four coronary arteries.
  ii. Compared with passively scattered proton therapy (PSPT), intensity-modulated proton therapy (IMPT) resulted in significantly lower heart V20, V30, and V40 but not MHD or heart V5 or V10. IMPT also resulted in significantly lower radiation doses to the left atrium, right atrium, left main coronary artery, and left circumflex artery, but not the left ventricle, right ventricle, left anterior descending artery, or right coronary artery. Factors associated with lower MHD included PBT ($P < .001$).
- Definitive chemoradiation using proton beam therapy versus IMRT for esophageal cancer improves survival outcomes[3]
  i. Compared with IMRT, PBT had significantly better overall survival (OS; $P = .011$), progression-free survival (PFS; $P = .001$), distant metastasis-free survival (DMFS; $P = .031$), as well as marginally better locoregional failure-free survival (LRFFS; $P = .075$).
  ii. No significant differences in rates of treatment-related toxicities were observed between groups.
  iii. On multivariate analysis, IMRT had worse OS (hazard ratio [HR]: 1.454; $P = .01$), PFS (HR: 1.562; $P = .001$), and LRFFS (HR: 1.461; $P = .041$) than PBT. Subgroup analysis by clinical stage revealed considerably higher 5-year OS (34.6% vs. 25.0%; $P = .038$) and PFS rates (33.5% vs. 13.2%; $P = .005$) in the PBT group for patients with stage III disease.
- **Inclusion criteria**
  i. All resectable or unresectable esophageal cancer patients with nonmetastatic esophageal cancers.
  ii. Adenocarcinoma or squamous cell carcinoma.
  iii. Eligible to receive definitive or preoperative chemoradiation.
  iv. Involves any part of the proximal thoracic to distal esophagus, the gastroesophageal junction, and the cardia of the stomach.

2) **IMPT** is indicated for esophageal cancer.

SCIENTIFIC EVIDENCE

1. Lin SH, Merrell KW, Shen J, et al. Multi-institutional analysis of radiation modality use and postoperative outcomes of neoadjuvant chemoradiation for esophageal cancer. *Radiother Oncol.* 2017;123(3):376-381.
2. Shiraishi Y, Xu C, Yang J, Komaki R, Lin SH. Dosimetric comparison to the heart and cardiac substructure in a large cohort of esophageal cancer patients treated with proton beam therapy or intensity-modulated radiation therapy. *Radiother Oncol.* 2017;125(1):48-54.
3. Xi M, Xu C, Liao Z, et al. Comparative outcomes after definitive chemoradiotherapy using proton beam therapy versus intensity-modulated radiation therapy for esophageal cancer: a retrospective single-institutional analysis. *Int J Radiat Oncol Biol Phys.* 2017;99(3):667-676.
4. Lin SH, Komaki R, Liao Z, et al. Proton beam therapy and concurrent chemotherapy for esophageal cancer. *Int J Radiat Oncol Biol Phys.* 2012;83(3):e345-e351.
5. Ling TC, Slater JM, Nookala P, et al. Analysis of intensity-modulated radiation therapy (IMRT), proton and 3D conformal radiotherapy (3D-CRT) for reducing perioperative cardiopulmonary complications in esophageal cancer patients. *Cancers (Basel).* 2014;6(4):2356-2368.
6. Mizumoto M, Sugahara S, Nakayama H, et al. Clinical results of proton-beam therapy for locoregionally advanced esophageal cancer. *Strahlenther Onkol.* 2010;186(9):482-488.
7. Mizumoto M, Sugahara S, Okumura T, et al. Hyperfractionated concomitant boost proton beam therapy for esophageal carcinoma. *Int J Radiat Oncol Biol Phys.* 2011;81(4):e601-e606.
8. Pan X, Zhang X, Li Y, Mohan R, Liao Z. Impact of using different four-dimensional computed tomography data sets to design proton treatment plans for distal esophageal cancer. *Int J Radiat Oncol Biol Phys.* 2009;73(2):601-609.
9. Sugahara S, Tokuuye K, Okumura T, et al. Clinical results of proton beam therapy for cancer of the esophagus. *Int J Radiat Oncol Biol Phys.* 2005;61(1):76-84.
10. Wang J, Wei C, Tucker SL, et al. Predictors of postoperative complications after trimodality therapy for esophageal cancer. *Int J Radiat Oncol Biol Phys.* 2013;86(5):885-891.
11. Wang SL, Liao Z, Vaporciyan AA, et al. Investigation of clinical and dosimetric factors associated with postoperative pulmonary complications in esophageal cancer patients treated with concurrent chemoradiotherapy followed by surgery. *Int J Radiat Oncol Biol Phys.* 2006;64(3):692-699.
12. Wei X, Liu HH, Tucker SL, et al. Risk factors for pericardial effusion in inoperable esophageal cancer patients treated with definitive chemoradiation therapy. *Int J Radiat Oncol Biol Phys.* 2008;70(3):707-714.
13. Welsh J, Gomez D, Palmer MB, et al. Intensity-modulated proton therapy further reduces normal tissue exposure during definitive therapy for locally advanced distal esophageal tumors: a dosimetric study. *Int J Radiat Oncol Biol Phys.* 2011;81(5):1336-1342.
14. Zhang X, Zhao KL, Guerrero TM, et al. Four-dimensional computed tomography-based treatment planning for intensity-modulated radiation therapy and proton therapy for distal esophageal cancer. *Int J Radiat Oncol Biol Phys.* 2008;72(1):278-287.
15. Wang J, Palmer M, Bilton SD, et al. Comparing proton beam to intensity-modulated radiation therapy planning in esophageal cancer. *Int J Particle Ther.* 2015;1(4):866-877.

Recommended Gastrointestinal Cancer Proton Therapy Indications

INDICATIONS

1) **Hepatocellular carcinoma**
   - Proton therapy with ablative doses for inoperable disease leads to prolongation of survival.[5,7,9,16,23,24]

2) **Intrahepatic cholangiocarcinoma**
   - Proton therapy with ablative doses for inoperable disease leads to prolongation of survival.[1,2]
3) **Isolated colorectal liver metastases** when liver constraints cannot be met with intensity-modulated radiation therapy (IMRT).
   - If all known disease can be covered, it is curative. Patients with stable and responding disease have a better prognosis, but treatment of all liver-confined colorectal metastases prolongs overall survival (OS), and some will be cured.
     - SBRT to ablative doses results in 90% local control.[6,26]
     - Surgical series demonstrating curative results in metastatic colorectal cancer with liver-dominant disease.[3,19]
4) **Recurrent, previously irradiated disease**
5) **Any patient younger than 40 years old with localized, surgically curable disease** where radiation is indicated.
6) **Intensity-modulated proton therapy (IMPT)** is recommended for the indications listed above only in conjunction with respiratory gating.

Inclusion criteria:

1. **Curative treatment:** For indications 1 to 3, ablative doses must be given to provide curative treatment. Three-dimensional conformal radiation therapy (3DCRT) or IMRT may be used if lower doses are prescribed. There may be exceptions, but the appeals process can address them.
2. Ablative doses:
   - 70 Gy in 10 fractions
   - 60 to 67.5 Gy in 15 fractions
   - 62.5 to 75 Gy in 25 fractions

SCIENTIFIC EVIDENCE

1. Hong TS, Wo JY, Yeap BY, et al. Multi-institutional phase II study of high-dose hypofractionated proton beam therapy in patients with localized, unresectable hepatocellular carcinoma and intrahepatic cholangiocarcinoma. *J Clin Oncol.* 2016;34(5):460-468.
2. Tao R, Krishnan S, Bhosale PR, et al. Ablative radiotherapy doses lead to a substantial prolongation of survival in patients with inoperable intrahepatic cholangiocarcinoma: a retrospective dose response analysis. *J Clin Oncol.* 2016;34(3):219-226.
3. Brouquet A, Abdalla EK, Kopetz S, et al. High survival rate after two-stage resection of advanced colorectal liver metastases: response-based selection and complete resection define outcome. *J Clin Oncol.* 2011;29:1083-1090.
4. Bush DA, Hillebrand DJ, Slater JM, Slater JD. High-dose proton beam radiotherapy of hepatocellular carcinoma: preliminary results of a phase II trial. *Gastroenterology.* 2004;127 (5 suppl 1):S189-S193.
5. Bush DA, Kayali Z, Grove R, et al. The safety and efficacy of high-dose proton beam radiotherapy for hepatocellular carcinoma: a phase 2 prospective trial. *Cancer.* 2011;117: 3053-3059.
6. Chang DT, Swaminath A, Kozak M, et al. Stereotactic body radiotherapy for colorectal liver metastases: a pooled analysis. *Cancer.* 2011;117:4060-4069.
7. Chiba T, Tokuuye K, Matsuzaki Y, et al. Proton beam therapy for hepatocellular carcinoma: a retrospective review of 162 patients. *Clin Cancer Res.* 2005;11:3799-3805.
8. Dionisi F, Ben-Josef E. The use of proton therapy in the treatment of gastrointestinal cancers: liver. *Cancer J.* 2014;20(6):371-377.

9. Fukumitsu N, Sugahara S, Nakayama H, et al. A prospective study of hypofractionated proton beam therapy for patients with hepatocellular carcinoma. *Int J Radiat Oncol Biol Phys.* 2009;74:831-836.
10. Hashimoto T, Tokuuye K, Fukumitsu N, et al. Repeated proton beam therapy for hepatocellular carcinoma. *Int J Radiat Oncol Biol Phys.* 2006;65(1):196-202.
11. Hata M, Tokuuye K, Sugahara S, et al. Proton beam therapy for aged patients with hepatocellular carcinoma. *Int J Radiat Oncol Biol Phys.* 2007;69(3):805-812.
12. Hata M, Tokuuye K, Sugahara S, et al. Proton beam therapy for hepatocellular carcinoma patients with severe cirrhosis. *Strahlenther Onkol.* 2006;182(12):713-720.
13. Hata M, Tokuuye K, Sugahara S, et al. Proton beam therapy for hepatocellular carcinoma with limited treatment options. *Cancer.* 2006;107(3):591-598.
14. Hata M, Tokuuye K, Sugahara S, et al. Proton beam therapy for hepatocellular carcinoma with portal vein tumor thrombus. *Cancer.* 2005;104(4):794-801.
15. Hong TS, DeLaney TF, Mamon HJ, et al. A prospective feasibility study of respiratory-gated proton beam therapy for liver tumors. *Pract Radiat Oncol.* 2014;4(5):316-322.
16. Kawashima M, Furuse J, Nishio T, et al. Phase II study of radiotherapy employing proton beam for hepatocellular carcinoma. *J Clin Oncol.* 2005;23:1839-1846.
17. Kim TH, Park JW, Kim YJ, et al. Phase I dose-escalation study of proton beam therapy for inoperable hepatocellular carcinoma. *Cancer Res Treat.* 2015;47(1):34-45.
18. Komatsu S, Fukumoto T, Demizu Y, et al. Clinical results and risk factors of proton and carbon ion therapy for hepatocellular carcinoma. *Cancer.* 2011;117(21):4890-4904.
19. Kopetz S, Chang GJ, Overman MJ, et al. Improved survival in metastatic colorectal cancer is associated with adoption of hepatic resection and improved chemotherapy. *J Clin Oncol.* 2009;27:3677-3683.
20. Lee SU, Park JW, Kim TH, et al. Effectiveness and safety of proton beam therapy for advanced hepatocellular carcinoma with portal vein tumor thrombosis. *Strahlenther Onkol.* 2014;190(9):806-814.
21. Ling TC, Kang JI, Bush DA, Slater JD, Yang GY. Proton therapy for hepatocellular carcinoma. *Chin J Cancer Res.* 2012;24(4):361-367.
22. Mizumoto M, Tokuuye K, Sugahara S, et al. Proton beam therapy for hepatocellular carcinoma adjacent to the porta hepatis. *Int J Radiat Oncol Biol Phys.* 2008;71(2):462-467.
23. Mizumoto M, Okumura T, Hashimoto T, et al. Proton beam therapy for hepatocellular carcinoma: a comparison of three treatment protocols. *Int J Radiat Oncol Biol Phys.* 2011;81(4):1039-1045.
24. Nakayama H, Sugahara S, Tokita M, et al. Proton beam therapy for hepatocellular carcinoma: the University of Tsukuba experience. *Cancer.* 2009;115:5499-5506.
25. Petersen JB, Lassen Y, Hansen AT, Muren LP, Grau C, Høyer M. Normal liver tissue sparing by intensity-modulated proton stereotactic body radiotherapy for solitary liver tumours. *Acta Oncol.* 2011;50(6):823-828.
26. Rusthoven KE, Kavanagh BD, Cardenes H, et al. Multi-institutional phase I/II trial of stereotactic body radiation therapy for liver metastases. *J Clin Oncol.* 2009;27:1572-1578.
27. Skinner HD, Hong TS, Krishnan S. Charged-particle therapy for hepatocellular carcinoma. *Semin Radiat Oncol.* 2011;21(4):278-286.
28. Sugahara S, Nakayama H, Fukuda K, et al. Proton-beam therapy for hepatocellular carcinoma associated with portal vein tumor thrombosis. *Strahlenther Onkol.* 2009;185(12):782-788.
29. Sugahara S, Oshiro Y, Nakayama H, et al. Proton beam therapy for large hepatocellular carcinoma. *Int J Radiat Oncol Biol Phys.* 2010;76(2):460-466.
30. Taddei PJ, Howell RM, Krishnan S, Scarboro SB, Mirkovic D, Newhauser WD. Risk of second malignant neoplasm following proton versus intensity-modulated photon radiotherapies for hepatocellular carcinoma. *Phys Med Biol.* 2010;55(23):7055-7065.

31. Toramatsu C, Katoh N, Shimizu S, et al. What is the appropriate size criterion for proton radiotherapy for hepatocellular carcinoma? A dosimetric comparison of spot-scanning proton therapy versus intensity-modulated radiation therapy. *Radiat Oncol.* 2013;8:48.
32. Qi WX, Fu S, Zhang Q, Guo XM. Charged particle therapy versus photon therapy for patients with hepatocellular carcinoma: a systematic review and meta-analysis. *Radiother Oncol.* 2014;114(3):289-295.

Recommended Head and Neck Cancer Proton Therapy Indications

INDICATIONS

1) **Nasal cavity** and **paranasal sinus tumors**
   - **Inclusion criteria**
     i. Ethmoid sinus tumors
        a. Histologies include sinonasal undifferentiated carcinoma (SNUC), small cell neuroendocrine carcinoma, sarcoma, lymphoma
        b. T1–T4a: Newly diagnosed, nonsurgical candidate or refuses surgery
        c. T2–T4a: Postoperative with perineural invasion (PNI), bone invasion, or positive margin
        d. T4b: Newly diagnosed or patient declines surgery
        e. Diagnosed after incomplete resection and gross residual disease
        f. Doses to optic apparatus structures exceed tolerance with photon therapy and may lead to blindness
        g. No evidence of metastatic disease
        h. Reirradiation in a site of recurrent disease
        i. Reirradiation in a site of secondary primary
     ii. Paranasal sinus tumors
        a. Histologies include squamous cell carcinoma, adenocarcinoma, minor salivary gland tumor, esthesioneuroblastoma, undifferentiated carcinoma, sarcoma, mucosal melanoma, lymphoma
        b. T1–T2: Postoperative with PNI, bone invasion, or positive margin
        c. T1–T4a: Newly diagnosed, nonsurgical candidate or refuses surgery
        d. T2–T4a: Postoperative with PNI, bone invasion, or positive margin
        e. T4b: Newly diagnosed or patient declines surgery
        f. Diagnosed after incomplete resection and gross residual disease
        g. Doses to optic apparatus structures exceed tolerance with photon therapy and may lead to blindness
        h. No evidence of metastatic disease
        i. Reirradiation in a site of recurrent disease
        j. Reirradiation in a site of secondary primary
   - For nasal cavity and paranasal sinus tumors, the preferred treatment algorithm includes surgery followed by postoperative external beam radiation therapy (EBRT). Even with this potentially disfiguring therapy, cure rates are poor, and treatment-related toxicities are common, severe, and can even be fatal. Control rates as low as 30% prompted investigation into new methods of treatment, particularly when tumors were situated near the skull base, and critical structures limit effective dose delivery to the tumor. Conventional EBRT to tumors of the paranasal sinuses has resulted in 24% to 41% incidence of blindness as a result of retinopathy or optic neuropathy. Treatment plans for proton beam radiation (PBR) compare favorably to photon EBRT, techniques such as intensity-modulated radiation therapy (IMRT) or 3D conformal radiation. A systemic review and

metaanalysis by Patel et al.[3] demonstrated a greater overall survival (OS) at 5 years with charged particle therapy over photon therapy and a higher disease-free survival and locoregional control (LRC) with proton therapy over IMRT. Investigators at the Massachusetts General Hospital (MGH) have had extensive experience with using proton therapy for nasal cavity and paranasal sinus cancer. In one such study, of 102 patients were treated between 1991 and 2002 with either PBR or combination proton-photon EBRT for locally advanced sinonasal cancers either with or without surgery.[4] Although that analysis showed that a complete resection improved DFS and OS, high-dose radiation provided excellent local control (LC) regardless of the extent of resection. Another MGH study of 23 patients with adenoid cystic carcinomas that invaded the skull base treated with combined proton-photon RT reported a 5-year LC of 93%, despite the fact that 87% of patients had gross tumor remaining at the time of radiation, and 48% of patients received biopsy only before RT.[5] The 5-year rates of freedom from distant metastasis were 62%; disease-free survival (DFS), 56%; and OS, 77%. These studies show good local control can be achieved with dose escalation using combined photon EBRT and PBR. The median doses used were 71.6 CGE and 75.9 CGE, respectively. However, the radiation delivery schedules were quite heterogeneous, with patients receiving conventional fractionation or twice-daily accelerated fractionation with or without concomitant boost. Truong et al.[6] published the MGH experience with PBR for locally advanced tumors of the sphenoid sinus. This group was also heterogeneous in terms of histology, extent of surgery, and receipt of chemotherapy. Some patients also received photon radiation therapy for the neck, if indicated by histology. At 2 years, the LC rate was 86% the rate of freedom from metastases was 50%, the DFS rate was 31%, and the OS rate was 53%. In an early MGH experience with 19 prospectively treated patients with neuroblastoma and neuroendocrine tumors of the paranasal sinus, the patients underwent either biopsy, subtotal resection, or gross total resection with positive margins and then went on to receive two cycles of cisplatin-etoposide followed by combination photon and proton radiation therapy.[7] A large field was treated with 1.8 Gy once daily using photons. A smaller field was supplemented with 1.6 CGE using protons on a twice-daily basis. The LC rate was good, with only two patients experiencing recurrence in the radiation field, both of which could be salvaged with surgery. No patients experienced radiation-induced vision loss, potentially because the chiasm and optic nerves were constrained to less than 55 CGE or less than 2 CGE per day and a stereotactic setup was used. At the Proton Medical Research Center in Tsukuba, Japan, 17 patients with T4 or recurrent nasal cavity or paranasal sinus carcinoma were treated with PBR to a median dose of 78 CGE in 36 fractions (range: 22–82.5 CGE).[16] The 2- and 5-year LC were 35% and 18%, respectively, and the 2- and 5-year OS were 47% and 16%, respectively. Four patients experienced grade 3 to 4 toxicity, but there were no treatment-related deaths, potentially because of the strict dose constraint of 50 CGE to both the brainstem and optic chiasm. Another Japanese group used PBR for unresectable head and neck malignancies including nasal cavity and paranasal sinus or skull base tumors.[9] The median dose of PBR was 65 CGE in 26 fractions, and 10 patients received neoadjuvant chemotherapy. At 1 year, they reported a 77% LC rate, with 3-year PFS and OS rates of 50% and 60%, respectively. The 5-year OS rate was 55%. In contrast to the MGH experience, however, treatment-related toxicities were not trivial. Cerebrospinal fluid leakage caused treatment-related death in one patient, and four other patients experienced grade 3 to 4 toxicities, including cataract, visual impairment, cranial nerve palsy, and osteonecrosis. However, because none the patients in this retrospective review were candidates for surgery, the inability to achieve LC of tumors in this area may very well have led to similar symptoms, and thus, the authors found this safety profile acceptable. With further improvements in technology to deliver PBR, such as intensity-modulated proton therapy (IMPT), the incidence of severe toxicities should be even lower in the future.

2) Nasopharyngeal tumors

- **Inclusion criteria**:
  - i. Histology including:
  - ii. Carcinoma (World Health Organization [WHO] I–III), adenoid cystic carcinoma, sarcoma, lymphoma
  - iii. T1–T4: Definitive treatment with radiation therapy alone or with concurrent chemotherapy
- Lin et al.[17] presented outcomes for patients with recurrent nasopharyngeal carcinoma initially treated at Loma Linda University Medical Center (LLUMC) with photon radiation therapy who were then reirradiated to doses of 59.4 to 70.2 CGE. Their OS and locoregional PFS were both 50% at 2 years but varied widely by how well the target was covered. Dose-volume histograms were analyzed for "optimal" (2-year OS: 83%) versus "suboptimal coverage" (2-year OS: 17%), where "optimal" was conservatively defined as 90% of the target volume receiving 90% of the prescribed dose Chan et al.[18] reported outcomes of 19 patients with T4 nasopharyngeal cancer treated with conformal photon-proton radiation therapy to a medial total dose of 73.6 CGE in either twice-daily or conventional fractionation. Ten patients also received induction or concurrent chemotherapy with docetaxel, cisplatin, carboplatin, or paclitaxel. Three-year rates of LC, PFS, and OS were 92%, 75%, and 74%, respectively, with one patient hospitalized for acute toxicities and five patients noted to have late toxicities, including temporal lobe radiographic changes, mandibular osteonecrosis, and endocrine dysfunction. A phase II study at MGH evaluated combined proton-photon radiation therapy to 70 CGE in 35 daily fractions given with concurrent cisplatin and fluorouracil (NCT00592501). The primary outcomes are acute toxicity, treatment compliance, and health-related quality of life at 3 years. Preliminary results from 23 consecutive patients with stage III to IVB nasopharyngeal cancer were presented at the 2014 meeting of the American Society for Radiation Oncology.[19] The LRC rate at 28 months was 100%; 2-year DFS and OS rates were 90% and 100%, respectively. Toxicities included hearing loss in 29%, weight loss in 38%, and gastrostomy tube placement in 48% but no grade 3 or greater xerostomia.

3) Oropharyngeal tumors

- **Inclusion criteria**
  - i. Histologies include squamous cell carcinoma, adenoid cystic carcinoma, sarcoma
  - ii. T1–T4a: Definitive treatment with radiation therapy alone or with concurrent chemotherapy
  - iii. T1–T4a: Postoperative with high-risk features (i.e., positive margins, extracapsular extension [ECE], PNI)
  - iv. Coverage of the retropharyngeal nodes required to the skull base
  - v. T4b: unresectable advanced stage disease with the treatment volume extending to the skull base
  - vi. Unknown primary with cervical nodal disease requiring coverage of the pharyngeal axis to the skull base
- Oropharyngeal cancer is often treated with radiation therapy alone or in combination with chemotherapy. In the 10 years since this book was written, IMRT has become the standard treatment technique for head and neck malignancies because of its ability to reduce dose to the parotids and minimize the risk of xerostomia. However, additional dose is now delivered to the oral cavity, larynx, brainstem, and muscle of mastication that can cause dysgeusia (loss of taste), dysphagia, xerostomia, and trismus. The unnecessary radiation dose to the head and neck outside of the tumor from IMRT results in nausea,

vomiting, anterior oral mucositis, oral pain, dysphagia, fatigue, loss of weight, gastrostomy tubes, emergency room visits with intravenous (IV) fluids, and hospitalization. After LLUMC opened the first proton treatment facility in the hospital-based environment in 1990, they opened a prospective protocol to treat patients with stage II–IV oropharyngeal cancer with a combination of photon and proton therapy. In 2005, Slater et al.[23] published the LLUMC experience using a concomitant boost technique, which consisted of 50.4 Gy in 1.8-Gy fractions to the primary disease volume, involved lymph nodes, and areas at risk with lateral opposed photon fields. Concomitant boost proton fields encompassed gross primary and nodal disease, which was delivered during the last 3.5 weeks of photon treatment in a twice-daily fashion, bringing the total tumor dose to 75.9 CGE. They achieved 92% 2-year LRC compared with 55% in the Radiation Therapy Oncology Group (RTOG) concomitant boost arm with standard radiation therapy, suggesting that higher doses could improve outcomes without an increase in toxicity. In an MD Anderson case-control study by Frank et al.[24] of IMPT versus IMRT, IMPT-treated patients had a gastrostomy tube rate of 19% compared with an IMRT rate of 46% and a lower rate of grade 3 dysphagia. The most recent data from MD Anderson on the first 50 patients treated with IMPT and a median follow-up of 25 months demonstrates one local treatment failure and one regional treatment failure with no grade 4 or 5 toxicities.[25]

4) **Periorbital tumors**
   - **Inclusion criteria**
     i. Medial canthal tumors (i.e., squamous cell carcinoma, basal cell carcinoma, Merkel cell carcinoma)
     ii. Tumors of the lacrimal sac/duct
     iii. Lacrimal gland tumors
     iv. Eyelid tumors
     v. Histologies include squamous cell carcinoma, basal cell carcinoma, adenoid cystic carcinoma, sarcoma
     vi. T1–T4a: Definitive treatment with radiation therapy alone or with concurrent chemotherapy
     vii. T1–T4a: Postoperative with high-risk features (i.e., positive margins, ECE, PNI)
     viii. T4b: Unresectable advanced stage disease with the treatment volume extending to the skull base
     ix. Orbit-sparing approach to prevent blindness
   - For orbit-sparing approaches to preserve the eye from enucleation or total exenteration, proton therapy is necessary to avoid long-term ophthalmologic complications that can affect many portions of the eye, including the lacrimal glands, eyelids, conjunctiva, sclera, cornea, lens, retina, optic nerves, and optic chiasm. Complications from radiation therapy include decreased tear production and dry eye, lacrimal duct atrophy and epiphora, eyelid or corneal ulceration, telangiectasis, conjunctiva neovascularization, keratinization, cataracts, glaucoma, retinopathy, and optic neuropathy.
     - Medial canthal tumors (i.e., squamous cell carcinoma, basal cell carcinoma, Merkel cell carcinoma)
     - Tumors of the lacrimal sac/duct
     - Lacrimal gland tumors
     - Eyelid tumors

5) **Skull-base tumors**
   - **Inclusion criteria**
     i. Histologies at the skull base include, paragangliomas/schwannomas, salivary gland tumors, chordomas and chondrosarcomas, sarcomas, squamous cell carcinoma, and adenoid cystic carcinoma.

ii. T1–T2: Postoperative and high-risk features (PNI, grade, positive margins)
iii. T3–T4a: Patient declines surgery or disease is medically inoperable
iv. T2–T4a: Postoperative with high-risk features (PNI, positive margins)
v. T4b: No surgical resection possible or surgical resection not recommended
vi. No evidence of distant metastases
vii. Skin primary with perineural spread into the skull base via foramen rotundum, ovale, or Meckel's cave toward the cavernous sinus

- For tumors arising at the base of the skull, complete resection is often impossible. Unfortunately, the relative radioresistance of these tumors makes treatment with a curative dose difficult without exposing the surrounding tissues to unacceptable toxicity. Treatment with photon EBRT leads to high recurrence rates and a 5-year progression-free survival (PFS) rate of less than 25%. Doses of 60 Gy and lower were equally ineffective. Even though doses given were inadequate for durable LC, significant brainstem and cranial nerve toxicities were seen with doses of 60 Gy.
  - Paragangliomas/schwannomas at the skull base
  - Salivary gland tumors at the skull base
  - Chordomas and chondrosarcomas at the skull base
  - Sarcomas and carcinomas at the skull base

6) **Reirradiation for recurrent head and neck tumors or new primary malignancies in a radiated field**
7) **IMPT** is indicated for all head and neck malignancies.

General inclusion criteria

1. **Curative primary and adjuvant treatment where the tumor and target radiation volume extends to the base of the skull**
   - For any of these indications where doses of 60 to 70 Gy are required for curative intent, IMRT may be used if lower doses are prescribed. There may be exceptions, but the appeals process can address them.
2. **Advanced-stage head and neck disease** where concurrent chemotherapy is required to control the local or regional disease
3. **Periorbital tumors** where blindness, enucleation, or total exenteration are a risk from standard radiation therapy
4. **Reirradiation in the head and neck** where cumulative doses exceeding 100 Gy may result in significant acute and long-term toxicity and death from treatment

General exclusion criteria (or peer to peer required for specific special circumstances):

1. Cancer of the larynx, unless carotid artery sparing not achievable with IMRT or specific histology with unresectable disease such as adenoid cystic carcinoma.
2. Cancer of the skin without PNI requiring treatment coverage to the skull base.
3. Cancer of the lip without PNI requiring treatment coverage to the skull base.
4. Mucosal melanoma without skull base involvement.

SCIENTIFIC EVIDENCE

1. Colevas AD, Yom SS, Pfister DG, et al. NCCN Guidelines Head and Neck Cancers-Version 2.2018, June 20, 2018. *J Natl Compr Cancer Netw.* 2018;16(5).
2. Holliday EB, Frank SJ. Proton radiation therapy for head and neck cancer: a review of the clinical experience to date. *Int J Radiat Oncol Biol Phys.* 2014;89(2):292-302.
3. Patel SH, Wang Z, Wong WW, et al. Charged particle therapy versus photon therapy for paranasal sinus and nasal cavity malignant diseases: a systematic review and meta-analysis. *Lancet Oncol.* 2014;15(9):1027-1038.

4. Resto VA, Chan AW, Deschler DG, Lin DT. Extent of surgery in the management of locally advanced sinonasal malignancies. *Head Neck* 2008;31(2):222-229.
5. Pommier P, Liebsch NJ, Deschler DG, et al. Proton beam radiotherapy for skull base adenoid cystic carcinoma. *Arch Otolaryngol Head Neck Surg* 2006;132(11):1242-1249.
6. Truong MT, Kamat UR, Liebsch NJ, et al. Proton radiotherapy for primary sphenoid sinus malignancies: treatment outcomes and prognostic factors. *Head Neck* 2009;31(10):1297-1308.
7. Fitzek MM, Thornton AF, Varvares M, et al. Neuroendocrine tumors of the sinonasal tract. Results of a prospective study incorporating chemotherapy, surgery, and combined proton-photon radiotherapy. *Cancer*. 2002;94:2623-2634.
8. Okano S, Tahara M, Zenda S, et al. Induction chemotherapy with docetaxel, cisplatin and S-1 followed by proton beam therapy concurrent with cisplatin in patients with T4b nasal and sinonasal malignancies. *Jpn J Clin Oncol.* 2012;42:691-696.
9. Zenda S, Kohno R, Kawashima M, et al. Proton beam therapy for unresectable malignancies of the nasal cavity and paranasal sinuses. *Int J Radiat Oncol Biol Phys.* 2011;81:1473-1478.
10. Lavertu P, Roberts JK, Kraus DH, et al. Squamous cell carcinoma of the paranasal sinuses: the Cleveland Clinic experience 1977–1986. *Laryngoscope*. 1989;99:1130-1136.
11. Waldron JN, O'Sullivan B, Warde P, et al. Ethmoid sinus cancer: twenty-nine cases managed with primary radiation therapy. *Int J Radiat Oncol Biol Phys.* 1998;41:361-369.
12. Takeda A, Shigematsu N, Suzuki S, et al. Late retinal complications of radiation therapy for nasal and paranasal malignancies: relationship between irradiated-dose area and severity. *Int J Radiat Oncol Biol Phys.* 1999;44:599-605.
13. Katz TS, Mendenhall WM, Morris CG, et al. Malignant tumors of the nasal cavity and paranasal sinuses. *Head Neck*. 2002;24:821-829.
14. Lomax AJ, Goitein M, Adams J. Intensity modulation in radiotherapy: Photons versus protons in the paranasal sinus. *Radiother Oncol.* 2003;66:11-18.
15. Mock U, Georg D, Bogner J, et al. Treatment planning comparison of conventional, 3D conformal, and intensity-modulated photon (IMRT) and proton therapy for paranasal sinus carcinoma. *Int J Radiat Oncol Biol Phys.* 2004;58:147-154.
16. Fukumitsu N, Okumura T, Mizumoto M, et al. Outcome of T4 (International Union Against Cancer Staging System, 7th edition) or recurrent nasal cavity and paranasal sinus carcinoma treated with proton beam. *Int J Radiat Oncol Biol Phys.* 2012;83:704-711.
17. Lin R, Slater JD, Yonemoto LT, et al. Nasopharyngeal carcinoma: repeat treatment with conformal proton therapy—dose-volume histogram analysis. *Radiology*. 1999;213:489-494.
18. Chan A, Liebsch L, Deschler D, et al. Proton radiotherapy for T4 nasopharyngeal carcinoma. *J Clin Oncol.* 2004;22:5574.
19. Chan A, Adams JA, Weyman E, et al. A phase II trial of proton radiation therapy with chemotherapy for nasopharyngeal carcinoma. *Int J Radiat Oncol Biol Phys.* 2012;84:S151-S152.
20. Kam MKM, Leung S-F, Zee B, et al. Prospective randomized study of intensity-modulated radiotherapy on salivary gland function in early-stage nasopharyngeal carcinoma patients. *J Clin Oncol.* 2007;25:4873-4879.
21. Liu S-W, Li J-M, Chang J-Y, et al. A treatment planning comparison between proton beam therapy and intensity-modulated x-ray therapy for recurrent nasopharyngeal carcinoma. *J X-Ray Sci Technol.* 2010;18:443-450.
22. Taheri-Kadkhoda Z, Björk-Eriksson T, Nill S, et al. Intensity-modulated radiotherapy of nasopharyngeal carcinoma: a comparative treatment planning study of photons and protons. *Radiat Oncol.* 2008;3:4.
23. Slater JD, Yonemoto LT, Mantik DW, et al. Proton radiation for treatment of cancer of the oropharynx: early experience at Loma Linda University Medical Center using a concomitant boost technique. *Int J Radiat Oncol Biol Phys.* 2005;62:494-500.

24. Frank SJ, Rosenthal DI, Ang K, et al. Gastrostomy tubes decrease by over 50% with intensity modulated proton therapy (IMPT) during the treatment of oropharyngeal cancer patients: a case-control study. *Int J Radiat Oncol Biol Phys.* 2013;87(2):S144.
25. Kutcheson K, Lewin JS, Garden AS, et al. Early experience with IMPT for the treatment of oropharyngeal tumors: acute toxicities and swallowing-related outcomes. *Int J Radiat Oncol Biol Phys.* 2013;87:S604.
26. Parsons JT, Bova FJ, Fitzgerald CR, et al. Severe dry-eye syndrome following external beam irradiation. *Int J Radiat Oncol Biol Phys.* 1994;30:775-780.
27. Barabino S, Raghavan A, Loeffler J, et al. Radiation therapy-induced ocular surface disease. *Cornea.* 2005;24:909-914.
28. Van de Water TA, Bijl HP, Schilstra C, et al. The potential benefit of radiotherapy with protons in head and neck cancer with respect to normal tissue sparing: a systematic review of literature. *Oncologist.* 2011;16:366-377.
29. Catton C, O'Sullivan B, Bell R, et al. Chordoma: long-term follow-up after radical photon irradiation. *Radiother Oncol.* 1996;41:67-72.
30. Frank SJ, Cox JD, Gillin M, et al. Multifield optimization intensity modulated proton therapy for head and neck tumors: a translation to practice. *Int J Radiat Oncol Biol Phys.* 2014;89:846-853.
31. Gunn GB, Blanchard P, Garden AS, et al. Clinical outcomes and patterns of disease recurrence after intensity modulated proton therapy for oropharyngeal squamous carcinoma. *Int J Radiat Oncol Biol Phys.* 2016;95:360-367.
32. Holliday EB, Kocak-Uzel E, Feng L, et al. Dosimetric advantages of intensity-modulated proton therapy for oropharyngeal cancer compared with intensity-modulated radiation: a case-matched control analysis. *Med Dosim.* 2016;41:189-194.
33. Eekers DBP, Roelofs E, Jelen U, et al. Benefit of particle therapy in re-irradiation of head and neck patients. Results of a multicentric in silico ROCOCO trial. *Radiother Oncol.* 2016;121:387-394.
34. Sapir E, Tao Y, Feng F, et al. Predictors of dysgeusia in patients with oropharyngeal cancer treated with chemotherapy and intensity modulated radiation therapy. *Int J Radiat Oncol.* 2016;96:354-361.
35. Jakobi A, Bandurska-Luque A, Stützer K, et al. Identification of patient benefit from proton therapy for advanced head and neck cancer patients based on individual and subgroup normal tissue complication probability analysis. *Int J Radiat Oncol Biol Phys.* 2015;92:1165-1174.
36. Blanchard P, Wong AJ, Gunn GB, et al. Toward a model-based patient selection strategy for proton therapy: external validation of photon- derived normal tissue complication probability models in a head and neck proton therapy cohort. *Radiother Oncol.* 2016;121:381-386.
37. Blanchard P, Garden AS, Gunn GB, et al. Intensity-modulated proton beam therapy (IMPT) versus intensity-modulated photon therapy (IMRT) for patients with oropharynx cancer—a case matched analysis. *Radiother Oncol.* 2016;120:48-55.
38. Sio TT, Lin HK, Shi Q, et al. Intensity modulated proton therapy versus intensity modulated photon radiation therapy for oropharyngeal cancer: first comparative results of patient-reported outcomes. *Int J Radiat Oncol Biol Phys.* 2016;95:1107-1114.
39. Romesser PB, Cahlon O, Scher ED, et al. Proton beam reirradiation for recurrent head and neck cancer multi-institutional report on feasibility and early outcomes. *Int J Radiat Oncol Biol Phys.* 2016;95:386-395.
40. Phan J, Sio TT, Nguyen TP, et al. Reirradiation of head and neck cancers with proton therapy: outcomes and analyses. *Int J Radiat Oncol Biol Phys.* 2016;96:30-41.
41. Esmaeli B, Yin VT, Hanna EY, et al. Eye-sparing multidisciplinary approach for the management of lacrimal gland carcinoma. *Head Neck.* 2016;38:1258-1262.

42. Holliday EB, Esmaeli B, Pinckard J, et al. A multidisciplinary orbit-sparing treatment approach that includes proton therapy for epithelial tumors of the orbit and ocular adnexa. *Int J Radiat Oncol Biol Phys.* 2016;95:344-352.
43. Bhattasali O, Holliday E, Kies MS, et al. Definitive proton radiation therapy and concurrent cisplatin for unresectable head and neck adenoid cystic carcinoma: a series of 9 cases and a critical review of the literature. *Head Neck.* 2016;38(suppl 1):E1472-E1480.
44. Romesser PB, Cahlon O, Scher E, et al. Proton beam radiation therapy results in significantly reduced toxicity compared with intensity-modulated radiation therapy for head and neck tumors that require ipsilateral radiation. *Radiother Oncol.* 2016;118:286-292.
45. Thaker NG, Frank SJ, Feeley TW. Comparative costs of advanced proton and photon radiation therapies: lessons from time-driven activity-based costing in head and neck cancer. *J Comp Eff Res.* 2015;4:297-301.
46. Verma V, Mishra MV, Mehta MP. A systematic review of the cost and cost- effectiveness studies of proton radiotherapy. *Cancer.* 2016;122:1483-1501.
47. Russo AL, Adams JA, Weyman EA, et al. Long-term outcomes after proton beam therapy for sinonasal squamous cell carcinoma. *Int J Radiat Oncol Biol Phys.* 2016;95:368-376.
48. Dagan R, Bryant C, Li Z, et al. Outcomes of sinonasal cancer treated with proton therapy. *Int J Radiat Oncol Biol Phys.* 2016;95:377-385.
49. Holliday EB, Garden AS, Rosenthal DI, et al. Proton therapy reduces treatment-related toxicities for patients with nasopharyngeal cancer: a case-match control study of intensity-modulated proton therapy and intensity modulated photon therapy. *Int J Part Ther.* 2015;2:19-28.
50. McDonald MW, Zolali-Meybodi O, Lehnert SJ, et al. Reirradiation of recurrent and second primary head and neck cancer with proton therapy. *Int J Radiat Oncol Biol Phys.* 2016;96:808-819.

Recommended Hematologic Cancer Proton Therapy Indications

INDICATIONS

1) **Mediastinal lymphoma**
   - **Inclusion criteria**
     i. Lymphoma located in the mediastinum with the following pathologies: Hodgkin lymphoma, diffuse large B-cell, lymphoblastic lymphoma, lymphoblastic leukemia of T, B, pre-T, or pre-B type, and primary mediastinal lymphoma
     ii. Lymphoma located behind the heart
     iii. Lymphoma in a patient who previously received radiation to the same area
   - For this young population that survives for decades, treating the critical organs to even low doses will result in second malignancies and heart disease 15 to 25 years later.
   - Studies of radiation-related heart disease strongly suggest that increasing dose to the heart increases the risk of cardiac complications,[4,5] with some suggesting that there is no threshold below which there is no risk.
   - In addition, our goal is to decrease the volume of lung receiving a low radiation dose with proton therapy compared with intensity-modulated radiation therapy (IMRT). Our recent work showed that a mean lung dose of as low as 13 Gy is associated with a higher rate of pneumonitis. This is different than the threshold for other oncologic sites because most of our patients receive one or more types of chemotherapy that cause lung toxicity (examples include bleomycin, gemcitabine, busulfan, brentuximab).

2) **Craniospinal irradiation**
- **Inclusion criteria**
  i. Definitive therapy OR
  ii. Conditioning before allogeneic transplant
- Our main goal is not to exit through critical organs primarily the vertebral bodies that contain more than 50% of the bone marrow (using proton therapy). Avoiding the marrow will prevent pancytopenia as well as permanent damage to a large part of the bone marrow that receives 30 Gy, which is the usual dose of radiation given.
- In the setting of autologous or allogeneic transplant, proton therapy will help to avoid the following critical organs: lungs, heart, thyroid, and bowel. This will decrease the side effects to these organs and substantially reduce the hospital stay, transfusions, and infection.

3) **Lymphoma near the paraspinal region along the whole vertebral body**
- **Inclusion criteria**
  i. Paraspinal masses of any type of lymphoma that need treatment with radiation as definitive therapy or as a consolidation
  ii. Sacral masses of any type of lymphoma
  iii. Posterior thoracic spinal masses that are located in the vicinity of the heart
  iv. Sternal masses
- Proton therapy will eliminate the risk of excess dose to the organs anterior to the mass, including thyroid, lungs, heart, bilateral kidneys, ovaries, and bowels
- Will also avoid dose to the bone marrow

SCIENTIFIC EVIDENCE

1. Brenner H, Gondos A, Pulte D. Ongoing improvement in long-term survival of patients with Hodgkin disease at all ages and recent catch-up of older patients. *Blood.* 2008; 111(6):2977-2983.
2. Carr ZA, Land CE, Kleinerman RA, et al. Coronary heart disease after radiotherapy for peptic ulcer disease. *Int J Radiat Oncol Biol Phys.* 2005;61:842-850.
   a. A statistically significant relationship was observed between coronary heart disease average dose to the heart in the 0 to 7.6 Gy range. The study is important in that it shows that even very low doses (≥2 Gy) may be associated with increased risk of coronary artery heart disease.
3. Chera BS, Rodriguez C, Morris CG, et al. Dosimetric comparison of three different involved nodal irradiation techniques for stage II Hodgkin's lymphoma patients: Conventional radiotherapy, intensity-modulated radiotherapy and three-dimensional proton radiotherapy. *Int J Radiat Oncol Biol Phys.* 2009;75(4):1173-1180.
   - Mean breast dose was highest (1.94 Gy) for conformal radiotherapy, 3.74 Gy for IMRT, 1.59 Gy for three-dimensional proton radiotherapy.
   - Mean lung doses: 4.83 Gy conformal radiotherapy, 5.38 Gy IMRT, and 30.4 Gy 3D proton therapy.
   - In general, the advantage for protons is seen in volume receiving relatively low dose (<15 Gy).
4. Darby SC, Ewertz M, McGale P, et al. Risk of ischemic heart disease in women after radiotherapy for breast cancer. *N Engl J Med.* 2013;11:987-998.
   - Cardiac risk strongly related to cardiac dose with no obvious threshold.
5. Hancock SL, Tucker MA, Hoppe RT. Factors affecting late mortality from heart disease after treatment of Hodgkin's disease. *JAMA.* 1993;270(16):1949-1955.

6. Heidenreich PA, Hancock SL, Vagelos RH, Lee BK, Schnittger I. Diastolic dysfunction after mediastinal irradiation. *Am Heart J.* 2005;150(5):977-982.
7. Heidenreich PA, Schnittger I, Strauss HW, et al. Screening for coronary artery disease after mediastinal irradiation for Hodgkin's disease. *J Clin Oncol.* 2007;25(1):43-49.
8. Hoppe BS, Flampouri S, Zaiden R, et al. Involved-node proton therapy in combined modality therapy for Hodgkin lymphoma: results of a phase 2 study. *Int J Radiat Oncol Biol Phys.* 2014;89(5):1053-1059.
   a. Progressively lower average integral dose and average dose to heart, lungs, breast, thyroid, and esophagus when 3D, IMRT, and proton plans were compared in 15 patients treated with involved-node proton therapy after chemotherapy. Three-year event-free survival rate 93%.
9. Hoppe BS, Flampouri S, Su Z, et al. Effective dose reduction to cardiac structures using protons compared with 3DCRT and IMRT in mediastinal Hodgkin lymphoma. *Int J Radiat Oncol Biol Phys.* 2012;84(2):449-455.
   a. Highly significant decrease in dose with comparison of proton therapy versus 3D or IMRT to multiple critical organs with proton therapy, including heart, left ventricle, right ventricle, left atrium, mitral valve, tricuspid valve, aortic valve (significant only for 3D vs. proton therapy), left anterior descending artery, left circumflex, right circumflex (significant only for 3D vs. proton therapy), pulmonary artery (significant only for 3D vs. proton therapy), and ascending aorta (significant only for IMRT vs. proton therapy).
10. Hoppe BS, Flampouri S, Su Z, et al. Consolidative involved-node proton therapy for stage IA–IIIB mediastinal Hodgkin lymphoma: preliminary dosimetric outcomes from a phase II study. *Int J Radiat Oncol Biol Phys.* 2012;83(1):260-267.
   a. "PT provided the lowest mean dose to the heart, lungs, and breasts for all 10 patients compared with either 3D-CRT or IMRT."
11. Jørgensen AY, Maraldo MV, Brodin NP, et al. The effect on esophagus after different radiotherapy techniques for early stage Hodgkin's lymphoma. *Acta Oncol.* 2013;52: 1559-1565.
   a. "Mean dose to the esophagus was 16.4 Gy with 3DCRT, 16.4 Gy with VMAT, 14.7, Gy with proton therapy and 34.2 Gy with mantle field treatment ($P<0.001$). No differences were seen in the estimated risk of developing esophagitis, stricture or cancer with 3DCRT compared with VMAT. Proton therapy performed significantly better with the lowest risk estimates for all parameters compared with the photon treatments, except compared with 3DCRT for stricture ($P = 0.066$)."
12. Li J, Dabaja B, Reed V, et al. Rationale for and preliminary results of proton beam therapy for mediastinal lymphoma. *Int J Radiat Oncol Biol Phys.* 2011;81(1):167-174.
   a. In 10 patients, "PBT delivered lower mean doses to the lung (6.2 vs. 9.5 Gy), esophagus (9.5 vs. 22.3 Gy), and heart (8.8 vs. 17.7 Gy) but not the breasts (5.9 vs. 6.1 Gy) than did conventional RT."
13. Maraldo MV, Brodin NP, Aznar MC, et al. Estimated risk of cardiovascular disease and secondary cancers with modern highly conformal radiotherapy for early-stage mediastinal Hodgkin lymphoma. *Ann Oncol.* 2013;24:2113-2118.
   a. Compared with arc IMRT (VMAT) or 3D conventional therapy, highly significant estimated benefit for protons as measured by cardiac mortality, cardiac morbidity, myocardial infarction, valvular disease (only VMAT vs. PT significant), lung cancer, breast cancer, and life years lost.

14. Mulrooney DA, Yeazel MW, Kawashima T, et al. Cardiac outcomes in a cohort of adult survivors of childhood and adolescent cancer: retrospective analysis of the Childhood Cancer Survivor Study cohort. *BMJ.* 2009;339:b4606.

15. Ng AK, Bernardo MP, Weller E, et al. Long-term survival and competing causes of death in patients with early-stage Hodgkin's disease treated at age 50 or younger. *Clin Oncol.* 2002;20(8):2101-2108.

16. Pinnix CC, Smith GL, Milgrom S, et al. Predictors of radiation pneumonitis in patients receiving intensity-modulated radiation therapy for Hodgkin and non-Hodgkin lymphoma. *Int J Radiat Oncol Biol Phys.* 2015;92(1):175-182.

17. Schneider U, Lomax A, Lombriser N. Comparative risk assessment of secondary cancer incidence after treatment of Hodgkin's disease with photon and proton radiation. *Radiat Res.* 2000;154:382-388.

a. This is basically a case report in which the risk of secondary cancer is calculated for several different kinds of plans (two field photons, IMRT, and two different proton plans). "Irradiation with protons using the spot scanning technique decreases the avoidable cancer incidence compared with photon treatment by a factor of about two."

18. Seppenwoolde Y, Lebesque JV, de Jaeger K, et al. Comparing different NTCP models that predict the incidence of radiation pneumonitis. *Int J Radiat Oncol Biol Phys.* 2003;55:724-735.

a. The risk of radiation pneumonitis in 382 patients with breast cancer, lymphoma, and lung cancer was assessed in relation to a variety of measures of radiation dose to the lungs. The risk of pneumonitis was estimated to be more than 5% if the mean lung dose was greater than approximately 12 Gy or if the volume of lung receiving more than 13 Gy (V13) was more than 23%.

Recommended Pediatric Cancer Proton Therapy Indications

INDICATIONS

1) Curative treatment of pediatric brain, nonbrain solid, and hematologic tumors

The *Stockholm Pediatric Proton Therapy Conference Consensus Report* in 2016 provides recommendations on which pediatric cancer patients may benefit from proton therapy.

Inclusion criteria

i. Brain tumors, such as medulloblastoma, ependymoma, low-grade glioma, craniopharyngioma, germ cell tumor, atypical teratoid rhabdoid tumor, choroid plexus tumor, anaplastic oligodendroglioma, meningioma, and cases requiring craniospinal irradiation. Spinal tumors for which anterior thoracic or abdominopelvic organs would be spared from radiation.

ii. Solid tumors, such as rhabdomyosarcoma, nonrhabdomyosarcoma soft tissue sarcoma, Ewing sarcoma, osteosarcoma, retinoblastoma, neuroblastoma, Wilms and other renal tumors, germ cell tumors, nasopharyngeal carcinoma, salivary gland tumor, and other head and neck cancer.

iii. Hematologic tumors, such as Hodgkin lymphoma, extranodal, nasal-type natural killer lymphoma. Also, leukemia or lymphoma requiring craniospinal irradiation.

General exclusion criteria

i. Definitive treatment of noncurable cases such as diffuse intrinsic pontine glioma, malignant gliomas other than anaplastic oligodendroglioma

ii. Whole brain, whole lung, and whole abdominal radiotherapy where the target volume is purposely not sparing any critical structure
iii. Total body irradiation

2) Reirradiation to spare critical structures/organs next to the target volume

SCIENTIFIC EVIDENCE

1. Antonini TN, Ris MD, Grosshans DR, et al. Attention, processing speed, and executive functioning in pediatric brain tumor survivors treated with proton beam therapy. *Radiother Oncol.* 2017;124(1):89-97.
2. Bishop AJ, Greenfield B, Mahajan A, et al. Proton beam therapy versus conformal photon radiation therapy for childhood craniopharyngioma: multi-institutional analysis of outcomes, cyst dynamics, and toxicity. *Int J Radiat Oncol Biol Phys.* 2014;90(2):354-361.
3. Eaton BR, Chowdhry V, Weaver K, et al. Use of proton therapy for re-irradiation in pediatric intracranial ependymoma. *Radiother Oncol.* 2015;116(2):301-308.
4. Eaton BR, Esiashvili N, Kim S, et al. Endocrine outcomes with proton and photon radiotherapy for standard risk medulloblastoma. *Neuro Oncol.* 2016;18(6):881-887.
5. Greenfield BJ, Jaramillo S, Abboud M, et al. Outcomes for pediatric patients with central nervous system germ cell tumors treated with proton therapy. *Clin Transl Radiat Oncol.* 2016;1:9-14.
6. Hattangadi JA, Rombi B, Yock TI, et al. Proton radiotherapy for high-risk neuroblastoma: early outcomes and dose comparison. *Int J Radiat Oncol Biol Phys.* 2012;83(3):1015-1022.
7. Hess CB, Indelicato DJ, Paulino AC, et al. An update from the Pediatric Proton Consortium Registry. *Front Oncol.* 2018;8:165.
8. Indelicato DJ, Merchant T, Laperriere N, et al. Consensus report from the Stockholm Pediatric Proton Therapy Conference. *Int J Radiat Oncol Biol Phys.* 2016;96(2):387-392.
9. Kahalley LS, Ris MD, Grosshans DR, et al. Comparing intelligence quotient change after proton versus photon radiotherapy for pediatric brain tumors. *J Clin Oncol.* 2016; 34(10):1043-1049.
10. Kamran SC, Goldberg SI, Kuhlthau KA, et al. Quality of life in patients with proton-treated medulloblastoma: results of a prospective assessment with 5 year follow-up. *Cancer.* 2018;124(16):3390-3400.
11. Ladra MM, Szymonifka JD, Mahajan A, et al. Preliminary results of a phase II trial of proton radiotherapy for pediatric rhabdomyosarcoma. *J Clin Oncol.* 2014;32(33): 3762-3770.
12. McGovern SL, Okcu MF, Munsell MF, et al. Outcomes and acute toxicities of proton therapy for pediatric atypical teratoid/rhabdoid tumor of the central nervous system. *Int J Radiat Oncol Biol Phys.* 2014;90(5):1143-1152.
13. Mouw KW, Yeap BY, Caruso P, et al. Analysis of patient outcomes following proton therapy for retinoblastoma. *Adv Radiat Oncol.* 2017;2(1):44-52.
14. Pulsifer MB, Duncanson H, Grieco J, et al. Cognitive and adaptive outcomes after proton radiation for pediatric patients with brain tumors. *Int J Radiat Oncol Biol Phys.* 2018;102(2):391-398.
15. Sato M, Gunther JR, Mahajan A, et al. Progression-free survival of children with localized ependymoma treated with intensity-modulated radiation therapy or proton-beam radiation therapy. *Cancer.* 2017;123(13):2570-2578.
16. Vern-Gross TZ, Indelicato DJ, Bradley JA, Rotondo RL. Patterns of failure in pediatric rhabdomyosarcoma after proton therapy. *Int J Radiat Oncol Biol Phys.* 2016;96(5): 1070-1077.
17. Yock TI, Yeap BY, Ebb DH, et al. Long-term toxic effects of proton radiotherapy for paediatric medulloblastoma: a phase 2 single-arm study. *Lancet Oncol.* 2016;17(3):287-298.

Recommended Prostate Cancer Proton Therapy Indications

INDICATIONS

1) **Definitive/curative treatment for men with intact localized or locally advanced prostate cancer**
   - **Inclusion criteria**
     i. Men with T1-2N0M0 with Gleason sum 7 (or higher) or prostate-specific antigen (PSA) levels of 10 ng/mL (or higher) prostate cancer who have elected to proceed with external beam radiation therapy for definitive therapy with or without hormone therapy and have a projected life expectancy of at least 10 years
       a. Doses ranges should be 76 to 80 Gy equivalents (GyE) at 1.8 to 2 GyE per fraction
       b. Some men (e.g., those with reasonable urinary function) can be considered for hypofractionated regimens of 70 to 72 GyE at 2.4 to 2.5 GyE per fraction
       c. Men with low-risk and select cases of intermediate-risk cancer (i.e., T1–2a, Gleason 7 in <50% cores, PSA <10) can be considered for clinical studies involving ultra-hypofractionation (e.g., 40 GyE at 8 GyE per fraction or 55.5 GyE at 3.7 GyE per fraction)
     ii. Men with T3–4 and/or Gleason 8 to 10 and/or PSA over 20 disease for which higher radiation doses are needed to maximize local control
       a. Conventional fractionation should typically be used (e.g., 76–82 GyE at 1.8–2 GyE per fraction)
       b. Pelvic nodal radiation (e.g., 44–50 GyE) may also be considered in some cases
       c. Given the increased target volumes and complexity of such cases, pencil beam proton delivery planning and delivery techniques may be required to optimize dosimetric constraints on normal tissues
   - Delivering a high radiation dose to the primary tumor in the prostate and/or seminal vesicles has become an important aspect of the optimal management of clinically localized prostate carcinoma. This is the result of multiple phase III studies demonstrating that a higher radiation dose reduces the risk of prostate cancer recurrence.
   - Proton therapy can be at least as effective as conventional external beam radiotherapy in treating clinically localized (encompassing low-risk, intermediate-risk, and high-risk) prostate cancer while reducing the risk of acute and late side effects of radiotherapy. When this book was written a phase III study (NCT 01617161) was in progress to compare proton therapy with conventional external beam radiotherapy using intensity-modulated radiotherapy (IMRT). Table 1 compares conventional external beam radiotherapy and proton therapy with respect to therapeutic effectiveness in terms of biochemical relapse-free rate, based on some of published manuscripts and abstracts. Biochemical relapse (also called *PSA relapse*) is a widely accepted surrogate representing prostate cancer recurrence. Table 2 compares the incidences of acute and late radiation toxicity between conventional external beam radiotherapy and proton therapy. Patient-reported quality of life data from two prospectively collected databases also suggest an approximately 50% reduction in problems with significant bowel urgency and frequency in patients treated with proton therapy compared with IMRT.
   - Clinical and laboratory studies have suggested that prostate cancer has a relatively slow rate of proliferation, characterized by a low α/β value (1.5–3 Gy) in a linear-quadratic model of cell survival after irradiation. This implies that a larger radiation dose per fraction (i.e., hypofractionation) is more effective for killing for prostate cancer cells than simply adding more fractions. Table 3 shows phase III studies comparing a conventional dose-fractionation regimen with a moderate hypofractionation regimen in a conventional external beam setting.

TABLE 1 ■ **Comparison Between Photon Versus Proton for Biochemical Relapse-Free Rate, Based on Some Prospective Studies**

Study	F/U (years)	*n*	Treatment	Biochemical Relapse-Free Rate
Photon				
RTOG 0126 (2015)	7	748	79.2 Gy in 44 fractions (intermediate risk)	84% at 5 years
Fox Chase Cancer Center (2013)	5.7	153	76 Gy in 38 fractions (mainly intermediate and high risk)	78.6% at 5 years
Italy (2012)	5.8	85	80 Gy in 40 fractions (intermediate and high risk)	79% at 5 years
Proton				
Univ. Florida (2014)	5.2	211	78 GyE (Gy): low risk 78-82 GyE (Gy): intermediate risk 78 GyE (Gy) + weekly docetaxel + 6-month ADT: high risk	99% at 5 years for low risk; 99% at 5 years for intermediate risk; 76% at 5 years for high risk
Japan (2011)	3.6	151	74 GyE in 37 fractions (low- and intermediate-risk)	94% at 3 years
Proton Radiation Oncology Group (2010)	8.9	197	28.8 GyE in 16 fractions (proton) + 50.4 Gy in 28 fractions (photon) (low and intermediate risk)	82.6% at 10 years

ADT, Androgen deprivation therapy *GyE,* Gray equivalents.

Moderate hypofractionation can be effective as conventional dose-fractionation without increasing the risk of radiation morbidity. The University of Florida reported outcomes of a prospective trial of hypofractionated proton therapy in 228 men with low- or intermediate-risk prostate cancer who had 5 years of follow-up. In that study, hypofractionated proton therapy (28–29 fractions over 5.5 weeks) yielded outcomes similar to those achieved with a standard-fractionation proton therapy (39–42 fractions over 8 weeks) in some patients. Men in this trial had prostate volumes less than 60 cc, IPSS (International Prostate Symptom Score) less than 15, and no previous treatment with either alpha reductase inhibitors (tamsulosin [Flomax], terazoxin Hcl [Hytrin], etc.) or anticoagulation (clopidogrel [Plavix], warfarin [Coumadin], etc.).

2) **Consolidative pelvic locoregional therapy** for men with isolated pelvic nodal metastases
   - **Inclusion criteria**
     i. Men with isolated nodal metastases (any T category) but without distant metastasis with good biochemical and radiographic responses to neoadjuvant hormone therapy
     ii. Men with good responses to upfront hormone therapy should be considered for radiation therapy to pelvic lymph nodes and prostate primary tumor
     iii. Doses should be as above for pelvic nodal therapy, but boost doses to the volumes of nodal involvement may be considered
     iv. Given the increased target volumes and complexity in such cases, pencil beam proton delivery planning and delivery techniques may be required to meet dosimetric constraints on normal tissues

TABLE 2 ■ **Comparison Between Photon Versus Proton for Radiation Toxicity**

					Acute Toxicity				Late Toxicity			
					GI		GU		GI		GU	
Study	**Tool for Toxicity Assessment**	**RT Dose**	**F/U (Years)**	***n***	**G2**	**≥G3**	**G2**	**≥G3**	**G2**	**≥G3**	**G2**	**≥G3**
Photon												
RTOG0126 (IMRT) (2013)	CTCAE v2.0 and RTOG/EORTC	79.2 Gy in 44 f	3.5	257	≥G2 GI or GU: 9.7%				≥G2: 15.1% at 3 yrs	≥G3: 2.6% at 3 yrs		
RTOG0126 (IMRT/3D-CRT) (2015)			7	748	≥G2 GI: 2.4%		≥G2 GU: 11.1%		≥ G2: 21% at 5 yrs	≥G3: 5% at 5 yrs	≥G2: 12% at 5 yrs	≥G3: 3% at 5 yrs
Fox Chase Cancer Center (IMRT) (2013)	LENT/RTOG (similar to CTCAE v4.0)	76 Gy in 38 f	5.7	153					20.5% at 5 yrs	2% at 5 yrs	≥G2: 37.9% at 5 yrs (or 13.4% with modified criteria)	
		70.2 Gy in 26 f		154					16.1% at 5 yrs	2% at 5 yrs	≥G2: 39.1% at 5 yrs (or 21.5% with modified criteria)	
Italy (3D-CRT) (2011)	RTOG/EORTC for acute toxicity; LENT-SOMA for late toxicity	80 Gy in 40 f	2.9	85	≥G2 GI: 21%		≥G2 GU: 40%		≥G2 rectal: 12%		≥G2 GU: 6%	
		62 Gy in 20 f	2.7	83	≥G2 GI: 35%		≥G2 GU: 47%		≥G2 rectal: 14%		≥G2 GU: 8%	
Proton												
Univ. Florida (2014)	CTCAE v3.0	78–82 GyE	5.2	211		0.5%		0.5%		1% at 5 yrs (0.5%, if CTCAE v4.0)		5.4% at 5 yrs (0.9%, if CTCAE v4.0)
Japan (2011)	CTCAE v2.0	74 GyE	3.6	151	0.7%	0%	12%	0%	2% at 2 yrs	0% at 2 yrs	4.1% at 2 yrs	0% at 2 yrs

CTCAE, Common Terminology Criteria for Adverse Events; *EORTC,* European Organisation for Research and Treatment of Cancer; *IMRT,* intensity-modulated radiation therapy; *GI,* gastrointestinal; *GU,* genitourinary; *LENT-SOMA,* Late Effects Normal Tissue Task Force Subjective, Objective, Management, Analytic; *RTOG,* Radiation Therapy Oncology Group; *yrs,* years.

TABLE 3 ■ **Phase III Studies Evaluating Hypofractionation Regimens: Photons**

Study	F/U (Years)	Patients	*n*	Treatment	Biochemical Relapse-Free Rate	
Fox Chase Cancer Center (2013)	5.7	Low to high risk (mainly intermediate and high risk); (ADT for intermediate and high risk)	153	76 Gy in 38 fractions (2 Gy/fraction)	78.6% at 5 years	*P* = .745
			154	70.2 Gy in 26 fractions (2.7 Gy/fraction)	76.7% at 5 years	
Italy (2012)	5.8	Intermediate and high risk (all had 9-month ADT)	85	80 Gy in 40 fractions (2 Gy/fraction)	79% at 5 years	*P* = .065
			83	62 Gy in 20 fractions over 5 weeks (4 fractions/week) (3.1 Gy/fraction)	85% at 5 years	

ADT, Androgen deprivation therapy; *F/U*, follow-up

3) **Adjuvant or salvage therapy** after radical prostatectomy
   - **Inclusion criteria**
     i. Men with prostate cancer with positive surgical margins or a detectable PSA level of 0.2 ng/mL or higher after radical prostatectomy
     ii. Adjuvant treatment to the prostatic bed and/or seminal vesicle bed for positive surgical margins to 64 to 66 GyE at 1.8 to 2 GyE per fraction
     iii. Salvage therapy to the prostatic bed to 68 to 72 GyE at 1.8 to 2 GyE per fraction for detectable PSA and/or clinical/radiographic recurrence after prostatectomy
     iv. Given the increased target volumes and complexity in such cases, pencil beam proton delivery planning and delivery techniques may be required to meet dosimetric constraints on normal tissues
4) **Intensity-modulated proton therapy (IMPT)** is indicated for high-risk prostate cancer

SCIENTIFIC EVIDENCE

1. Al-Mamgani A, van Putten WL, Heemsbergen WD, et al. Update of Dutch multicenter dose-escalation trial of radiotherapy for localized prostate cancer. *Int J Radiat Oncol Biol Phys.* 2008;72:980-988.
2. Arcangeli S, Strigari L, Gomellini S, et al. Updated results and patterns of failure in a randomized hypofractionation trial for high-risk prostate cancer. *Int J Radiat Oncol Biol Phys.* 2012;84:1172-1178.
3. Arcangeli G, Fowler J, Gomellini S, et al. Acute and late toxicity in a randomized trial of conventional versus hypofractionated three-dimensional conformal radiotherapy for prostate cancer. *Int J Radiat Oncol.* 2011;79:1013-1021.
4. Beckendorf V, Guerif S, Le Prise E, et al. 70 Gy versus 80 Gy in localized prostate cancer: 5-year results of GETUG 06 randomized trial. *Int J Radiat Oncol Biol Phys.* 2011;80:1056-1063.

5. Choi S, Amin M, Palmer M, et al. Comparison of intensity modulated proton therapy (IMPT) to passively scattered proton therapy (PSPT) in the treatment of prostate cancer. *Int J Radiat Oncol Biol Phys.* 2011;81:S154-S155.
6. Dearnaley DP, Sydes MR, Graham JD, et al. Escalated-dose versus standard-dose conformal radiotherapy in prostate cancer: first results from the MRC RT01 randomised controlled trial. *Lancet Oncol.* 2007;8:475-487.
7. Hoffman K, Voong K, Pugh T, et al. Risk of late toxicity in men receiving dose-escalated hypofractionated intensity modulated prostate radiation therapy: results from a Randomized Trial. *Int J Radiat Oncol Biol Phys.* 2014:1074-1084.
8. Hoppe B, Michalski J, Mendenhall N, et al. Comparative effectiveness study of patient-reported outcomes after proton therapy or intensity-modulated radiotherapy for prostate cancer. *Cancer.* 2014;20:1076-1082.
9. Hoppe BS, Michalski JM, Mendenhall NP, et al. Comparative effectiveness study of patient-reported outcomes after proton therapy or intensity-modulated radiotherapy for prostate cancer. *Cancer.* 2014;120:1076-1082.
10. Kim Y, Cho K, Pyo H, et al. A phase II study of hypofractionated proton therapy for prostate cancer. *Acta Oncol.* 2013;52:477-485.
11. Kole T, Nichols R, Lei S, et al. A dosimetric comparison of ultra-hypofractionated passively scattered proton radiotherapy and stereotactic body radiotherapy (SBRT) in the definitive treatment of localized prostate cancer. *Acta Oncol.* 2014:4(6):825-831.
12. Kuban DA, Tucker SL, Dong L, et al. Long-term results of the M. D. Anderson randomized dose-escalation trial for prostate cancer. *Int J Radiat Oncol Biol Phys.* 2008;70:67-74.
13. Mendenhall NP, Hoppe BS, Nichols RC, et al. Five-year outcomes from 3 prospective trials of image-guided proton therapy for prostate cancer. *Int J Radiat Oncol Biol Phys.* 2014;88:596-602.
14. Mendenhall NP, Li Z, Hoppe BS, et al. Early outcomes from three prospective trials of image-guided proton therapy for prostate cancer. *Int J Radiat Oncol Biol Phys.* 2012;82(1):213-221.
15. Michalski JM, Yan Y, Watkins-Bruner D, et al. Preliminary toxicity analysis of 3-dimensional conformal radiation therapy versus intensity modulated radiation therapy on the high-dose arm of the Radiation Therapy Oncology Group 0126 prostate cancer trial. *Int J Radiat Oncol Biol Phys.* 2013;87:932-938.
16. Michalski J, Moughan J, Purdy J, et al. Effect of standard vs dose-escalated radiation therapy for patients with intermediate-risk prostate cancer. The NRG Oncology RTOG 0126 randomized clinical trial. *JAMA Oncol.* 2018;4(6):e180039.
17. Nihei K, Ogino T, Onozawa M, et al. Multi-institutional phase II study of proton beam therapy for organ-confined prostate cancer focusing on the incidence of late rectal toxicities. *Int J Radiat Oncol Biol Phys.* 2011;81:390-396.
18. Nihei K, Ogino T, Onozawa M, et al. Multi-institutional phase II study of proton beam therapy for organ-confined prostate cancer focusing on the incidence of late rectal toxicities. *Int J Radiat Oncol Biol Phys.* 2011;81(2):390-396.
19. Pollack A, Walker G, Horwitz EM, et al. Randomized trial of hypofractionated external-beam radiotherapy for prostate cancer. *J Clin Oncol.* 2013;31:3860-3868.
20. Pollack A, Zagars GK, Starkschall G, et al. Prostate cancer radiation dose response: results of the M. D. Anderson phase III randomized trial. *Int J Radiat Oncol Biol Phys.* 2002;53(5):1097-1105.
21. Pollack A, Walker G, Buyyounouski MK, et al. Five Year results of a randomized external beam radiotherapy hypofractionation trial for prostate cancer. *Int J Radiat Oncol Biol Phys.* 2011;81(2):S1.
22. Pugh TJ, Munsell M, Choi S, et al. Quality of life and toxicity from passively scattered and spot-scanning proton beam therapy for localized prostate cancer. *Int J Radiat Oncol Biol Phys.* 2013;87:946-953.

23. Pugh TJ, Amos R, John-Baptiste S, et al. Multifield optimization intensity-modulated proton therapy (MFO-IMPT) for prostate cancer: robustness analysis through simulation of rotational and translational alignment errors. *Med Dosim*. 2013;38:344-350.
24. Pugh TJ, Lee A. Proton beam therapy for the treatment of prostate cancer. *Cancer J*. 2014:415-420.
25. Shipley WU, Tepper JE, Prout GR Jr, et al. Proton radiation as boost therapy for localized prostatic carcinoma. *JAMA*. 1979;241(18):1912-1915.
26. Shipley WU, Verhey LJ, Munzenrider JE, et al. Advanced prostate cancer: the results of a randomized comparative trial of high dose irradiation boosting with conformal protons compared with conventional dose irradiation using photons alone. *Int J Radiat Oncol Biol Phys*. 1995;32(1):3-12.
27. Slater JD, Rossi CJ Jr, Yonemoto LT, et al. Proton therapy for prostate cancer: the initial Loma Linda University experience. *Int J Radiat Oncol Biol Phys*. 2004;59:348-352.
28. Yonemoto LT, Slater JD, Rossi CJ Jr, et al. Combined proton and photon conformal radiation therapy for locally advanced carcinoma of the prostate: preliminary results of a phase I/II study. *Int J Radiat Oncol Biol Phys*. 1997;37(1):21-29.
29. Yu J, Cramer L, Herrin J, et al. Stereotactic body radiation therapy versus intensity-modulated radiation therapy for prostate cancer: comparison of toxicity. *J Clin Oncol*. 2014:1195-1201.
30. Zietman AL, DeSilvio ML, Slater JD, et al. Comparison of conventional-dose vs high-dose conformal radiation therapy in clinically localized adenocarcinoma of the prostate: a randomized controlled trial. *JAMA*. 2005;294(10):1233-1239.
31. Zietman AL, Bae K, Slater JD, et al. Randomized trial comparing conventional-dose with high-dose conformal radiation therapy in early-stage adenocarcinoma of the prostate: long-term results from Proton Radiation Oncology Group/American College of Radiology 95-09. *J Clin Oncol*. 2010;28(7):1106-1111.
32. Mendenhall NP, Hoppe BS, Nichols RC, et al. Five-year outcomes from 3 prospective trials of image-guided proton therapy for prostate cancer. *Int J Radiat Oncol Biol Phys*. 2014;88(3):596-602.
33. Bryant C, Smith TL, Henderson RH, et al. Five-year biochemical results, toxicity, and patient-reported quality of life after delivery of dose escalated image guided proton therapy for prostate cancer. *Int J Radiat Oncol Biol Phys*. 2016;95(1):422-434.
34. Henderson RH, Bryant C, Hoppe BS. Five-year outcomes from a prospective trial of image-guided accelerated hypofractionation proton therapy for prostate cancer. *Acta Oncol*. 2017;56(7):963-970.
35. Iwata H, Ishikawa H, Takagi M, et al. Long-term outcomes of proton therapy for prostate cancer in japan: retrospective analysis of a multi-institutional survey. *Int J Radiat Oncol Biol Phys*. 2017;(99):E241-E242.
36. Holtzman AL, Hoppe BS, Letter HP, et al. Proton therapy as salvage treatment for local relapse of prostate cancer following cryosurgery or high-intensity focused ultrasound. *Int J Radiat Oncol Biol Phys*. 2016;95(1):465-471.

Recommended Thoracic Cancer Proton Therapy Indications

INDICATIONS

1) **Non-small cell lung cancer (NSCLC)**
   - **Inclusion criteria**
     i. Stage II–IIIA disease
     ii. Stage IIIB disease

- Supraclavicular node, bilateral hila, and T4 tumors
- Treatment with curative intent, regardless of protocol

2) **Postoperative lung cancer patients** with bilateral N2 disease (hilum)
3) **Thymoma**
   - **Inclusion criteria**
     i. Anterior chest tumors
     ii. Preoperative and postoperative thymic carcinoma
4) **Mesothelioma**
5) **Recurrent, previously irradiated disease in** the chest: proton therapy will decrease the risk of overlap in normal organs during treatment planning for recurrent disease.
6) **Intensity-modulated proton therapy (IMPT)** is indicated for definitive treatment for locally advanced NSCLC with complicated anatomy or reirradiation.

Exclusion criteria

1. Patients treated for palliation alone (generally this is with doses < 60 Gy and often without chemotherapy)

SCIENTIFIC EVIDENCE

1. Nguyen QN, Ly NB, Komaki R, et al. Long-term outcomes after proton therapy, with concurrent chemotherapy, for stage II–III inoperable non-small cell lung cancer. *Radiother Oncol.* 2015;115(3):367-372.
2. Chang JY, Komaki R, Wen HY, et al. Toxicity and patterns of failure of adaptive/ablative proton therapy for early-stage, medically inoperable non-small cell lung cancer. *Int J Radiat Oncol Biol Phys.* 2011;80(5):1350-1357.
3. Gomez DR, Tucker SL, Martel MK, et al. Predictors of high-grade esophagitis after definitive three-dimensional conformal therapy, intensity-modulated radiation therapy, or proton beam therapy for non-small cell lung cancer. *Int J Radiat Oncol Biol Phys.* 2012;84(4):1010-1016.
4. Hoppe BS, Flampouri S, Henderson RH, et al. Proton therapy with concurrent chemotherapy for non-small-cell lung cancer: technique and early results. *Clin Lung Cancer.* 2012;13(5):352-358.
5. Koay EJ, Lege D, Mohan R, Komaki R, Cox JD, Chang JY. Adaptive/nonadaptive proton radiation planning and outcomes in a phase II trial for locally advanced non-small cell lung cancer. *Int J Radiat Oncol Biol Phys.* 2012;84(5):1093-1100.
6. Wink KC, Roelofs E, Solberg T, et al. Particle therapy for non-small cell lung tumors: where do we stand? A systematic review of the literature. *Front Oncol.* 2014;4:292
7. McAvoy S, Ciura K, Wei C, et al. Definitive reirradiation for locoregionally recurrent non-small cell lung cancer with proton beam therapy or intensity modulated radiation therapy: predictors of high-grade toxicity and survival outcomes. *Int J Radiat Oncol Biol Phys.* 2014;90(4):819-827.
8. Oshiro Y, Okumura T, Kurishima K, et al. High-dose concurrent chemo-proton therapy for stage III NSCLC: preliminary results of a Phase II study. *J Radiat Res.* 2014;55(5):959-965.
9. Bush DA, Cheek G, Zaheer S, et al. High-dose hypofractionated proton beam radiation therapy is safe and effective for central and peripheral early-stage non-small cell lung cancer: results of a 12-year experience at Loma Linda University Medical Center. *Int J Radiat Oncol Biol Phys.* 2013;86(5):964-968.
10. Berman AT, Teo BK, Dolney D, et al. An in-silico comparison of proton beam and IMRT for postoperative radiotherapy in completely resected stage IIIA non-small cell lung cancer. *Radiat Oncol.* 2013;8:144.

11. Gomez DR, Gillin M, Liao Z, et al. Phase 1 study of dose escalation in hypofractionated proton beam therapy for non-small cell lung cancer. *Int J Radiat Oncol Biol Phys.* 2013;86(4):665-670.
12. Lopez Guerra JL, Gomez DR, Zhuang Y, et al. Changes in pulmonary function after three-dimensional conformal radiotherapy, intensity-modulated radiotherapy, or proton beam therapy for non-small-cell lung cancer. *Int J Radiat Oncol Biol Phys.* 2012;83(4): e537-e543.
13. Chang JY, Komaki R, Lu C, et al. Phase 2 study of high-dose proton therapy with concurrent chemotherapy for unresectable stage III nonsmall cell lung cancer. *Cancer.* 2011;117(20):4707-4713.
14. Sejpal S, Komaki R, Tsao A, et al. Early findings on toxicity of proton beam therapy with concurrent chemotherapy for nonsmall cell lung cancer. *Cancer.* 2011;117(13):3004-3013.
15. Chang JY, Jabbour SK, Ruysscher DD, et al. Consensus statement on proton therapy in early-stage and locally advanced non-small cell lung cancer. *Int J Radiat Oncol Biol Phys.* 2016;95(1):505-516.
16. Berman AT, James SS, Rengan R, et al. Proton beam therapy for non-small cell lung cancer: current clinical evidence and future directions. *Cancer.* 2015;7(3):1178-1190.
17. Higgins KA, O'Connell K, Liu Y, et al. National Cancer Database analysis of proton versus photon radiation therapy in non-small cell lung cancer. *Int J Radiat Oncol Biol Phys.* 2017;97(1):128-137.
18. Liao ZX, Lee JJ, Komaki R, et al. Bayesian randomized trial comparing intensity modulated radiation therapy versus passively scattered proton therapy for locally advanced non-small cell lung cancer. *J Clin Oncol.* 2018;36(18):1813-1822.

INDEX

Page numbers followed by "*f*" indicate figures and "*t*" indicate tables.

R

S

T